AF711820

MRI—ARTHROSCOPY CORRELATIVE ATLAS

MRI–ARTHROSCOPY CORRELATIVE ATLAS

Mark D. Miller, MD, Lt Col (Sel) USAF MC
Clinical Associate Professor of Surgery
Uniformed Services University of Health Sciences
Bethesda, Maryland
Assistant Clinical Professor of Orthopaedic Surgery
University of Colorado Health Sciences Center
Associate Team Physician
Department of Orthopaedic Surgery
United States Air Force Academy Hospital
United States Air Force Academy, Colorado

John R. Osborne, MD, Lt Col USAF MC
Clinical Assistant Professor of Radiology and
Nuclear Medicine
Uniformed Services University of Health Sciences
Bethesda, Maryland
Chief, Radiology Services
United States Air Force Academy Hospital
United States Air Force Academy, Colorado

Jon J.P. Warner, M.D.
Associate Professor of Orthopaedic Surgery
University of Pittsburgh School of Medicine
Director, Shoulder Service Center for Sports Medicine
and Rehabilitation
Pittsburgh, Pennsylvania

Freddie H. Fu, M.D.
Blue Cross of Western Pennsylvania
Professor and Executive Vice Chairman
Department of Orthopaedic Surgery
University of Pittsburgh Medical Center
Musculoskeletal Institute
Pittsburgh, Pennsylvania

Suzanne Merrick Edmonds
Medical Illustrator
Colorado Springs, Colorado

W. B Saunders Company
A Division of Harcourt Brace & Company
Philadelphia London Toronto
Montreal Sydney Tokyo

W.B. SAUNDERS COMPANY
A Division of Harcourt Brace & Company
The Curtis Center
Independence Square West
Philadelphia, Pennsylvania 19106

Library of Congress Cataloging-in-Publication Data

MRI—arthroscopy correlative atlas / Mark D. Miller . . . [et al.].

p. cm.
Includes index.

ISBN 0–7216–6054–1

1. Joints—Magnetic resonance imaging—Atlases. 2. Arthroscopy—Atlases. I. Miller, Mark D. [DNLM: 1. Arthroscopy—methods—atlases. 2. Joint Diseases—diagnostic—atlases. WE 17 M9392 1997]

RC932.M75 1997 616.7′207548—dc21

DNLM/DLC 96–44085

MRI–ARTHROSCOPY CORRELATIVE ATLAS ISBN 0–7216–6054–1

Copyright © 1997 by W.B. Saunders Company

All rights reserved. No part of this publication may be reproduced or transmitted in any form or by any means, electronic or mechanical, including photocopy, recording, or any information storage and retrieval system, without permission in writing from the publisher.

Printed in the United States of America.

Last digit is the print number: 9 8 7 6 5 4 3 2 1

To our patients,
in the hope that a better understanding of
what we see
will result in a greater appreciation of
what we do.

MDM
JRO
JJPW
FHF

Foreword

With regard to diagnostic techniques that in recent years have been applied to the assessment of internal derangements of joints, magnetic resonance (MR) imaging and arthroscopy have been dominate. Review of recent radiology literature underscores the considerable interest in and benefit of MR imaging in the evaluation of a variety of problems affecting the articulations of the peripheral skeleton. A similar review of recent orthopaedic literature reveals more information regarding the application of arthroscopy to this evaluation and, furthermore, the importance of arthroscopy as both a diagnostic and therapeutic method. What is lacking in the available literature, however, is a work detailing how MR imaging and arthroscopy can be used as complementary, rather than competitive, techniques. How refreshing, indeed, to find a text authored by specialists and recognized experts in both orthopaedic surgery and radiology, who not only have emphasized this complementary role, but also have correlated the findings derived from one method with those from the other.

The editors of this text have also organized the material in a very logical fashion. A useful introduction first to MR imaging and then to arthroscopy is followed by a trip about the human body, with stops at each of the important appendicular skeletal sites: knee, hip, ankle, shoulder, elbow, and wrist. In each location, an analysis of both techniques is included using concise text, vivid images and drawings, and references to appropriate articles in the literature. Subsequently, in each chapter, cases are included in the form of an atlas, in which important findings derived by both MR imaging and arthroscopy are detailed.

What impresses me most about this text is not that orthopaedic surgeons may be encouraged to ". . . carefully consider the preoperative images prior to surgery," although this clearly is important, nor that radiologists ". . . consider what their interpretations mean," although surely this too is important, but rather that work such as this indicates in no uncertain terms that two specialties (orthopaedic surgery and radiology), by working closely together, can produce information that is more useful and more relevant clinically than that possible by working independently. They have also done so without bias.

At a time when new books appear at an ever increasing rate, it is satisfying to find one that clearly has a message. I suggest that you find room on your bookshelf for this text, even if it means discarding some other work.

DONALD RESNICK, M.D.

Foreword

Magnetic resonance imaging (MRI) has afforded unparalleled high resolution definition of the musculoskeletal soft tissues. This advance in imaging has resulted in a greater ability to diagnose a wide variety of abnormalities. The clinical usefulness of MRI is based upon a thorough understanding of the best techniques for obtaining these images, the normal anatomy and its variations, as well as the pathologic anatomy. The anatomy defined by MRI must be correlated with the pathology noted at the time of surgery, the preoperative clinical symptoms, and the physical examination findings. Clinical correlation is necessary to understand the significance of any of the MRI abnormalities. This correlation is particularly important when the findings are of an asymptomatic nature or are related to the normal aging process.

The authors of this text have considered all these issues and present an excellent correlation of MRI findings with normal surgical anatomy, surgical pathology, and clinical findings. This book provides a strong foundation for understanding of the clinical importance and clinical significance of MRI in a variety of musculoskeletal disorders. The arthroscopic images are correlated with the MRI findings and are enhanced with line drawings, which place the arthroscopic images into complete anatomic perspective. The book is a valuable source for the education of the practicing clinician.

JOSEPH IANOTTI, M.D.

Preface

MRI–Arthroscopy Correlative Atlas was written primarily to give orthopaedic surgeons better insight into the implications of magnetic resonance imaging findings in the diagnosis and treatment of their patients. It is also intended to offer radiologists a better understanding of the clinical manifestations of the images they are interpreting. We hope to encourage the orthopaedist to carefully consider the preoperative images prior to surgery, and the radiologist to consider what their interpretations mean. Taking this one step further, we encourage both disciplines to share their findings with each other, and, in this way, truly learn.

This project began as a direct result of the cooperation between surgeons and radiologists: A casual "sidewalk consult follow-up" in the hallway, an informal review of the day's cases, a sharing of images and arthroscopic photographs in conference, and a compilation of all material that could be gathered into this volume.

We are indebted to those surgeons and radiologists who were willing to share their cases. This project could not have been accomplished without them. However, much like Franz Shubert's *Unfinished Symphony*, this work remains incomplete. We need your input, your cases, your findings. Please send us MRI images and arthroscopic photographs of your interesting cases to the address given.* If we use them in the second edition, we will send you a free copy of the text when it is published.

MDM
JRO
JJPW
FHF

Address

*Department of Orthopaedic Surgery
10 MDG/SGOSO
4102 Pinion Drive, Suite 100
USAF Academy, CO 80840

Acknowledgments

We wish to thank the following individuals for the use of their cases in this atlas:

William P. Abraham, MD, Lt Col USAF MC
Clinical Assistant Professor of Radiology and Nuclear Medicine
Uniformed Services University of Health Sciences, Bethesda, Maryland
Department of Radiology,
United States Air Force Academy Hospital
United States Air Force Academy, Colorado

J.W. Thomas Byrd, MD, FACS
Southern Sports Medicine and Orthopaedic Center
Department of Orthopaedics and Rehabilitation
Vanderbilt University School of Medicine
Nashville, Tennessee

Steven F. Conti, MD
Assistant Professor, Orthopaedic Surgery
Chief, Foot and Ankle Service
University of Pittsburgh School of Medicine
Pittsburgh, Pennsylvania

William B. Geissler, MD
Associate Professor, Division of Hand and Upper Extremity
Head, Department of Arthroscopic Surgery and Sports Medicine
Department of Orthopaedics
University of Mississippi
Jackson, Mississippi

James M. Glick, MD
Senior Attending Orthopaedic Surgery
Mt. Zion Hospital
Associate Clinical Professor of Orthopaedic Surgery
University of California Medical Center San Francisco
San Francisco, California

Christopher D. Harner, MD
Associate Professor of Orthopaedics
Associate Director, Center for Sports Medicine
University of Pittsburgh
Pittsburgh, Pennsylvania

Daniel T. Hinkin, MD, Lt Col USAF MC
Clinical Assistant Professor of Surgery
Uniformed Services University of Health Sciences
Bethesda, Maryland
Chief of Sports Medicine and Head Team Physician
United States Air Force Academy Hospital
United States Air Force Academy, Colorado

Ronald Jones, MD, Lt Col USAF MC
Chief of Sports Medicine
Wilford Hall, United States Air Force Medical Center
Lackland Air Force Base, Texas

Michael G. Maday, MD
Midland Orthopedic Associates
Medical Director, SCORE Sports Medicine
Attending Orthopaedic Surgeon
Mercy Hospital and Medical Center
Chicago, Illinois

John McBride, MD, Lt Col MC USA
Chief of Sports Medicine
Fitzsimmons Army Medical Center
Aurora, Colorado

J. Serge Parisien, MD
Chief, Arthroscopic Surgery Service
Attending Orthopaedic Surgeon
Hospital for Joint Diseases
Associate Professor of Clinical Orthopaedic Surgery
New York University Medical School, New York, New York

Scott M. Smith, MD, Lt Col USAF MC
Assistant Chief, Department of Orthopaedics
United States Air Force Academy Hospital
United States Air Force Academy, Colorado

Steven M. Topper, MD, Maj USAF MC
Clinical Assistant Professor of Surgery
Uniformed Services University of Health Sciences, Bethesda, Maryland
Assistant Clinical Professor of Orthopaedic Surgery
University of Colorado Health Sciences Center
Chief of Hand Surgery
United States Air Force Academy Hospital
United States Air Force Academy, Colorado

Steven F. Viegas, MD
Professor and Chief, Division of Hand Surgery
Department of Orthopaedic Surgery and Rehabilitation
University of Texas Health Sciences Center
Galveston, Texas

G. Bradford Wright, MD, Maj USAF MC
Department of Orthopaedic Surgery
United States Air Force Academy Hospital
United States Air Force Academy, Colorado

Table of Contents

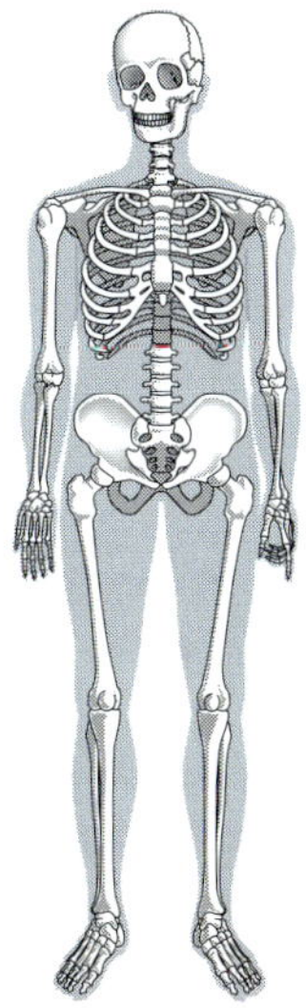

CHAPTER

1

Introduction

Introduction to Magnetic Resonance Imaging

Magnetic resonance imaging (MRI) is a sensitive, noninvasive method for evaluating musculoskeletal disease (Fig. 1–1). High-resolution imaging of normal body tissues and pathologic processes is possible because of the extraordinary tissue contrast achieved through a variety of techniques. This attribute is perhaps the single greatest advantage of MRI over plain radiography, computed axial tomography, and bone scintigraphy.

MRI generates contrast differently from radiography. The black-and-white regions of a plain radiograph are determined by the number of x-rays penetrating through the bone and soft tissue to the image receptor. In MRI, on the other hand, the gradations of black to white (plain radiography terminology) or bright to dark (MRI terminology) depend on the complex interplay of many factors that can be categorized into two principal groups. First, there are factors derived from the inherent biophysical properties characteristic of the tissue. Factors that reflect tissue intensity (brightness or darkness) are hydrogen proton density, T1 relaxation time, T2 relaxation time, T2* relaxation time, and flow. Second, there are factors from the imaging system and technique. Factors that reflect the system and technique are pulse sequence type (e.g., spin-echo, fast spin-echo, gradient-recalled echo, short tau inversion recovery [STIR]), timing parameters (e.g., repetition time/echo time [TR/TE]), flip angle, slice thickness and gap, and matrix size and field of view. Table 1–1 offers a helpful glossary of terms. Knowledge of the capabilities of pulse sequences and the trade-off considerations regarding spatial and contrast determinants is critical to the successful application of this diagnostic method.[7, 10, 11]

BASIS OF THE MAGNETIC RESONANCE IMAGE

Magnetic resonance is defined as the absorption and release of energy by nuclei in an external magnetic field when stimulated by radiofrequency (RF) energy at a specific frequency called the Larmor, or resonance, frequency. MRI uses the principles of this resonance to create body images. The natural abundance and strength with which it

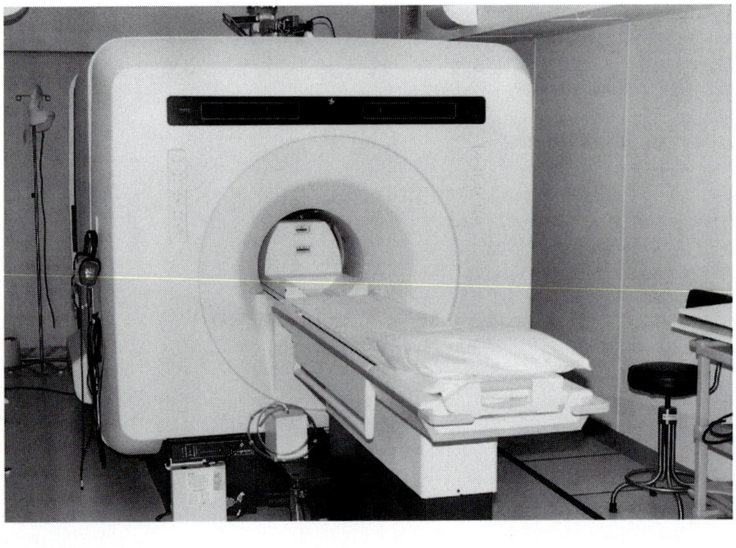

Figure 1–1
1.5 Tesla Field Strength Superconducting Magnet. (Courtesy of General Electric, Milwaukee, Wisconsin.)

Table 1–1 • Glossary of Basic MRI Terms

T1:	Time constant of exponential growth of magnetization. T1 measures how fast a tissue gains magnetization (and hence signal). A tissue with short T1, like fat, will gain signal quickly and be bright on a T1-weighted image.
T2:	Time constant of exponential decay of signal after an excitation pulse. T2 measures how long a tissue maintains its signal. A tissue with long T2, like water, will maintain its signal and be bright on a T2-weighted image.
T2*:	Similar to T2, but includes effects of magnetic field in homogeneity.
TR:	Repetition time. The time between successive excitation pulses.
TE:	Echo time. The time that an echo is formed (by a refocusing pulse given at TE/2).
NEX:	Number of excitations. The number of times a sequence is repeated and averaged. Higher NEX results in decreased noise and a less grainy image, but also longer scan times.
FOV:	Field of view. The dimension of the square area that is being imaged. FOV must be large enough to include all of the areas of interest. Larger FOV means more spins are being imaged, hence the signal is increased and the image is less grainy. Smaller FOV will increase the resolution.
Spin echo:	A standard scan sequence in which a series of one or more echoes are formed after an initial excitation pulse. This is often performed with two echoes, the first giving a proton-density–weighted image and the second a T2-weighted image.
FSE:	Fast-spin echo. A new technique to generate spin-echo images in much shorter times.
GRE:	Gradient-recalled echo. A generic term for a scan sequence that uses changes in the gradients, rather than refocusing pulses, to generate echoes. The exact scan sequence available depends on the manufacturer (GRASS, SPGR, MPGR, FLASH, FISP, etc.).

From Hardin CW, Gilley JS. The armchair adventurer's guide to magnetic resonance imaging: Theory and clinical applications. Oper Tech Sports Med 1995; 3:11.

interacts with magnetic fields makes hydrogen the most suitable of all nuclei for clinical imaging.

In MRI, the static external magnetic field establishes equilibrium between hydrogen protons aligned parallel and antiparallel to the external field. RF energy pulses are used to excite protons from the lower-energy parallel alignment into the higher-energy antiparallel alignment. Upon discontinuation of the radiowaves, the excited protons lose this extra energy through T1 (longitudinal) relaxation and T2 (transverse) relaxation mechanisms. The intensity of the magnetic resonance signal that results is determined by these two factors as well as a third factor, the number of hydrogen protons, or proton density. These parameters are then exploited to make significant differences in signal intensity from various sorts of tissues. The positions of the nuclei are localized during the process by the application of spatially dependent magnetic fields called gradients. The x,y,z coordinate system is represented by slice selection, frequency-encoding, and phase-encoding gradients to resolve two-dimensional images spatially. Finally, the information is transformed by the computer into an image using a mathematical process called the Fourier transform.[1] Sketched briefly, then, these are the basic steps involved in the production of a magnetic resonance image (Fig. 1–2).

The goal in designing an imaging sequence is to highlight differences between tissues based on the previously mentioned three parameters. This suggests three basic types of sequences, namely T1-weighted, proton density–weighted, and T2-weighted sequences and resultant images. TR and TE are prime variables in this highlighting process (Table 1–2). The spin-echo sequence is the most common sequence utilized in MRI of the musculoskeletal system. The T1-weighted (short TR/short TE) sequence reveals areas of short T1 relaxation time as bright signal and areas of long T1 relaxation time as dark signal.

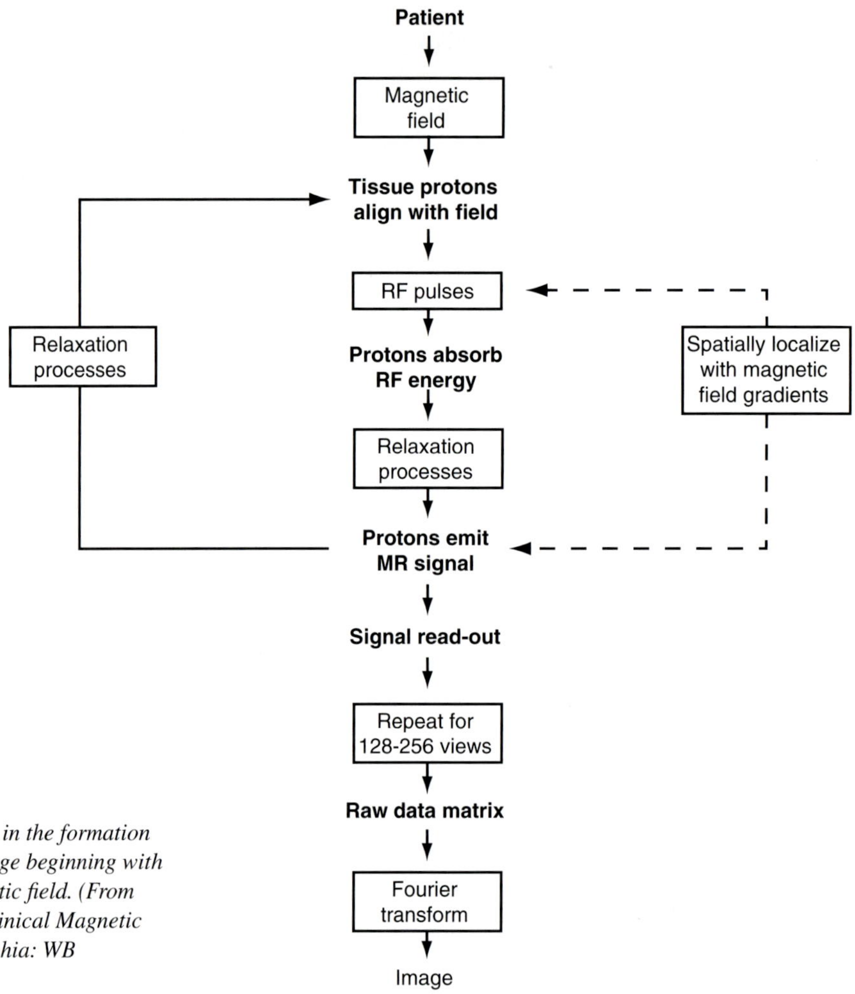

Figure 1–2
Summary of the steps involved in the formation of the magnetic resonance image beginning with the patient entering the magnetic field. (From Edelman RR, Hesselink JR. Clinical Magnetic Resonance Imaging. Philadelphia: WB Saunders, 1990, p 5.)

Because fat is the most common tissue within the body that has a short T1 relaxation time, fat is bright on the T1-weighted image. Similarly, a spin-echo sequence that is T2-weighted (long TR/long TE) reveals areas of long T2 relaxation time as high signal intensity and areas of short T2 relaxation time as low signal intensity. Therefore, areas of the body containing excess amounts of free water such as a bone contusion are bright on a T2-weighted image. Regions that contain liquid such as a cyst are bright on T2-weighted images. Most disease processes that are associated with excess free water, such as inflammation and neoplasia, also tend to be bright on T2-weighted images (Table 1–3).[7, 10, 11]

Table 1–2 • Image Weighting as Determined by TR and TE

	Short TE	Long TE
Short TR	T1-weighted	Not useful
Long TR	Proton-density–weighted	T2-weighted

From Hardin CW, Gilley JS. The armchair adventurer's guide to magnetic resonance imaging: Theory and clinical applications. Oper Tech Sports Med 1995; 3:5.

Table 1–3 • Tissue Signal Intensities on T1-, T2-, and T2*-Weighted Images

	T1-Weighted	T2-Weighted	T2*-Weighted
Cortical bone	Low	Low	Low
Marrow—yellow	High	Intermediate	Low
Marrow—red	Low/intermediate	Low/intermediate	Low
Marrow edema	Low	High	Intermediate
Hyaline cartilage	Intermediate	Intermediate	Intermediate/high
Meniscus	Low	Low	Low
Meniscal tear	High	Intermediate	High
Ligament	Low	Low	Low
Tendon	Low	Low	Low
Fluid	Low	High	High
Fat	High	Intermediate	Low
Blood—acute	Low/intermediate	Low	Mixed
Blood—chronic	High	High	Mixed

From Hardin CW, Gilley JS. The armchair adventurer's guide to magnetic resonance imaging: Theory and clinical applications. Oper Tech Sports Med 1995; 3:5.

PULSE SEQUENCES

The standard spin-echo T1-weighted and T2-weighted sequences have remained the gold standard in MRI of the musculoskeletal system. The spin-echo pulse sequence utilizes a 90-degree RF pulse followed by a 180-degree refocusing pulse. The TR and TE, as mentioned earlier, determine the type of contrast. The T1-weighted sequence uses a short TR/TE and provides superb anatomic definition in a short time relative to other sequences. It particularly helps distinguish normal bone marrow from pathology. The proton density–weighted sequence uses a long TR/short TE and has excellent signal-to-noise characteristics, though contrast resolution is limited. The T2-weighted sequence uses a long TR/TE and best highlights most pathologic lesions with excellent contrast between the lesion and normal tissue. Despite the excellent contrast and versatility, spin-echo limitations do exist and include relatively long imaging times (especially the T2-weighted sequence), thick image slices, and the inability to perform three-dimensional imaging and dynamic studies.[7, 10, 11]

Fast spin-echo is not simply "fast" spin-echo imaging. The sequence utilizes multiple 180-degree pulses during each TR in order to collect more information in a given time. Typical acquisition times in practice are one half to one fourth that of spin-echo with comparable contrast. The length of the echo train, the inter-echo interval, and the effective TE are all new variables that can be modified to optimize the type of contrast desired. The real contribution is the increased speed, which enables modification of the imaging parameters to optimize spatial resolution. The field of view can be decreased as the NEX (number of excitations) is increased, and the matrix can be made finer with imaging of smaller voxels. A voxel is that volume element in the body that corresponds to one picture element (pixel) in the image. The resultant images do differ from conventional spin-echo images. There is edge-enhancement, and fat remains bright on the T2-weighted images. Blurring is the major artifact in the phase-encoding direction. Choosing a shorter echo train length and inter-echo interval helps to minimize this problem.[11]

A variety of gradient recalled-echo sequences utilize smaller flip angles (less than 90 degrees), short TRs, and gradient reversal (versus the 180-degree refocusing pulse used in conventional spin-echo) to refocus the spinning hydrogen nuclei. The real difference between the variety of sequences is whether or not the residual transverse magnetization that exists following the administration of the small-flip-angle RF pulse is "spoiled" or "rewound." A spoiled sequence creates T1-weighted and proton density–weighted images. A rewound sequence creates T2-weighted images. The common advantages include high signal-to-noise ratio per unit of time, short imaging times, the ability to obtain thin (less than 1-mm) slices, and three-dimensional imaging with subsequent multiplanar reconstruction. Short imaging time helps minimize patient-motion artifacts. Dynamic imaging such as might be used in a patellar tracking study can be easily performed. Radial imaging is also a spin-off that can better define meniscal or labral abnormalities. This sequence, however, is sensitive to magnetic susceptibility effects ("blooming") from ferromagnetic and paramagnetic substances. Hemorrhage and calcification are more readily detectable in some circumstances.[10, 11]

Three concepts of MRI are closely related: chemical shift, bandwidth, and fat suppression. These relationships are beyond the scope of this discussion, and the reader is referred to an excellent review by Brateman.[5] Fat-suppression techniques, however, can be broadly divided into two major categories: chemical shift techniques and inversion recovery techniques. Chemical shift exploits differences between fat and water-containing tissues. Inversion recovery, known as short tau inversion recovery (STIR), exploits differences in the T1 relaxation times between fat and other tissues.

An appreciation of the basis for each fat-suppression method helps one to use them appropriately. A good example is that STIR is not useful for distinguishing between fat and blood because STIR suppresses fat owing to its T1 relaxation time. Fat and blood sometimes have the same T1 relaxation times; therefore, both would be suppressed. The STIR sequence utilizes a 180-degree RF pulse to invert longitudinal magnetization, followed by the conventional spin-echo pulses. An appropriate inversion time, which is the time between the initial 180-degree pulse and the subsequent 90-degree pulse, nulls out signal from fat. This results in images with selective suppression of fat and allows for an additive effect of T1, proton density, and T2. Normally these have opposing effects on image contrast. The prolonged T1 and T2 features of most pathologic processes are then highlighted against normal tissue. This technique is exquisitely sensitive in the detection of bone-marrow abnormalities because the normal fat marrow is nulled. STIR images have significant limitations, including decreased signal-to-noise ratio, decreased spatial coverage, and loss of anatomic detail. Contrast agents are not useful with this sequence because their T1 relaxation times may be shortened to that of fat and, therefore, the signal is nulled as with fat.

Chemical shift techniques to suppress fat (e.g., fat-saturation: "Fat Sat") can utilize frequency-selective excitation, phase contrast, or a hybrid combination of the two techniques. The Fat Sat technique takes advantage of an intrinsic difference of resonance frequencies of fat and water protons by applying a frequency-selective presaturation pulse immediately prior to the imaging sequence. The pulse effectively eliminates the longitudinal magnetization of hydrogen in fat, allowing for a "water-only" image. Fat-saturation sequences have proved useful in assessing cartilage, imaging bone-marrow abnormalities, and detecting pathology following intravenous contrast enhancement. The absence or presence of true cortical thinning can be assessed with this technique better than it can with conventional spin-echo imaging. Contrast enhancement with conventional spin-echo imaging may actually mask pathology in the bone marrow. The Fat Sat technique makes the pathology more conspicuous because the normal marrow signal is suppressed. Fat suppression can be non-uniform; thus it is important to evaluate normal fat signal in the region of interest to see whether suppression has been adequate.[12]

A series of sagittal and coronal MRIs of the knee demonstrates the varying appearance of osseous, articular, vascular, and soft tissue structures when the knee is studied with these various sequences and techniques (Figs. 1–3 through 1–11).

Text continued on page 10

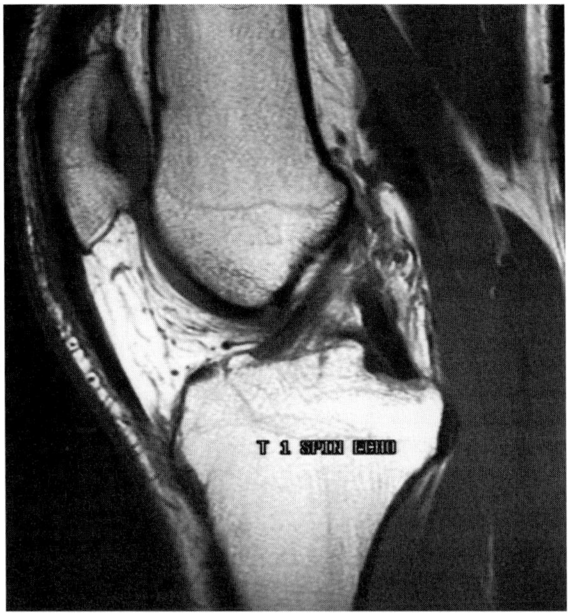

Figure 1–3
Sagittal T1 spin-echo image. *Bone marrow and subcutaneous fat are bright signal. Ligaments and tendons are dark signal. Muscle is intermediate to low signal.*

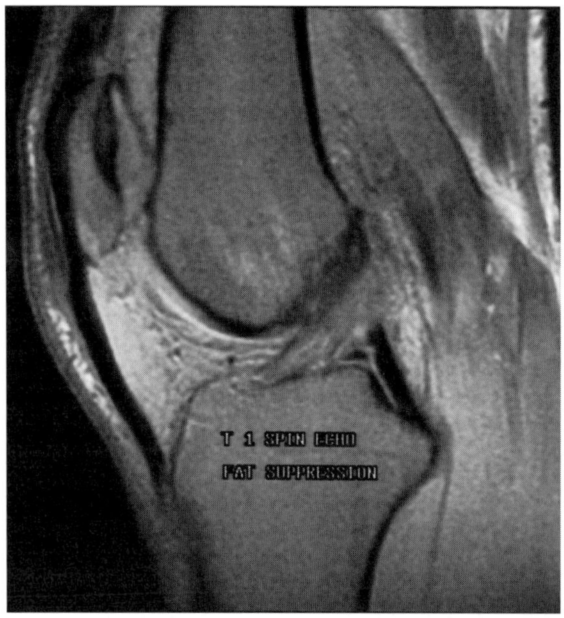

Figure 1–4
Sagittal T1 spin-echo image with fat saturation. *The bone marrow and subcutaneous fat signal is now suppressed. Any enhancing process after gadolinium administration would easily stand out on this low-contrast image.*

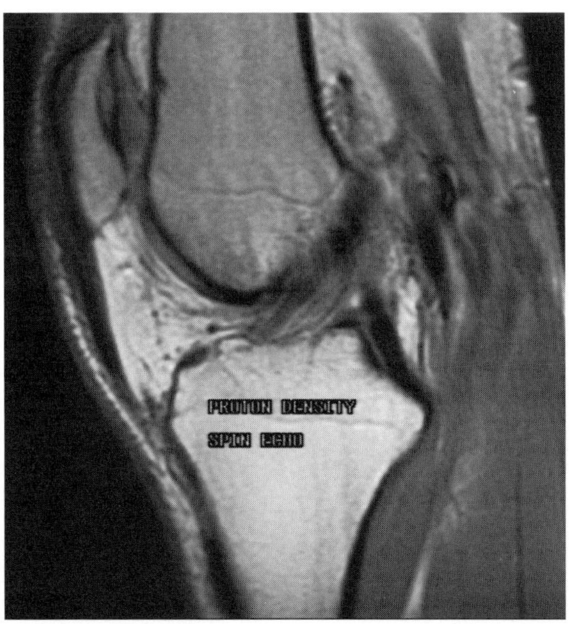

Figure 1–5
Sagittal proton-density spin-echo image. *Minor contrast resolution loss is evident compared with the T1 spin-echo image.*

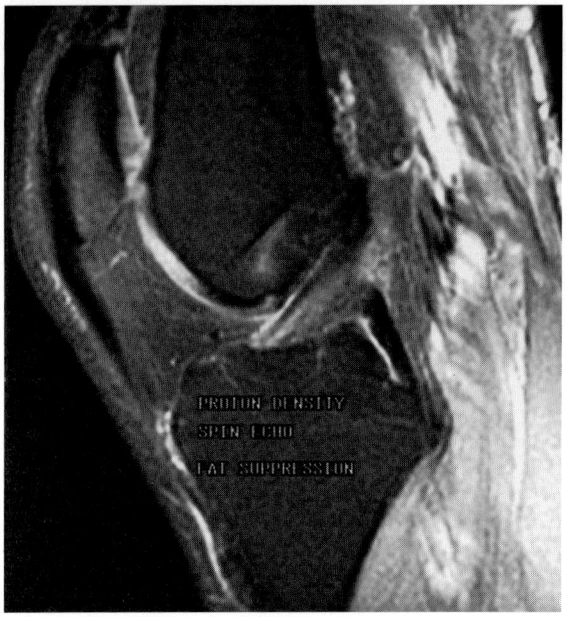

Figure 1–6
Sagittal proton-density spin-echo image with fat saturation. *Fluid and cartilage are bright with this technique. Bone contusions, when present, are particularly well seen on this low-contrast image.*

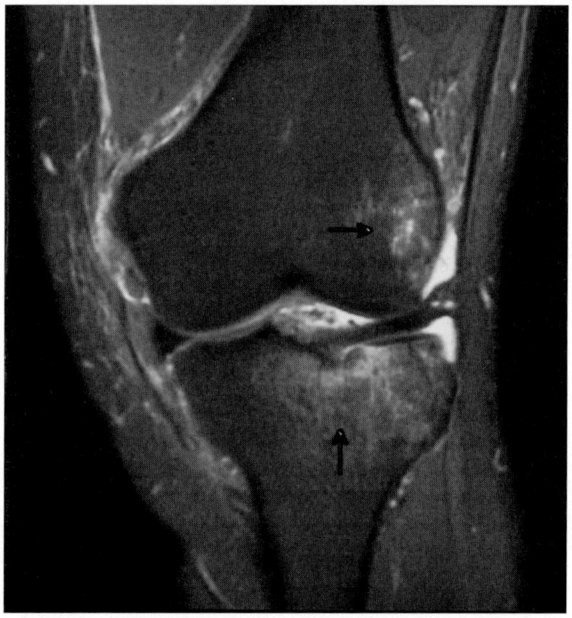

Figure 1–7
Coronal proton-density fast spin-echo image with fat saturation. *Contrast is similar to that of Figure 1–6, although imaging time is considerably faster and visualization of bone contusions* (arrows) *is excellent.*

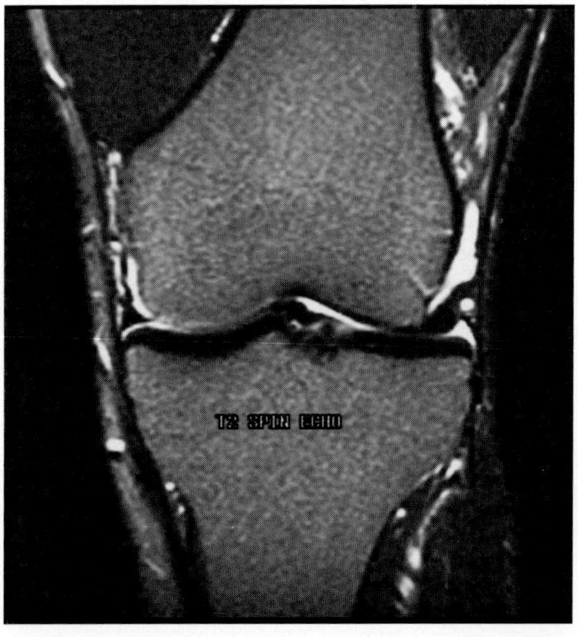

Figure 1–8
Coronal T2 spin-echo image. *Bone marrow and subcutaneous fat signal is diminished compared with the T1 spin-echo image. Joint fluid is bright signal.*

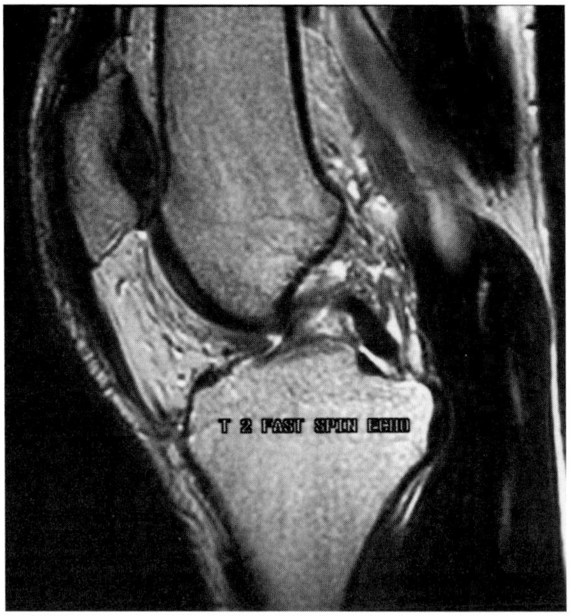

Figure 1–9
Sagittal T2 fast spin-echo image. *Note that bone marrow and subcutaneous fat signal is weaker than in the T1 spin-echo image (Fig. 1–3) but greater than in the T2 spin-echo image (Fig. 1–8).*

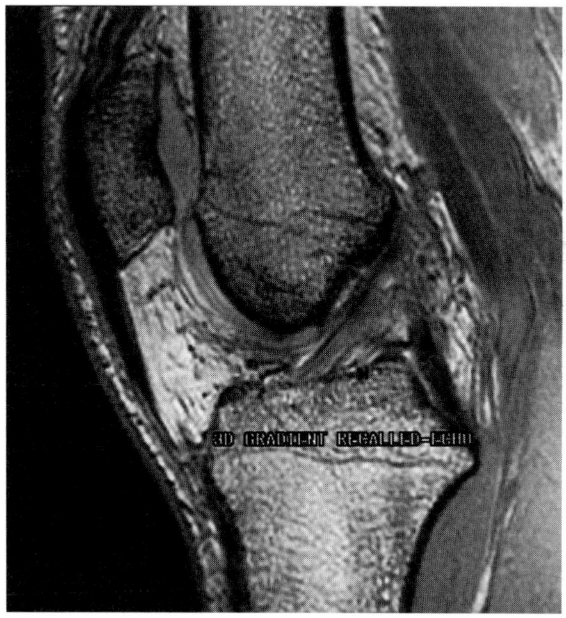

Figure 1–10
Sagittal three-dimensional gradient recalled-echo image. *This sequence is a volume acquisition. Slice thickness is less than on the other sequences to allow reconstruction in other imaging planes, but imaging time is also relatively longer. The weighting of the image is similar to that of the T2 sequence, but this image is not as sensitive to bone-marrow pathology.*

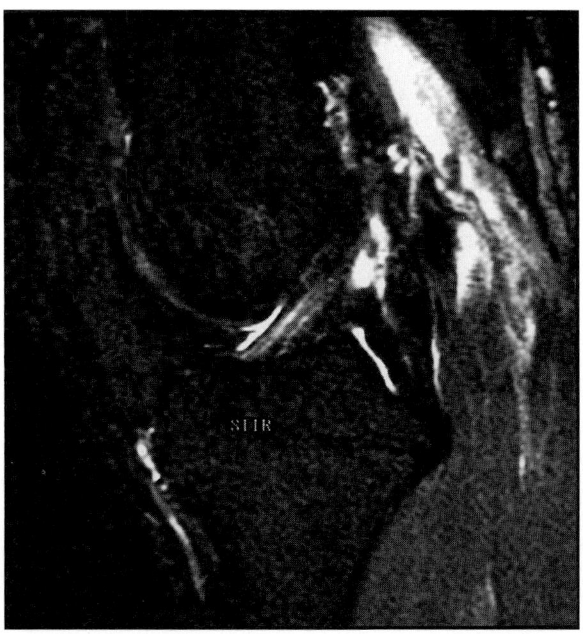

Figure 1–11
Sagittal STIR image. *Fluid is bright. Bone marrow and subcutaneous fat are dark, as are other soft tissue structures. This sequence is sensitive to bone marrow and soft tissue disorders such as bone contusions or osteomyelitis.*

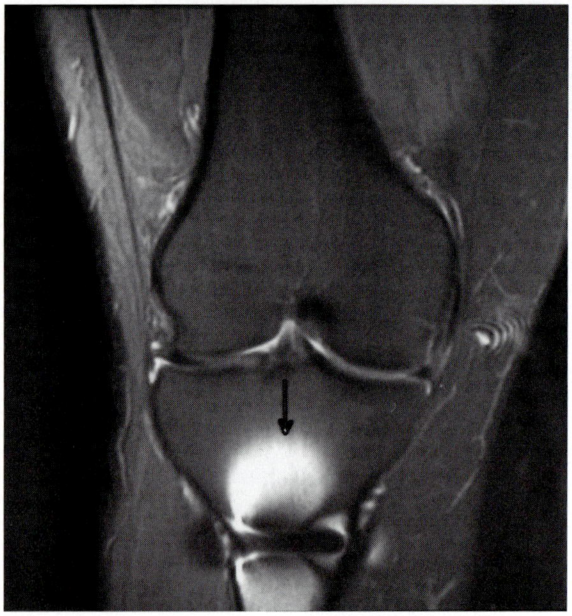

Figure 1–12
Coronal proton-density fast spin-echo image with fat saturation. *Note the distortion produced by metal as an area of signal void is surrounded by a bright signal inflection zone* (arrow).

MAGNETIC RESONANCE ARTIFACTS

The process of creating magnetic resonance images frequently gives rise to artifacts in the final display. Many can be corrected or improved through an understanding of their cause. Some artifacts are obvious and totally degrade the image. Other artifacts are regional or subtle. The various artifacts may be conveniently considered under the following headings: sequence, reconstruction algorithm, field, and noise. Each category can in turn be subdivided into system-related and patient-related artifacts. Bellon and coworkers present an excellent review of artifacts in spin-echo imaging.[2] Such review is beyond the scope of this chapter, but the following paragraph briefly comments on and illustrates several artifacts to indicate the nature of such problems.

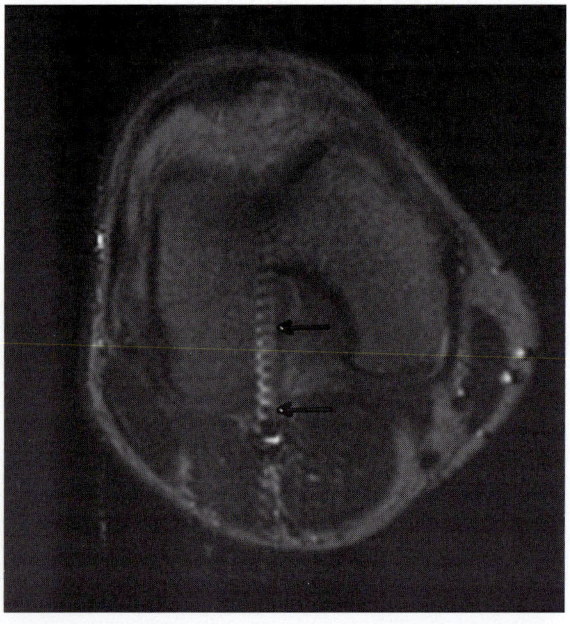

Figure 1–13
Axial gradient recalled-echo image. *Note the vertically oriented artifact resulting from popliteal artery pulsation* (arrows). *The artifact can be horizontally oriented by switching the phase-encoding and frequency-encoding directions.*

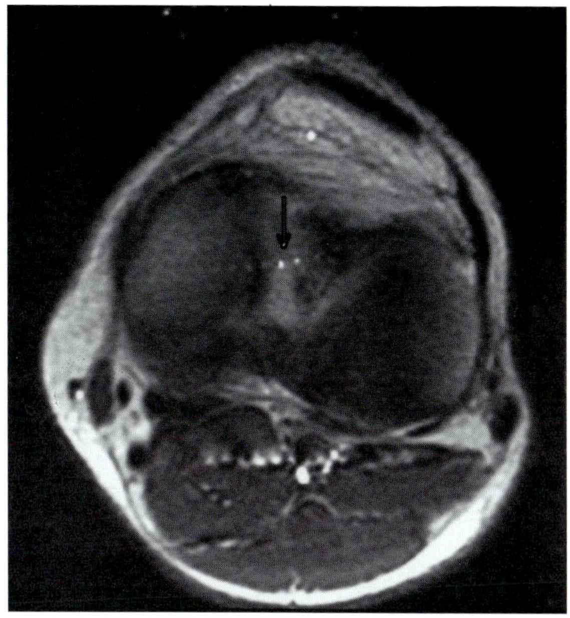

Figure 1–14
Axial gradient recalled-echo image. *Note the bright, linearly oriented artifact* (arrow) *from extraneous radiofrequency noise.*

Focal disturbances due to the presence of paramagnetic or ferromagnetic substances are an example of a patient-related field artifact. They are difficult to rectify because they often originate from within the patient. The distortion produces a signal void, often surrounded by a rim of increased signal known as the inflection zone (Fig. 1–12). Another patient-related artifact is related to pulsatile flow in a vessel (Fig. 1–13). The system-related effect of RF interference is due to detection of extraneous broadcast energy by the receiver coils of the scanner if the RF energy resonates with the Larmor frequency. When the bandwidth of the extraneous RF noise is narrow, a linear artifact perpendicular to the frequency encoding gradient becomes visible (Fig. 1–14).

CONTRAST

The only intravenous MRI contrast agents currently approved for general use by the Food and Drug Administration (FDA) are chelates containing gadolinium, a rare-earth element. They are potent promoters of T1 and T2 relaxation. The biodistribution of gadolinium chelates into the vascular and interstitial compartments is similar to that of iodine contrast agents. The major difference, however, between paramagnetic contrast agents, which contain no iodine, and conventional iodinated contrast agents is their mechanism of action. Unlike iodinated contrast for x-ray film, which improves tissue contrast directly by opacification, paramagnetic contrast agents operate indirectly to provide contrast enhancement by facilitating T1 and T2 relaxation through alteration of the magnetic environment of tissue. Both T1 and T2 relaxation times are shortened. The major advantage of gadolinium chelates is their better safety margin compared with radiographic contrast agents. Severe reactions are rare (approximately 1 in 350,000). Another advantage is the absence of nephrotoxicity in patients with impaired renal function. The improved contrast enhancement is best seen on T1 images.[3, 4, 6]

The role of gadolinium is extensive in the musculoskeletal system. The definition of tumor margins and the identification of cystic or necrotic components of osseous or soft tissue tumors is improved, although the sensitivity is not necessarily improved. In combination with fat-suppression techniques, gadolinium provides greater sensitivity to osteomyelitis. Identification of focal rim-enhancing inflammatory fluid collections maintains considerable clinical importance, because these sites represent targets for aspiration and drainage. Gadolinium enhancement is helpful in distinguishing the specific features of inflammatory arthritis, such as pannus formation, synovitis, effusions, and subchondral abnormalities. Diffusion of gadolinium into joint fluid following intravenous administration can be exploited for its arthrographic effect.

Although gadolinium is not currently FDA-approved for intra-articular administration, magnetic resonance arthrography has many reported potential applications. The knee and shoulder have been explored the most with regard to magnetic resonance arthrography. In the knee, imaging following intra-articular injection of gadolinium may better delineate meniscal re-tears and meniscocapsular separations, assess the thickness of articular cartilage, and evaluate communications between a cyst and the joint. Magnetic resonance arthrography increases the sensitivity to partial rotator-cuff tears, as well as to injuries to the glenoid labrum and glenohumeral ligaments.[1, 3, 4, 6, 12, 13]

CONTRAINDICATIONS AND SAFETY GUIDELINES

Absolute contraindications to MRI are few. Cardiac pacemakers, older ferromagnetic intracranial aneurysm clips, metal in the eye, implanted neurostimulators, and cochlear implants are seriously influenced in a magnetic field. Numerous publications address these safety matters.[14] Approximately 5% of patients experience claustrophobia during MRI; anxiolytic agents usually work well in this situation. Young children often require sedation. Although there is no convincing evidence to suggest a risk to the fetus, pregnancy is considered a relative contraindication to MRI, particularly in the first trimester.[8, 9]

CONCLUSION

The complexity of MRI is a mixed blessing. The physics and complex interplay of variables are at times intimidating, and yet they are important in the optimal utilization of the technique and interpretation of magnetic resonance images. Fortunately, the complexity also allows the technique to probe many subtle aspects of tissue biochemistry in response to disease. When properly interpreted, these complicated tissue effects allow MRI to display unprecedented sensitivity and characterization of human anatomy and pathology non-invasively.

References

1. Adam G, Dammer M, Bohndorf K, et al. Rheumatoid arthritis of the knee: Value of gadopentetate dimeglumine–enhanced MR imaging. AJR 1991; 156:457-466.
2. Bellon EM, Haacke EM, Coleman PE. MR artifacts: A review. AJR 1986; 147:1271-1281.
3. Beltran J, Chandnani V, McGhee RA, et al. Gadopentetate dimeglumine–enhanced MR imaging of the musculoskeletal system. AJR 1991; 156:457-466.
4. Bloem JL, Reiser MF, Vanel D. Magnetic resonance contrast agents in the evaluation of the musculoskeletal system. Magnet Res Q 1990; 6:136-163.
5. Brateman L. Chemical shift imaging: A review. AJR 1986; 146:971-980.
6. Drape J, Thelen P, Gay-Depassier P, et al. Intraarticular diffusion of Gd-DOTA after intravenous injection in the knee: MR imaging evaluation. Radiology 1993; 188:227-234.
7. Edelman RR, Kleefield J, Wentz KU, et al. Basic principles of magnetic resonance imaging. *In* Edelman RR, Hessilink JR, eds. Clinical Magnetic Resonance Imaging. 1990. Philadelphia: WB Saunders, 1990.
8. Edelman RR, Warach S. Magnetic resonance imaging (part one). N Engl J Med 1993; 328:708-716.
9. Edelman RR, Warach S. Magnetic resonance imaging (part two). N Engl J Med 1993; 328:785-791.
10. Griffey RH, Harms SE. General manipulation of magnetic resonance images. *In* Stoller DW, ed. Magnetic Resonance Imaging in Orthopaedics and Sports Medicine. Philadelphia: JB Lippincott, 1994.
11. Hardin CW, Gilley JS. The armchair adventurer's guide to magnetic resonance imaging: Theory and clinical applications. Oper Tech Sports Med 1995; 3:2-13.
12. Morrison WB, Schweitzer ME, Bock GW, et al. Diagnosis of osteomyelitis: Utility of fat-suppressed contrast-enhanced MR imaging. Radiology 1993; 189:251-257.
13. Palmer WE, Caslowitz PL, Chew FS. MR arthrography of the shoulder: Normal intraarticular structures and common abnormalities. AJR 1995; 164:141-146.
14. Shellock FG, Morisoli S, Kanal E. MR procedures and biomedical implants, materials, and devices: 1993 update. Radiology 1993; 189:587-599.

Introduction to Arthroscopy

Arthroscopy has come a long way since the introduction of the first practical arthroscope by Wantanabe and Takeda in 1960.[26] What was first a diagnostic tool, used only in the knee, soon became an operative device that could be used for a variety of procedures in numerous joints. O'Connor is credited with the development of operative knee arthroscopy,[20] although numerous pioneers—-including Johnson,[14] McGinty,[17] Jackson,[12] and others—have contributed greatly to the development of this field. Arthroscopy has become the standard of care for many problems. Fellowships, societies, textbooks, and journals have blossomed, and although controversy continues about its application in the treatment of various disorders, arthroscopy is clearly here to stay.

Arthroscopy has many advantages over open arthrotomy. It can be done with small incisions, increased accuracy, lower complication rates, decreased hospital time, and often shorter recovery periods.[2] Additionally, arthroscopy can dramatically increase diagnostic accuracy.[1, 5] Disadvantages of arthroscopy include the "steep learning curve" associated with its use. Finally, although indications continue to be proposed, there are limitations to its use, and equipment costs can be high.[2] Arthroscopy as a therapeutic tool is not a panacea.[7] Pathology that is *visualized* arthroscopically can not always be *treated* arthroscopically. Many procedures involve a combination of arthroscopic and open techniques. The effective use of arthroscopy lies in understanding its limitations.

In the inaugural issue of its journal, the Arthroscopy Association of North America presented guidelines for the practice of arthroscopic surgery[25]:

1. The arthroscopist should perform an adequate history and physical examination as well as obtaining radiographs or other pertinent laboratory evaluations of the patient; or determine that they have already been performed.
2. The risks, benefits, alternatives of treatment, and potential complications should be carefully outlined to each patient before an arthroscopic evaluation.
3. The arthroscopist should exercise due consideration in selecting the correct arthroscopic procedure for a particular condition.
4. A detailed report of the procedure should be prepared, including the arthroscopic findings and description of the operation.

OPERATIVE SUITE

Arthroscopy is most commonly performed in a standard surgical suite in either a hospital or an ambulatory surgical facility. Office arthroscopy, although advocated by some, may have significant limitations and is used primarily for diagnosis in selected patients. Newer flexible fiberoptic catheter systems resulted in under-recognition and underestimation of the severity of intra-articular knee pathology in one study.[18] A relatively large room that can accommodate the bulky arthroscopic equipment is preferred. Storage space for video equipment, shaver blades, instruments, and other equipment should be available in the room or nearby. Dedicated, well-trained operating room personnel are a must. Adequate electrical support, lighting, suction, and other logistic concerns should be considered.

Equipment sterilization is also important. Standard autoclaving is not appropriate for arthroscopes, cables, and many of the instruments used in arthroscopy. Gas sterilization with ethylene oxide is effective, but because of the long turnover times associated with this method, instruments can not be re-used during the same operative day.[14] Because of these concerns, most centers have elected to accept high-level disinfection in lieu of sterilization. This is accomplished by cold-soaking the equipment for 10 minutes in a 2% aqueous solution of glutaraldehyde.[15] Unfortunately, this solution can produce synovitis in patients,[10] as well as cause harmful effects in health care workers.[8, 27] A newer system that uses peracetic acid (Steris, Mentor, Ohio) is convenient and efficacious, and it may ultimately replace other methods of sterilization.[4]

ARTHROSCOPIC EQUIPMENT

Arthroscopy requires an arthroscope, a camera, a light source and fiberoptic cable, an irrigation system, cannulas, and various hand and motorized instruments.

An arthroscope is a small-diameter fiberoptic instrument that allows direct visualization of joints[2] (Fig. 1–15). It is designed to fit into a sleeve, or cannula. The cannula is first inserted into the joint with a sharp or blunt rod called a trocar, and then the trocar is exchanged for the arthroscope. A fiberoptic cable and camera is attached to the arthroscope, and irrigation fluid is attached to one or more cannulas. A specially adapted video camera is usually attached to the eyepiece of the arthroscope, and images can be recorded directly onto video or onto an accompanying printer (Fig. 1–16).

Arthroscopes are classified according to their diameter and viewing angle. The most commonly used arthroscope is 4 mm with a 25- to 30-degee angle. Smaller arthroscopes (2.5 mm and 1.9 mm) can be used for smaller joints (e.g., wrist). Different angles (70 or 90 degrees) are sometimes useful when visualization can be difficult (e.g., posterior knee).

Instruments used during arthroscopy include both hand-operated instruments (e.g., probes, baskets, grabbers) and motorized instruments (shavers) (Fig. 1–17). Commercially available shavers of various sizes, shapes, angles, and blades are useful in a variety of situations (Fig. 1–18). Intra-articular cautery also can be useful, and specially adapted tips that can be used with normal irrigating systems are available.

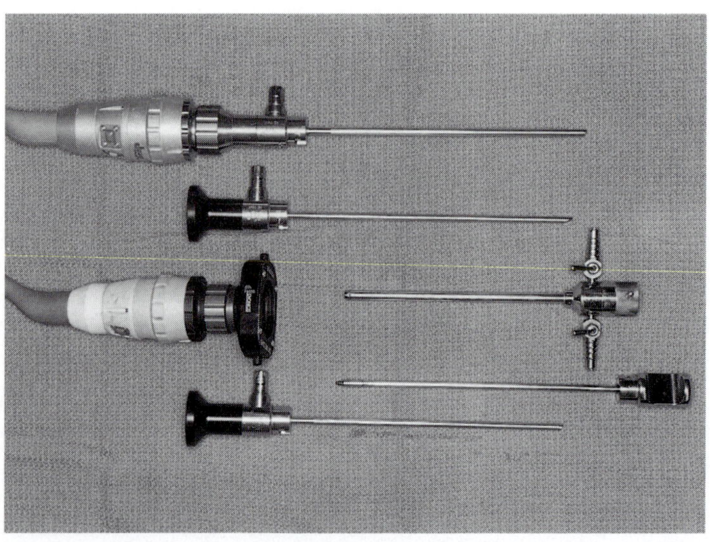

Figure 1–15
Top to bottom: 30-degree arthroscope with attached cable, 70-degree detached arthroscope, detachable camera cable (left) *and sleeve (cannula)* (right), *trocar for introduction of sleeve, and 30-degree detached arthroscope. (From DiGiovine NM, Bradley JP. Arthroscopic equipment and setup.* In *Fu FH, Harner CD, Vince KG, eds. Knee Surgery. Baltimore: Williams & Wilkins, 1994, pp 543–556.)*

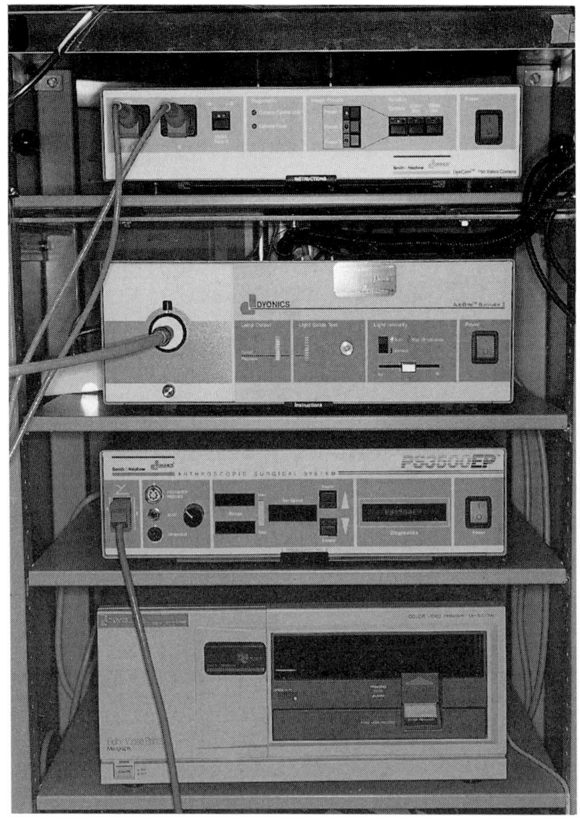

Figure 1–16
Top to bottom: Arthroscopic cart demonstrating camera, light source with cable, video, and printer. Monitor (not shown) can be placed on top of the cart. (From DiGiovine NM, Bradley JP. Arthroscopic equipment and setup. In *Fu FH, Harner CD, Vince KG, eds. Knee Surgery. Baltimore: Williams & Wilkins, 1994, pp 543–556.)*

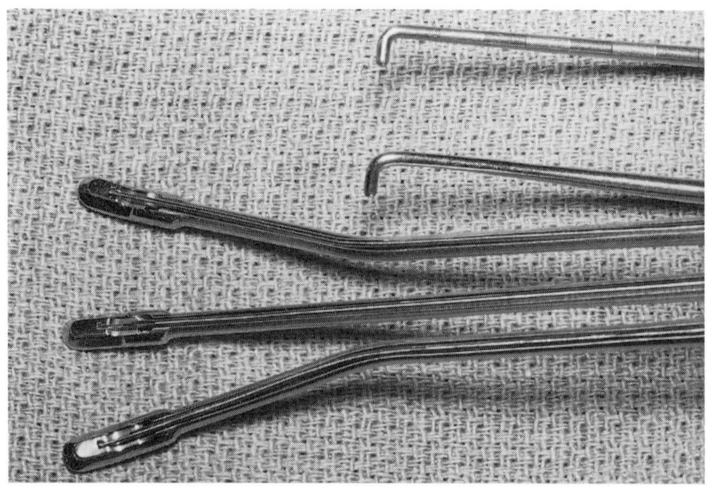

Figure 1–17
Probes (top two instruments) *and baskets* (bottom three instruments) *come in a variety of sizes and angles. (From Ciccotti MG, Shields CL, El Attrache N. Meniscectomy.* In *Fu FH, Harner CD, Vince KG, eds. Knee Surgery. Baltimore: Williams & Wilkins, 1994, pp 591–613.)*

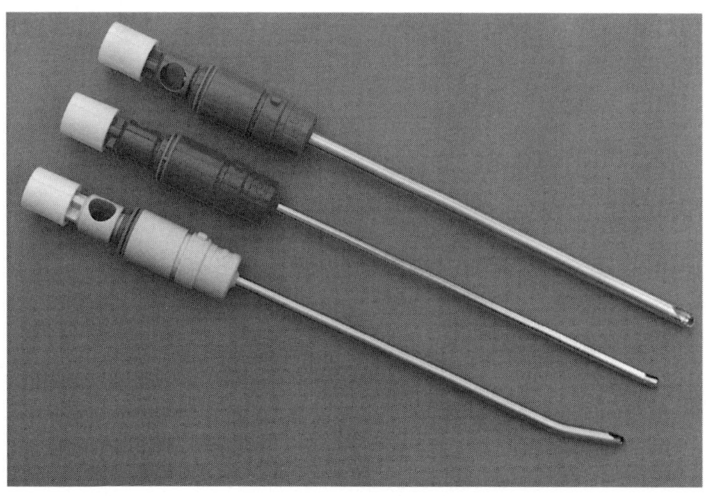

Figure 1–18
Arthroscopic shavers come in a variety of sizes, angles, and blades. (From Ciccotti MG, Shields CL, El Attrache N. Meniscectomy. In *Fu FH, Harner CD, Vince KG, eds. Knee Surgery. Baltimore: Williams & Wilkins, 1994, pp 591–613.)*

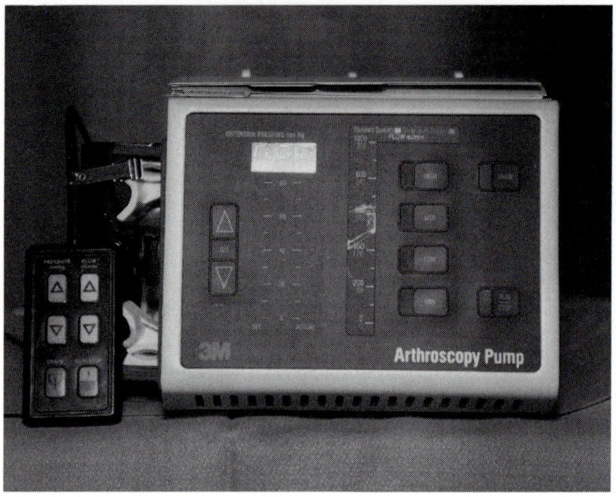

Figure 1–19
Commercially available arthroscopy pump allows precise control of flow rate and hydrostatic pressure. (From Ciccotti MG, Shields CL, El Attrache N. Meniscectomy. In *Fu FH, Harner CD, Vince KG, eds. Knee Surgery. Baltimore: Williams & Wilkins, 1994, pp 591–613.)*

Irrigation is used during arthroscopy for joint distention, improved visualization, and removal of debris. Lactated Ringer's solution is usually used because it is more physiologic than normal saline.[22] However, a 1995 study suggests that 5% mannitol may prevent excessive loss of proteoglycan from hyaline cartilage.[9] Cannulas are used for fluid egress or ingress. Hydrostatic pressure is necessary to maintain joint distention. This can be accomplished by gravity or via commercially available pumps (Fig. 1–19).

ARTHROSCOPIC VISUALIZATION

One must understand several fundamental concepts in order to accurately interpret arthroscopic images. First of all, the typical arthroscope does not "look" straight ahead but instead is directed at a 25- to 30-degree angle off the axis.[21] This allows greater visual control and improves the field. The arthroscopist can keep the arthroscope stationary and rotate the viewing angle, allowing a 60-degree view from a 30-degree scope (Fig. 1–20).[3]

Another consideration is that an object's size as seen on the monitor is magnified. The degree of magnification varies with the distance of the object from the lens of the arthroscope. Therefore, judging distances and size requires practice. Knowing the dimensions of an instrument, such as an arthroscopic probe, helps in determining the relative size of the object being visualized.

Finally, it is helpful to know about normal versus abnormal findings in each joint. We have included a section on the normal arthroscopic anatomy of each joint in order to provide a frame of reference for the cases that follow.

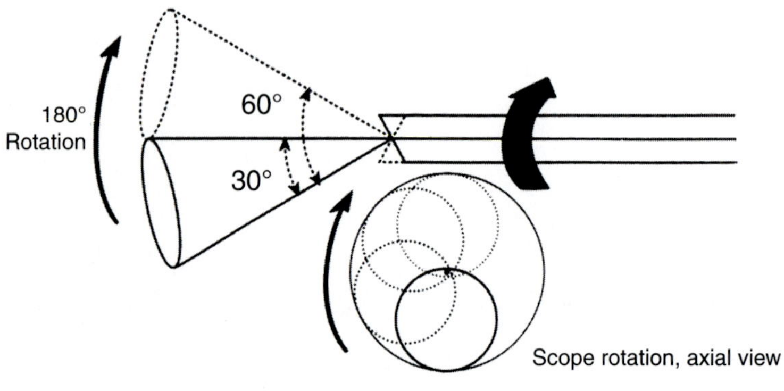

Figure 1–20
Rotation of a 30-degree arthroscope allows a 60-degree view. (From Crane L, Sullivan DJ. Instrumentation. In *McGinty JB, ed. Operative Arthroscopy. New York: Raven Press, 1991, p 6.)*

ARTHROSCOPIC TECHNIQUE

Arthroscopic technique is covered in more detail for the individual joints in the chapters to follow, but several principles apply. Extreme care should be taken in positioning the extremity for arthroscopy to avoid any compression that can result in neuropraxia. The nonoperative side is padded and protected, and excessive traction or unnecessary motion of the operative extremity is avoided. Numerous positioning and traction devices are commercially available and are often helpful. Tourniquets, when used, should be as wide as possible, and tourniquet time should be minimized. Surgical preparation and draping should be performed carefully to seal the operative field and create a sterile environment.

A joint-specific systematic diagnostic examination should be accomplished before any therapeutic procedures are performed. A complete arthroscopic examination can usually be performed in a few minutes, and then a complete operative plan can be confirmed or modified according to these findings.

ARTHROSCOPIC COMPLICATIONS

Any operation carries a risk of complications, and arthroscopy is no exception.[24] Perhaps the most common complication is inadvertent damage to intra-articular structures.[7] This risk is inversely proportional to the surgeon's experience and the care with which he or she performs the procedure. Proper portal placement, gentle technique, and attention to detail are critical. Instruments can break, especially when older, unserviced instruments are used.[16] Nerve or vessel injury can result from improper portal placement. One needs a thorough knowledge of local anatomy prior to performing arthroscopy. In joints at particular risk (such as the elbow), the "nick and spread" method is preferred. The skin only is cut with a blade, and a small hemostat is used to "clear the way" prior to inserting instruments with this method. Tourniquet paresis can be reduced with a wide cuff and by limiting tourniquet time to less than 90 minutes whenever possible.[23] Fluid extravasation has also been reported,[19] although the incidence of this complication can be reduced with careful placement of inflow cannulas and proper use of inflow pumps. Synovial fistula formation is a rare complication of arthroscopy and is usually remedied by 7 to 10 days of immobilization and, occasionally, delayed closure. Infection is an extremely rare complication of arthroscopy, usually the result of a break in sterile technique.[6] High-dose antibiotics and arthroscopic irrigation and debridement may be indicated in severe cases.[11]

ARTHROSCOPIC APPLICATIONS

Arthroscopy can be used for a variety of diagnostic and therapeutic purposes. It is useful in almost all major joints for irrigation and debridement, loose or foreign body removal, synovectomy, debridement of loose soft tissue, addressing osteoarticular lesions or fractures, and diverse other procedures. The use of arthroscopy in the knee and shoulder has steadily increased. It has become the standard treatment of meniscal tears. Applications continue to expand, and the future "scope" of arthroscopic applications is limited only by the imagination of the arthroscopist.

References

1. Cassells SW. Arthroscopy: Diagnostic and Surgical Practice. Philadelphia: Lea & Febiger, 1984.
2. Coward DB. General principles and instrumentation of arthroscopic surgery. *In* Chapman MW, ed. Operative Orthopaedics. Philadelphia: JB Lippincott, 1988, pp 1549-1559.
3. Crane L, Sullivan DJ. Instrumentation. *In* McGinty JB, ed. Operative Arthroscopy. New York: Raven Press, 1991, pp 5-10.
4. Crow S. Peracetic acid sterilization: A timely development for a busy healthcare industry. Infect Control Hosp Epidemiol 1992; 13:111-113.
5. Dandy D. Arthroscopic Surgery of the Knee. New York: Churchill Livingstone, 1981.

6. DeLee JC. Complications of arthroscopy and arthroscopic surgery: Results of a national survey. Arthroscopy 1988; 4:214-220.
7. DiGiovine NM, Bradley JP. Arthroscopic equipment and setup. *In* Fu FH, Harner CD, Vince KG, eds. Knee Surgery, Baltimore: Williams & Wilkins, 1994.
8. Fowler JF. Allergic contact dermatitis from glutaraldehyde exposure. J Occupat Med 1989; 31:852-853.
9. Gradiner R, Trager J, Klauser RJ. Influence of various irrigation fluids on articular cartilage. Arthroscopy 1995; 11(3):263-269.
10. Harner CD, Fu FH, Mason GC, Wissinger HA, Robin BS. Cidex-induced synovitis. Am J Sports Med 1989; 17:96-102.
11. Jackson RW. The septic knee: Arthroscopic treatment. Arthroscopy 1985; 1:194-197.
12. Jackson RW, Ovadin DN. Videoarthroscopy. Arthroscopy 1985; 1:108-115.
13. Johnson GM, Mancuso R, Whitbook C. Sterilization methods: Keeping up with health trends. Med Rev Outlook 1992; 3 (1).
14. Johnson LL. Arthroscopic Surgery: Principles and Practice, 3rd ed. St. Louis: CV Mosby, 1986.
15. Johnson LL, Shneider DA, Austin MD. Two per cent glutaraldehyde: A disinfectant in arthroscopy and arthroscopic surgery. J Bone Joint Surg [Am] 1982; 64:237-239.
16. Kieser C. A review of the complications of arthroscopic knee surgery. Arthroscopy 1992; 8:79-83.
17. McGinty JB, ed. Operative Arthroscopy. New York, Raven Press, 1991.
18. Meister K, Harris L, Indelicato PA, Miller G. A comparison of an optical catheter office arthroscope with a standard rigid rod-lens arthroscope in the evaluation of intra-articular pathology of the knee. American Academy of Sports Medicine Final Program. Book of Abstracts and Outlines, 21st Annual Meeting, Toronto, July 16-19, 1995.
19. Noyes FR, Spievack ES. Extraarticular fluid dissection in tissues during arthroscopy: A report of clinical cases and a study of intraarticular and thigh pressures in cadavers. Am J Sports Med 1982; 10:346-351.
20. O'Connor RL. Arthroscopy in the diagnosis and treatment of acute ligament injuries of the knee. J Bone Joint Surg [Am] 1974: 56:333-337.
21. Olsen EJ, King NA. Arthroscopic anatomy. *In* Fu FH, Harner CD, Vince KG, eds. Knee Surgery. Baltimore: Williams & Wilkins, 1994, pp 77-99.
22. Reagan BF, McInery VK, Treadwell BV, Zarins B, Mankin HJ. Irrigating solutions for arthroscopy: A metabolic study. J Bone Joint Surg [Am] 1983; 65:629-931.
23. Sapega AA, Heppenstall RD, Chance B, Park YS, Sokolow D. Optimizing tourniquet application and release times in extremity surgery: A biomechanical and ultrastructural study. J Bone Joint Surg [Am] 1985; 67:303-314.
24. Small NC. Complications in arthroscopy: The knee and other joints. Arthroscopy 1986; 2:253-258.
25. Suggested Guidelines for the Practice of Arthroscopic Surgery. [Editorial] Arthroscopy 1985; 1:74.
26. Wantanabe M, Takeda S. The number 21 arthroscope. J Jpn Orthop Assoc 1960; 34:1041.
27. Wiggins P, McCurdy SA, Zeidenberg W. Epistaxis due to glutaraldehyde exposure. J Occupat Med 1989; 31:854-856.

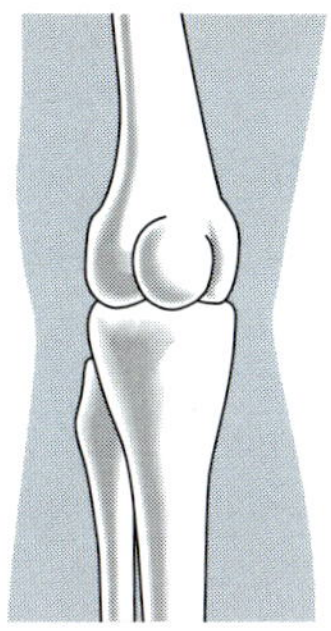

CHAPTER

2

Knee

MRI of the Knee

The greatest impact of musculoskeletal MRI has been in the evaluation of the knee. Reicher and coworkers[20] initiated a bright future for MRI of the knee in 1985 with their initial description of MRI used for meniscal tear detection and other knee disorders. The examination is highly accurate and has a high negative predictive value.[6] Although MRI is unlikely to replace arthroscopy as the standard examination for internal derangements of the knee, it is important in the evaluation of meniscal tears, discoid menisci, cruciate and collateral ligament tears, occult bone trauma, chondromalacia, anterior cruciate ligament reconstructions, and masses.[22]

TECHNIQUE

Techniques for imaging the knee vary greatly among imaging centers. Experience, individual preference, and equipment, such as the coil (Fig. 2–1) and magnetic field strength, affect the resulting protocol.[2] Specific imaging techniques can increase the sensitivity and specificity for particular knee disorders; therefore, a short, relevant clinical history greatly helps to optimize the protocol for maximum diagnostic information. If the appropriate sequences are obtained, MRI's accuracy in detecting meniscal tears is expected to be greater than 90%.[6] It is important to realize that the accuracy of arthroscopy is considered to be 95% in the best of hands; therefore, the diagnostic accuracy of MRI can be no better than the standard.[23]

One can use many common imaging sequences singularly or in combination. These include routine spin-echo (SE), fast scan techniques such as gradient recalled-echo (GRE) or fast spin-echo (FSE), and short tau inversion recovery (STIR).[17]

The three standard imaging planes are the direct coronal, sagittal, and axial views. We routinely examine the knee in these three planes using a field of view of 14 cm, 256 × 192 matrix, and 4-mm slice thickness. We obtain coronal FSE proton-density fat-saturation, sagittal SE T1, and FSE T2 sequences. The axial plane is evaluated with either a three-dimensional GRE or an FSE proton-density fat-saturation sequence to evaluate the patellar

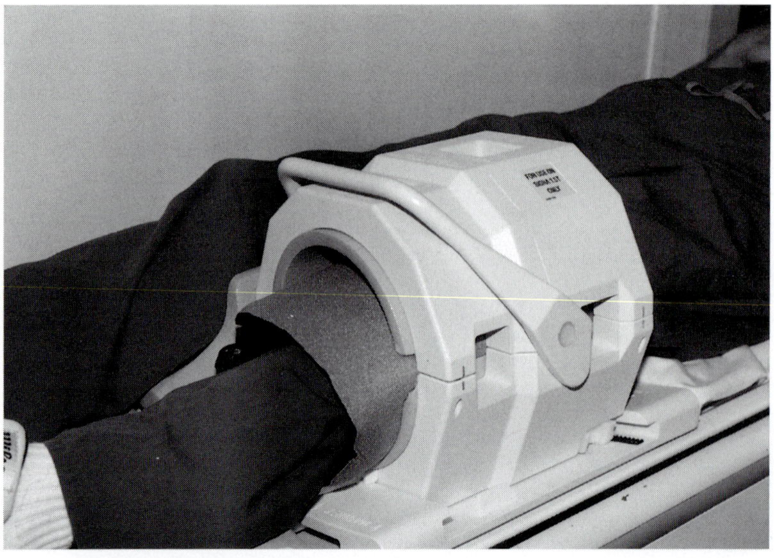

Figure 2–1
Knee phased array coil (receive only).

cartilage. An axial FSE T2 sequence is obtained for evaluation of masses such as a popliteal cyst, ganglion, or large meniscal cyst.

The coronal plane optimally evaluates the collateral ligaments and body of the menisci. The sagittal plane reveals the cruciate ligaments, anterior and posterior horns of the menisci, and the synovial anatomy, especially the suprapatellar pouch. Overall, the bones, muscles, tendons, and neurovascular structures are fully evaluated with the integration of all three planes.[30]

MRI ANATOMY

MRI anatomy of the knee is well displayed in the axial, coronal, and sagittal planes (Figs. 2–2, 2–3, 2–4, 2–5, and 2–6).

The knee is a complex joint allowing flexion, extension, anteroposterior gliding, and internal-external rotation. The major articular surfaces are the medial and lateral condyles of the femur and the patellar surface.

Two menisci are in the knee joint, one within the medial compartment and one within the lateral compartment. The medial meniscus is semicircular, and the lateral meniscus is almost a complete circle. The anterior and posterior horns of the lateral meniscus are equal in size. The medial meniscus has a larger posterior than anterior horn and is firmly attached to the deep aspect of the medial collateral ligament. The menisci are further attached to the tibia at their central and inferior, peripheral portions. The anterior horns are attached by the transverse ligament. The posterior horn of the lateral meniscus is traversed by the popliteus tendon, which courses posterior and inferior from the lateral femoral condyle. The posterior horn of the lateral meniscus is also secured to the medial femoral condyle by the ligament of Wrisberg, which passes posterior to the posterior cruciate ligament (PCL), and less constantly by the smaller ligament of Humphrey, which passes anterior to the PCL. The menisci serve the important functions of shock absorption, distribution of nutrient synovial fluid within the joint, load transmission, and stability. The normal adult meniscus is homogeneously low in signal on all pulse sequences. Children normally have intra-substance signal within their menisci.[11]

The anterior and posterior cruciate ligaments are important to knee stability. The two structures are intra-articular and extrasynovial. The anterior cruciate ligament (ACL) extends obliquely and anteriorly as numerous fascicles joined in two functional units (the anteromedial band and the posterolateral band) from the medial aspect of the lateral femoral condyle in the intercondylar notch to the anterior aspect of the tibia. MRI reveals the ACL as a straight, continuous, striated band of low to intermediate signal. The PCL passes from the lateral aspect of the medial femoral condyle in the intercondylar notch to the posterior edge of the tibial plateau. MRI shows the PCL as a gently convex, curving structure with uniform low signal.[5, 31]

The medial collateral ligament (MCL) is visualized on MRI as a thin curvilinear structure of low signal joining the medial femoral and tibial condyles. The MCL has superficial and deep components. The more superficial component arises from the medial femoral epicondyle and inserts on the medial tibial metaphysis just deep to the pes anserinus. The deep component is firmly attached to the medial meniscus. The two components join anteriorly to form the medial patellar retinaculum. Several identifiable structures reside laterally. The lateral collateral ligament arises from the lateral femoral condyle and attaches to the anterior and superior aspect of the fibular head. The biceps femoris tendon attaches just posterior to the lateral collateral ligament. The iliotibial track attaches to the anterior and lateral tibial tubercle.[21, 30]

The important tendons around the knee include the quadriceps tendon and the patellar tendon. The MRI appearance of these tendons is uniformly low in signal, although the quadriceps tendon has a striated appearance at its attachment to the patella on the T1 sequence. The patellar tendon may show buckling if the knee is positioned in slight hyperextension. The infrapatellar fat pad is a fibrofatty structure in the space between the patellar tendon and the femur and tibia.[5, 30]

Text continued on page 27

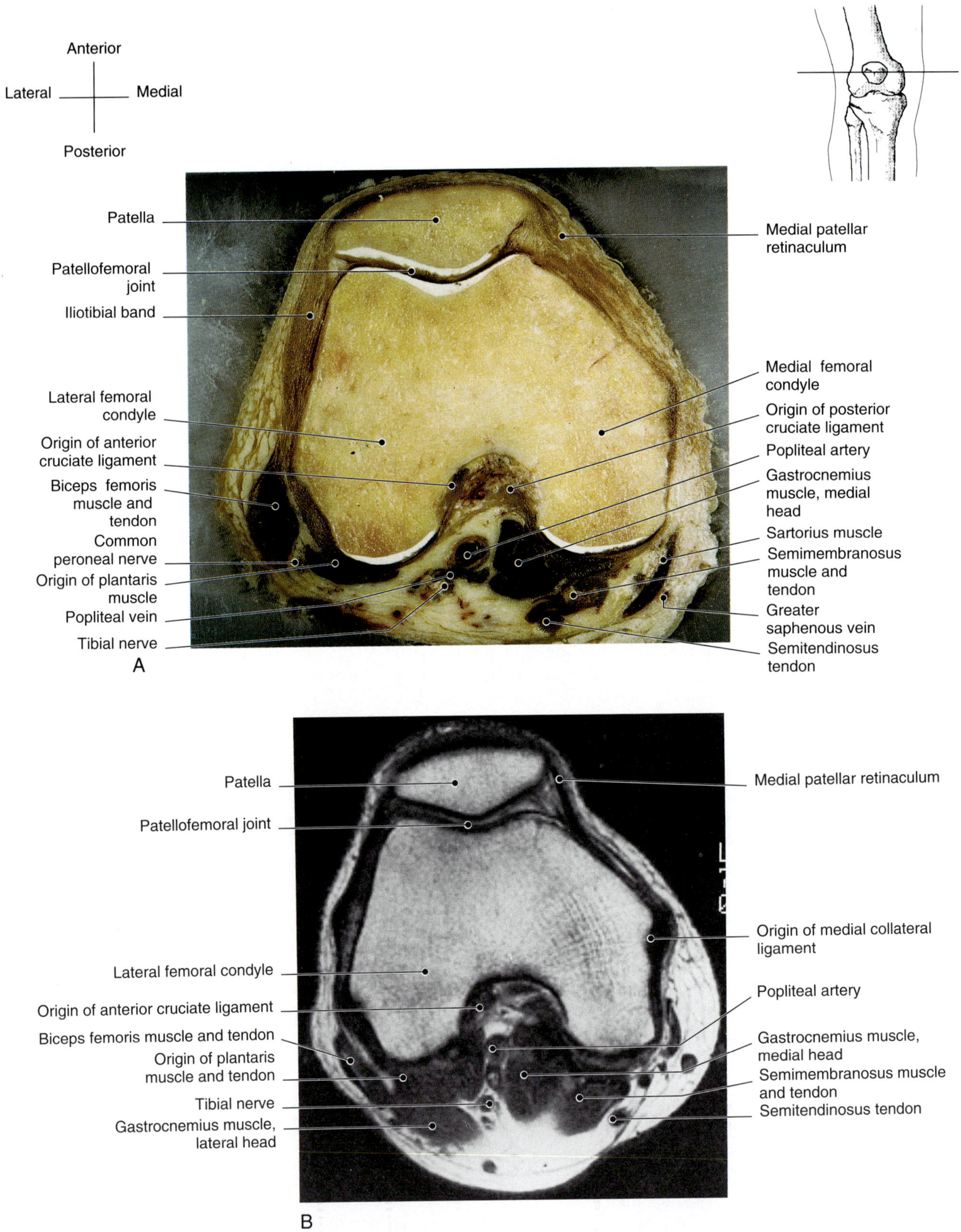

Figure 2–2

Axial cryoplaned section (A) *and magnetic resonance image (TR, 500ms; TE, 20 ms)* (B) *of the knee at the level of the patellofemoral joint. (From Chan WP, Rauschning W, Wu CY, et al. Magnetic resonance imaging anatomy and cryomicrotome atlas.* In *Chan WP, Lang P, Genant HK, eds. MRI of the Musculoskeletal System. Philadelphia: WB Saunders, 1994.)*

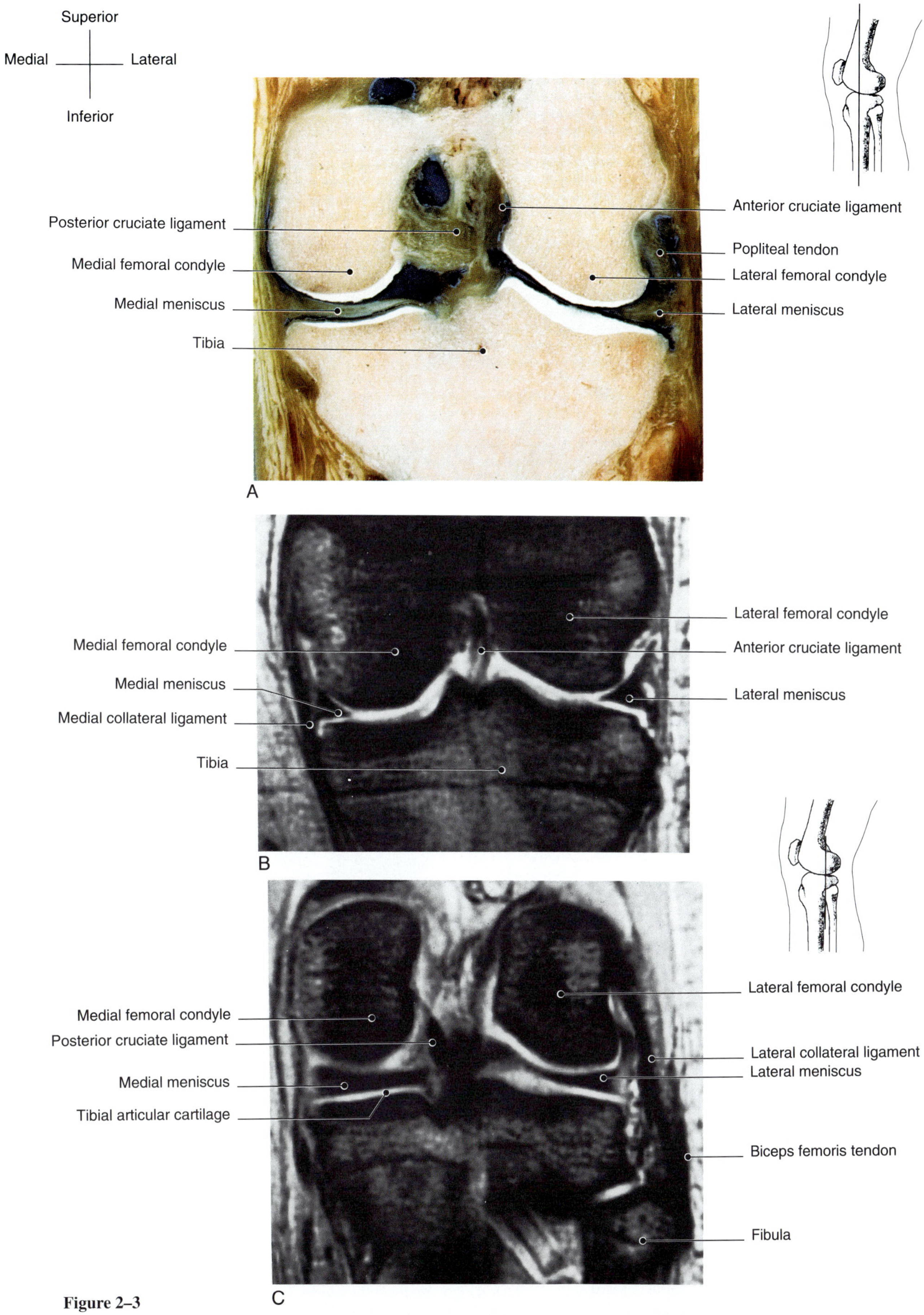

Figure 2–3
Midcoronal cryoplaned section of the knee (A) *and midcoronal* (B) *and posterior coronal* (C) *magnetic resonance images (TR, 400ms; TE, 15 ms; flip angle, 30 degrees) of the knee. (From Chan WP, Rauschning W, Wu CY, et al. Magnetic resonance imaging anatomy and cryomicrotome atlas.* In *Chan WP, Lang P, Genant HK, eds. MRI of the Musculoskeletal System. Philadelphia: WB Saunders, 1994.)*

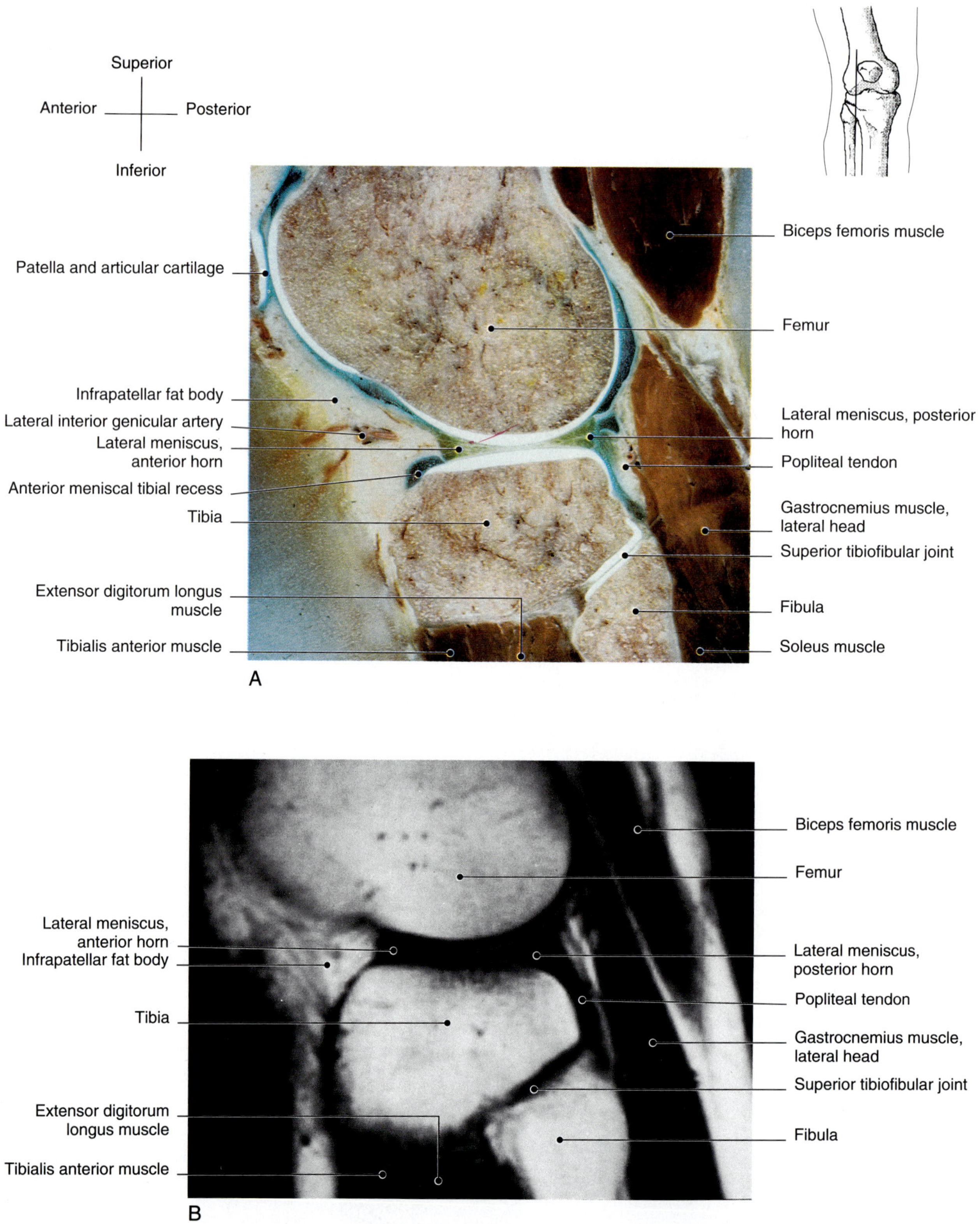

Figure 2–4

Paramedian sagittal cryoplaned section (A) *and magnetic resonance image (TR, 800ms; TE, 20 ms)* (B) *of the knee at the level of the lateral meniscus. (From Chan WP, Rauschning W, Wu CY, et al. Magnetic resonance imaging anatomy and cryomicrotome atlas.* In *Chan WP, Lang P, Genant HK, eds. MRI of the Musculoskeletal System. Philadelphia: WB Saunders, 1994.)*

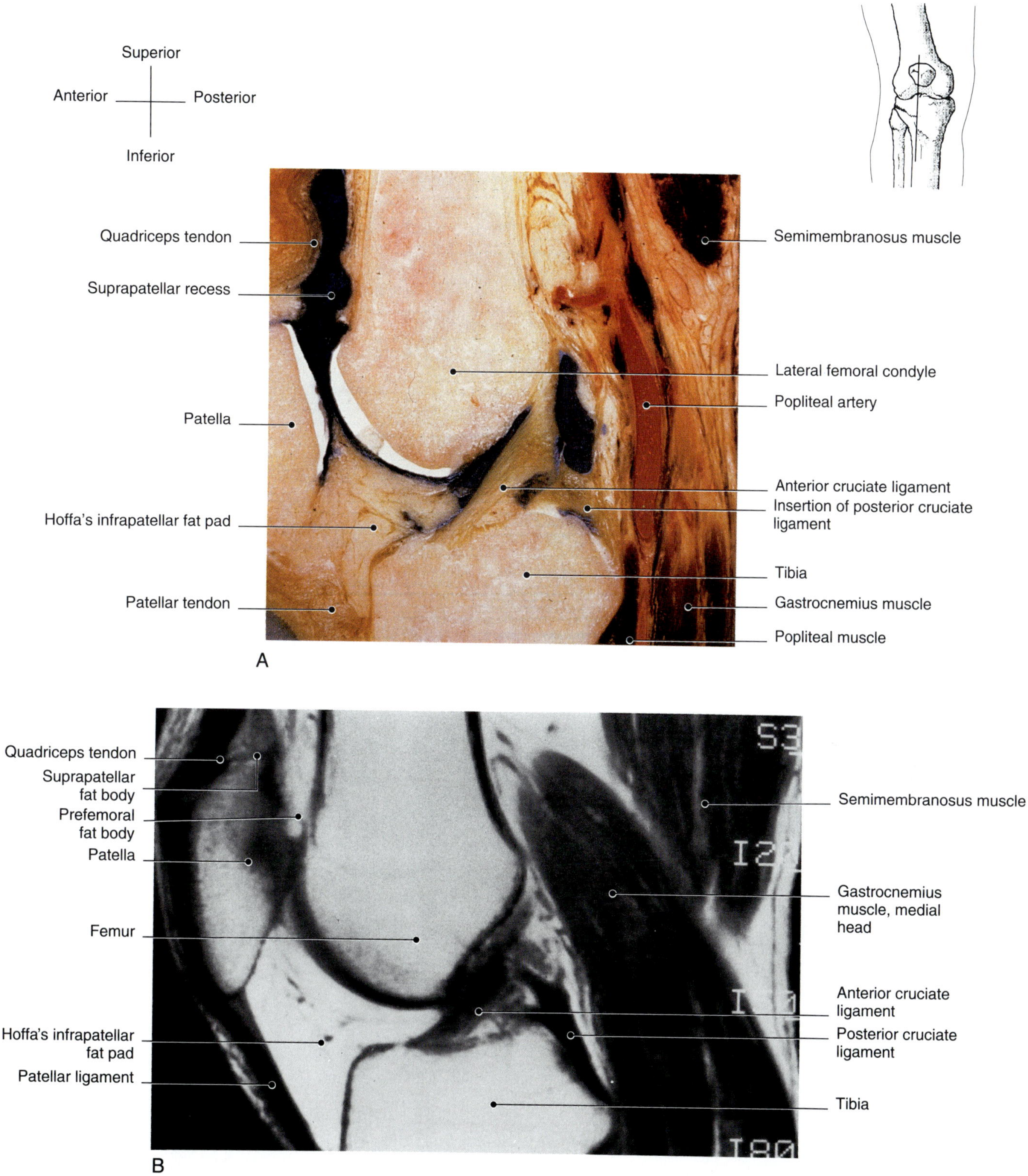

Figure 2–5
Sagittal cryoplaned section (A) *and magnetic resonance image (TR, 800ms; TE, 20 ms)* (B) *of the knee through the posterior cruciate ligament. (From Chan WP, Rauschning W, Wu CY, et al. Magnetic resonance imaging anatomy and cryomicrotome atlas.* In *Chan WP, Lang P, Genant HK, eds. MRI of the Musculoskeletal System. Philadelphia: WB Saunders, 1994.)*

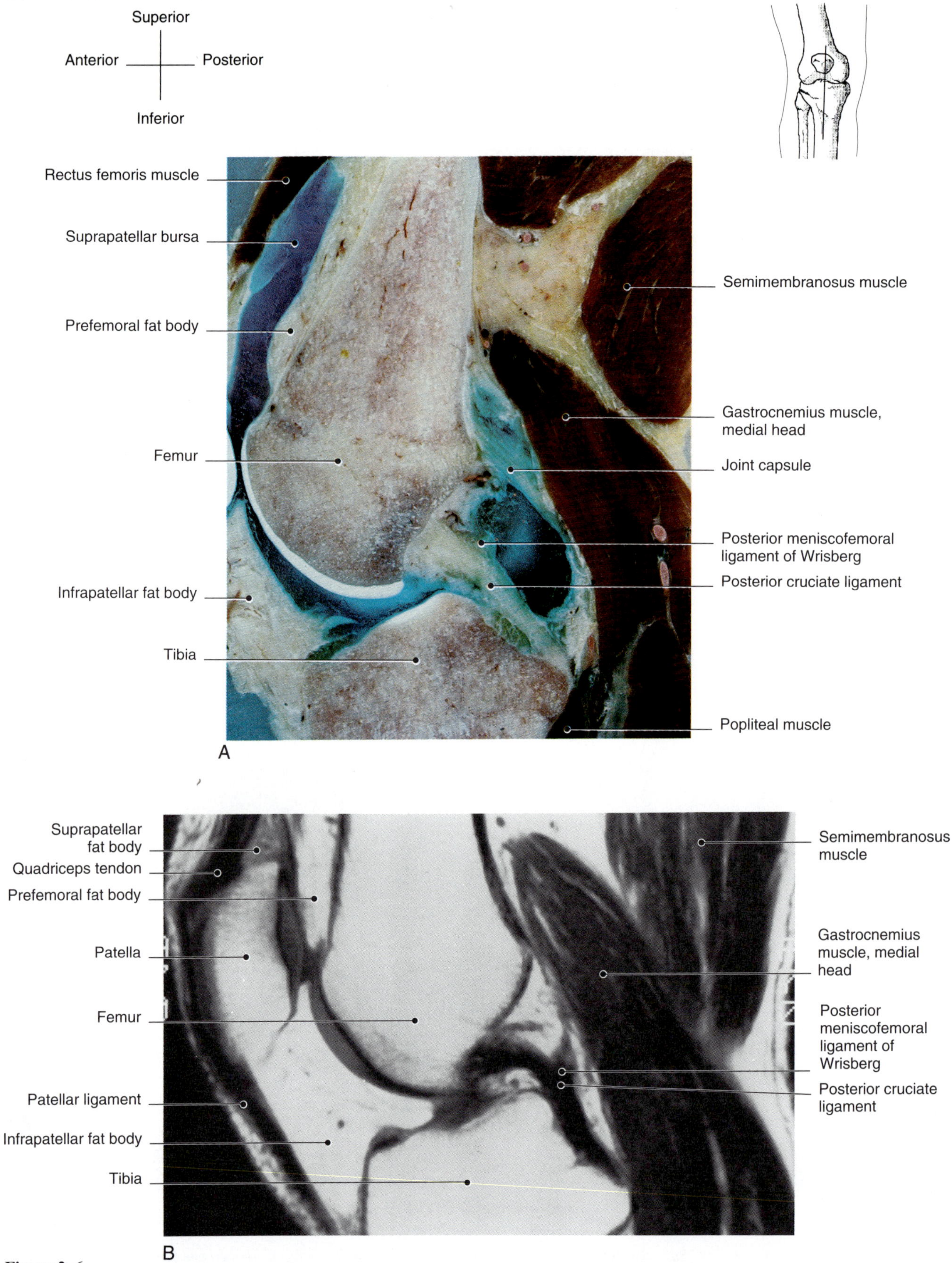

Figure 2–6

Sagittal cryoplaned section (A) *and magnetic resonance image (TR, 800ms; TE, 20 ms)* (B) *of the knee through the anterior cruciate ligament. (From Chan WP, Rauschning W, Wu CY, et al. Magnetic resonance imaging anatomy and cryomicrotome atlas.* In *Chan WP, Lang P, Genant HK, eds. MRI of the Musculoskeletal System. Philadelphia: WB Saunders, 1994.)*

Synovium lines the internal surface of the joint. There are several important bursae. The suprapatellar bursa develops as a separate structure and usually communicates with the joint as the suprapatellar pouch following atrophy of the plica from the lateral to medial aspects. The deep infrapatellar bursa is at the junction of the patellar tendon with the tibial tuberosity. Bursae also are anterior to the patella and patellar tendon. One other important bursa is the posterior medial bursa associated with the gastrocnemius and semimembranosus tendons. Communication between the joint and this bursa often produces popliteal cysts.[5, 30]

The femur, tibia, and patella are the major osseous structures of the knee joint. Bone marrow signal varies. Hematopoietic marrow gradually converts to fatty marrow from childhood to adult life. Adults, however, may continue to have hematopoietic activity, which appears patchy and lower in signal on the T1 sequence than the characteristic high signal of fatty bone marrow on this sequence. The patella is a large sesamoid bone with a thick articular cartilage.[5, 30]

Lateral, medial, and anterior muscle groups are visualized in the knee region. The lateral group comprises the biceps femoris, lateral gastrocnemius, popliteus, and plantaris; the medial group comprises the semimembranosus, medial gastrocnemius, sartorius, and gracilis; the anterior group comprises the vastus intermedius, medialis, medialis obliqui, lateralis, and the rectus femoris.[5, 30]

There are four major neurovascular structures: the popliteal artery, the vein, and the tibial and peroneal nerves.

PATHOLOGY

Normal Meniscus, Meniscal Degeneration, and Meniscal Tears

Lesions of the menisci are common injuries in orthopaedic practice. Since orthopaedic surgeons have increasingly employed meniscus-sparing treatments, MRI has become increasingly important in the diagnosis and evaluation of a suspected meniscal injury. Diagnostic arthroscopy is widely used and accepted as the standard against which all other methods are measured; however, as a new and noninvasive technique, MRI has proved highly accurate in the evaluation of the meniscus and has a high negative predictive value (approximating 95%).[23] A normal MRI examination of the knee is, therefore, highly accurate in excluding an internal derangement.[16]

Meniscal tears are represented by high signal in the meniscus, which contacts the superior or inferior articular surface.[7, 8, 15] Visualization is improved with narrowed-window and magnified photography.[3] There are a couple of exceptions, however: the "picture frame" meniscus (Fig. 2–7), which reveals high-signal replacement of the meniscus except

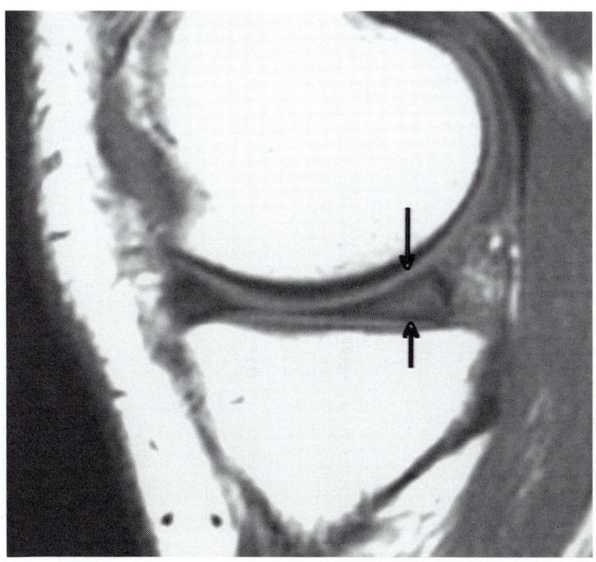

Figure 2–7
Sagittal T1 SE image, "picture-frame meniscus." *Note diffuse increased signal within the posterior horn of the medial meniscus framed with normal meniscal signal* (arrows).

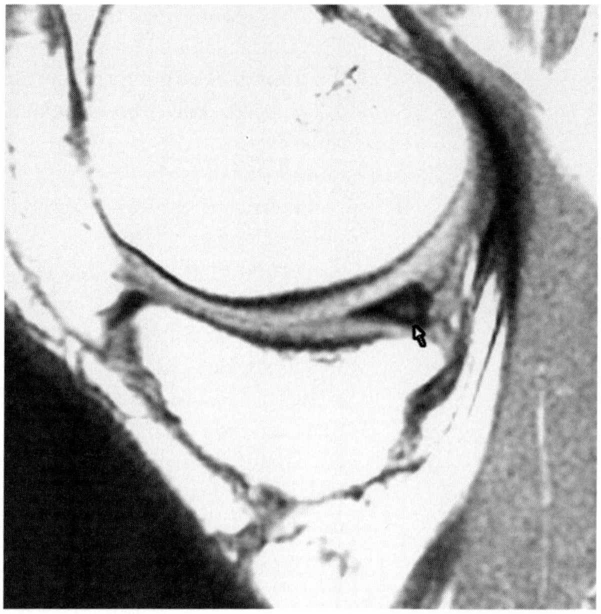

Figure 2–8
Sagittal T1 SE image, Grade-1 meniscal signal. *Note focal globular signal in the posterior horn of the lateral meniscus* (arrow), *which does not communicate with an articular surface.*

for the margins, and meniscal cysts, which by definition are associated with meniscal tears even though classic communication of abnormal meniscal signal to an articular surface occasionally is not identified. Conversely, extension of abnormal meniscal signal to an articular surface on only one image is often shown to be normal at arthroscopy.[13] Generally, medial meniscal tears are considerably more common than lateral meniscal tears, and posterior horn tears are more common than mid-body tears. An isolated anterior horn tear is rare.[16]

Meniscal tears should be characterized by location and direction. A familiar grading system consisting of three grades has been devised for intrameniscal signal.[13] Grade-1 sig-

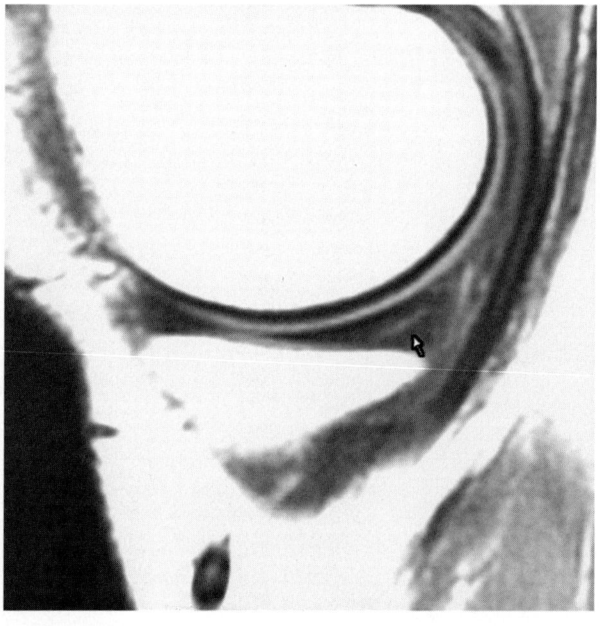

Figure 2–9
Sagittal T1 SE image, Grade-2 meniscal signal. *Note increased linear signal in the posterior horn of the medial meniscus* (arrow), *which does not communicate with an articular surface.*

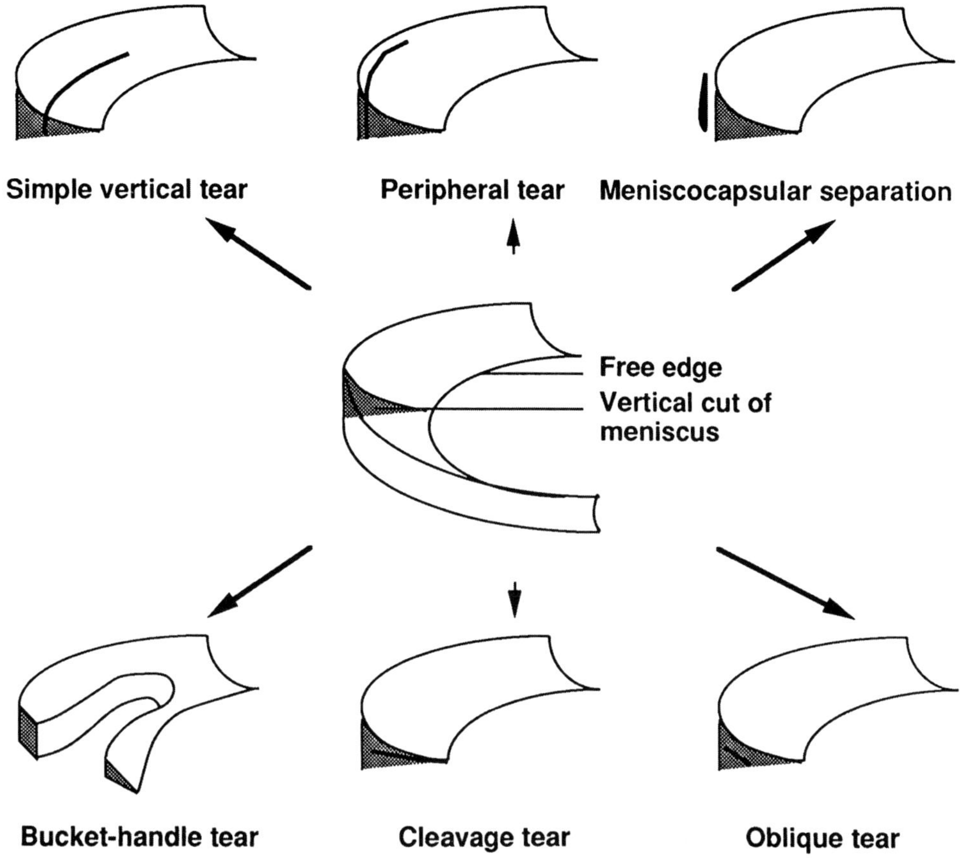

Figure 2–10

Types of meniscal tears. (From Chan WP, Fritz RC, Steinbach LS, et al. The knee: Internal derangements. In *Chan WP, Lang P, Genant HK, eds. MRI of the Musculoskeletal System. Philadelphia: WB Saunders, 1994.)*

nal has an ovoid or globular shape that does not communicate with any meniscal articular surface (Fig. 2–8). Grade-2 signal has a linear appearance that does not communicate with any meniscal articular surface (Fig. 2–9). Grade 1 and Grade 2 indicate intra-substance degeneration and should not be reported as tears. The term "tear," in these instances, might lead to an unnecessary arthroscopy. Grade-3 signal represents a definitive tear, either partial or full thickness, that communicates with an articular surface.[8] These tears frequently are symptomatic, unlike the Grade-1 and Grade-2 meniscal signal.[14]

Grade-3 meniscal tears can be classified in many ways[30] (Fig. 2–10). Basically, there are traumatic and degenerative meniscal tears. Their MRI appearance on the triangular cross-section of the meniscus can be divided into vertical and horizontal tears, which are the typical presentations of traumatic and degenerative tears, respectively. Both orientations may coexist and present as a complex tear.

If one visualizes the surface morphology, tears can be divided into longitudinal and radial (or transverse) tears. The longitudinal tear extends along the meniscus parallel to the free and peripheral margins either part way or for the whole length of the meniscus and may emerge to the superior or inferior articular surface. The radial (or transverse) tear radially extends perpendicular to these same margins of the meniscus. Such tears are common along the free margin of the lateral meniscus in the middle one third of the body (Fig. 2–11). They are vertically oriented without a horizontal component or flap. They are also more difficult to detect and should be deliberately sought during review of MRI results.[18, 30]

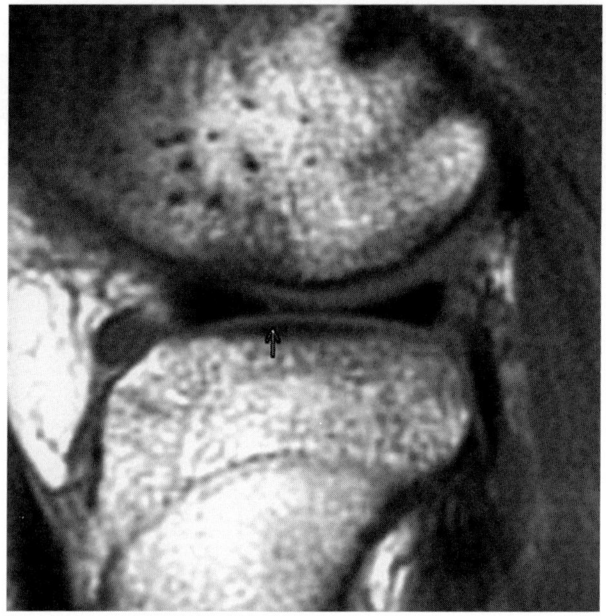

Figure 2–11
Sagittal T1 SE image, radial tear. *Note the small focus of increased signal* (arrow) *at the free margin of the middle one third of the lateral meniscus.*

A flap tear is an attached portion of the meniscus that has become unstable and relocates into the weight-bearing portion of the joint or turns superiorly on itself (Fig. 2–12). Flap tears are more common in the posterior horns. Flap tears are typically associated with degenerative tears. A parrot-beak tear begins at the free margin and extends into the meniscus at an oblique angle (a parrot-beak tear is a combination of a longitudinal and a radial tear).[18, 30]

The horizontal cleavage tear (Fig. 2–13) is empirically the most common tear pattern; it extends to the inferior surface more often than to the superior surface and is likely to be seen in the posterior horn of the medial meniscus.[18, 30]

The bucket-handle tear is a full-thickness longitudinal tear, usually of the medial meniscus, which can allow the free edge of the meniscus to become displaced into the intercondylar notch. It can be recognized on the sagittal image in that only one image has the "bow-tie" configuration when one has scanned from the periphery to the free margin. The

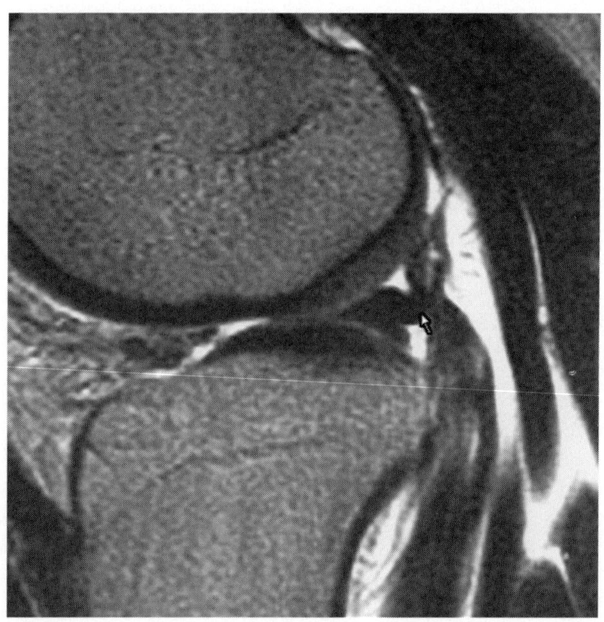

Figure 2–12
Sagittal T2 FSE image, flap tear. *Note evidence of a meniscal flap* (arrow) *in the posterior horn of the lateral meniscus that has turned superiorly on itself.*

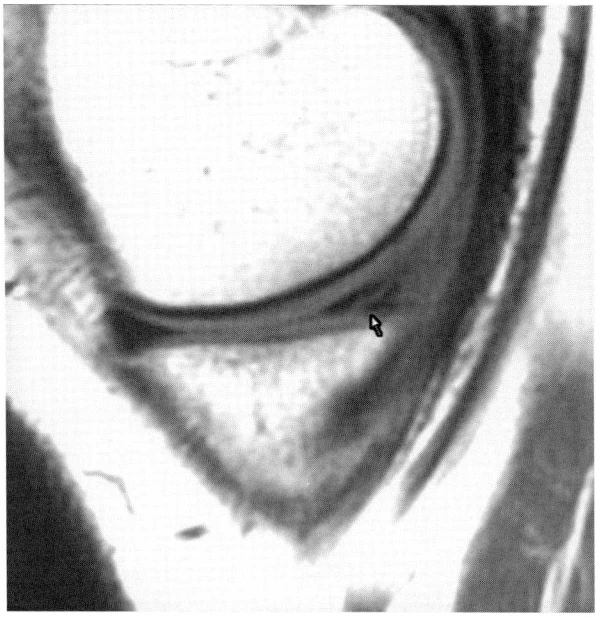

Figure 2–13
Sagittal T1 SE image, horizontal cleavage tear. *Note linear increased signal in the posterior horn of the medial meniscus* (arrow) *that communicates with the inferior articular surface.*

coronal image is excellent in showing this type of tear, which is likely to involve a shortened meniscus that is truncated at the apex of the triangular configuration. The medially displaced fragment of the bucket-handle tear is sometimes displayed on sagittal images as a band of low signal intensity parallel and anterior to the posterior cruciate ligament[33] (Fig. 2–14).

Discoid Meniscus

The discoid meniscus is a congenitally enlarged meniscus that occurs in a small percentage of the population. The lateral discoid meniscus is the most common presentation. The discoid meniscus tends to tear and occasionally is symptomatic in the absence of a frank tear. Such menisci are easily identified on coronal images because the meniscus extends to the intercondylar notch on multiple images. Sagittal imaging shows three or more consecutive images revealing the bow-tie appearance of the meniscus.[26]

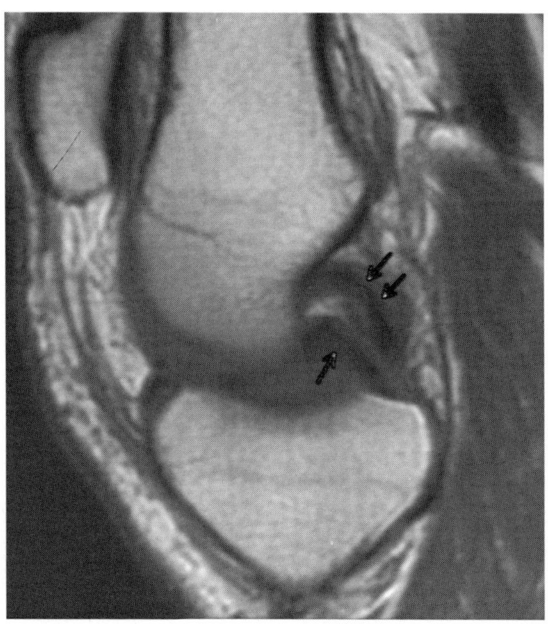

Figure 2–14
Sagittal T1 SE image, "double-PCL" sign. *Note a medially displaced meniscal fragment in the intercondylar area* (arrow) *that has decreased signal and runs parallel and anterior to the posterior cruciate ligament* (arrows).

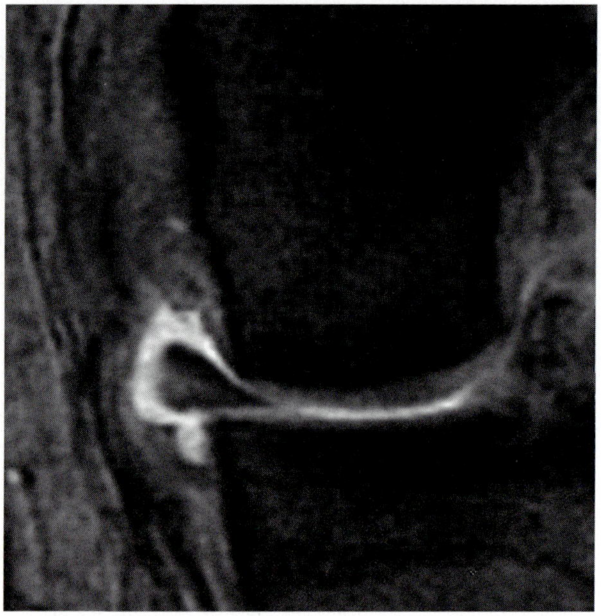

Figure 2–15
Coronal GRE image, menisco-capsular separation. *Bright fluid signal passes between the peripheral aspect of the medial meniscus and the capsule.*

Meniscocapsular Separation

A meniscocapsular separation usually involves the less mobile medial meniscus when it is torn from its attachment to the joint capsule. It commonly is associated with a medial collateral ligament injury. It is best visualized on a T2 or GRE coronal image where joint fluid is noted between the medial meniscus and the capsule (Fig. 2–15). On the sagittal image, the tibial plateau articular cartilage should be covered by the posterior horn of the medial meniscus without an exposed articular cartilage surface. Detachment also is suggested by displacement of this posterior horn of the medial meniscus by 5 mm or more, resulting in uncovered tibial articular cartilage, or by fluid between the peripheral edge of the meniscus and the capsule.[11]

Meniscal Cysts

Meniscal cysts are associated with either horizontal or complex meniscal tears and are more likely to have a degenerative rather than a traumatic etiology. These cysts form as synovial fluid is forced through the tear and then pushes its way through the meniscocapsular margin. Meniscal cysts are more common laterally and are usually contained by the joint capsule (Fig. 2–16). The weakest area is between the lateral collateral ligament and the iliotibial band, and most cysts are seen in relation to the lateral meniscus at this location. Medial meniscal cysts are usually found posteriorly in the weak area immediately posterior to the MCL. Medial meniscal cysts also can extend from the posterior horn and dissect peripherally to a more anterior location. On MRI these cysts are smooth-walled structures and are high in signal on T2 images. Septations, loculations, and dissections into the soft tissues distant from the meniscus are not uncommon.[4]

Postoperative Menisci

The same criteria used to diagnose tears in native menisci can be used for tears in a regenerated meniscus. In patients who have undergone partial meniscectomy, tears are likely at

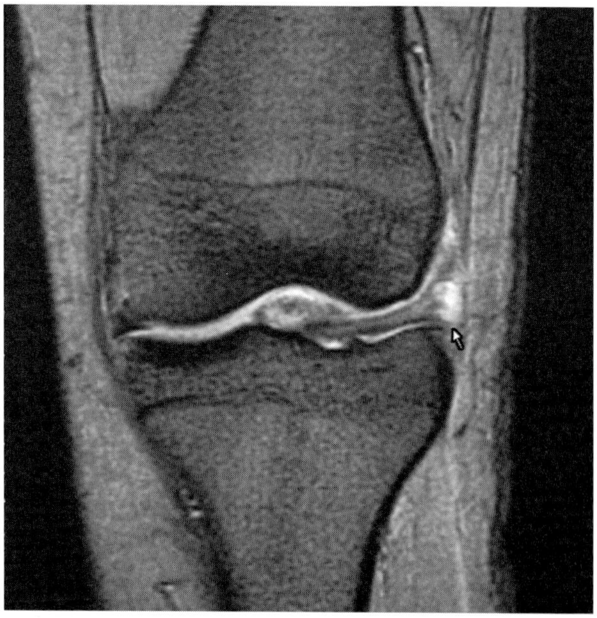

Figure 2–16
Coronal GRE image, meniscal cyst. *A small, fluid-filled cyst* (arrow) *communicates with a degenerative tear of the lateral meniscus.*

the junction of the remaining native meniscus with the regenerated meniscus. Grade-3 signal, however, can persist even with a healed or arthroscopically repaired tear.[9] Grade-3 signal in such patients may represent a surgical repair scar, nonhealing, or a new tear.[10] Correlation with the original tear pattern and knowledge of the arthroscopic surgery are certainly useful in accurately interpreting the MRI findings. Intra-articular gadolinium may help in identifying imbibed synovial fluid in menisci that have been re-torn after a primary repair (Fig. 2–17).[1]

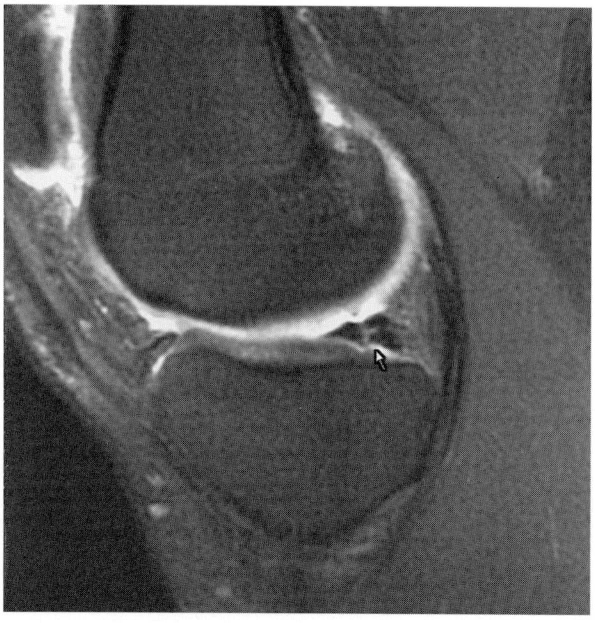

Figure 2–17
Sagittal T1 SE fat-suppressed image with intra-articular gadolinium. *Note a stellate area* (arrow) *of increased signal in the posterior horn of the medial meniscus consistent with a re-tear.*

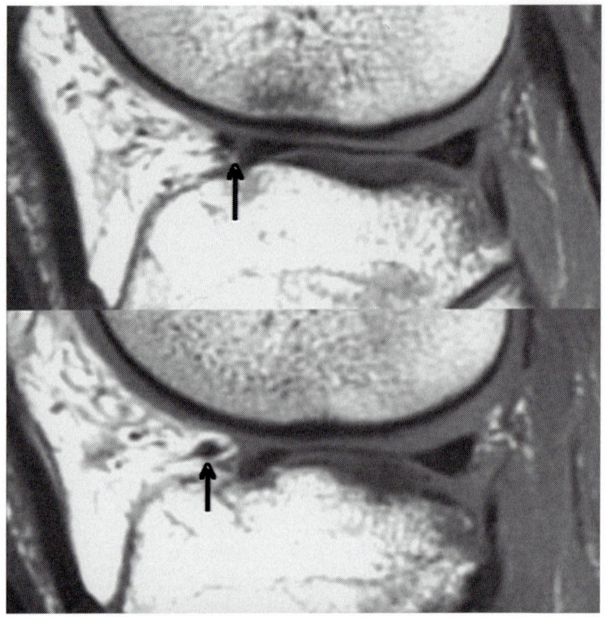

Figure 2–18
Sagittal T1 SE image. *Top, Pseudotear* (arrow) *of the anterior horn of the lateral meniscus secondary to insertion of the transverse ligament.* Bottom, *A sagittal image just medial to* A *reveals the transverse ligament* (arrow) *in cross-section prior to inserting on the meniscus.*

PITFALLS IN MRI OF MENISCAL TEARS

Many common pitfalls are encountered in MRI of the meniscus. A knowledge of such normal variants of the meniscus will avoid false-positive diagnoses.[15, 19, 30] Most of these pitfalls involve the lateral meniscus. One of the most common pitfalls is caused by the transverse ligament. This structure connects the anterior horns of medial and lateral menisci and can be appreciated in both coronal and sagittal imaging. High signal in the region of the confluence of the transverse ligament with the anterior horn of the lateral meniscus can mimic a meniscal tear (Fig. 2–18).

At the posterior horn of the lateral meniscus, the popliteus tendon sheath may be mistaken for Grade-3 signal and be falsely interpreted as a tear (Fig. 2–19). A joint effusion causes fluid in the popliteus sheath to have high signal intensity on T2 images. The thick-

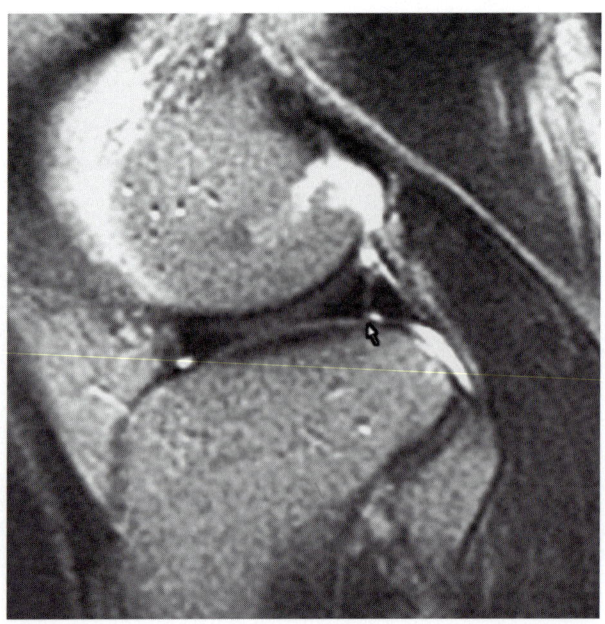

Figure 2–19
Sagittal T2 FSE image. *Pseudotear* (arrow) *in the posterior horn of the lateral meniscus created by fluid within the popliteal tendon sheath.*

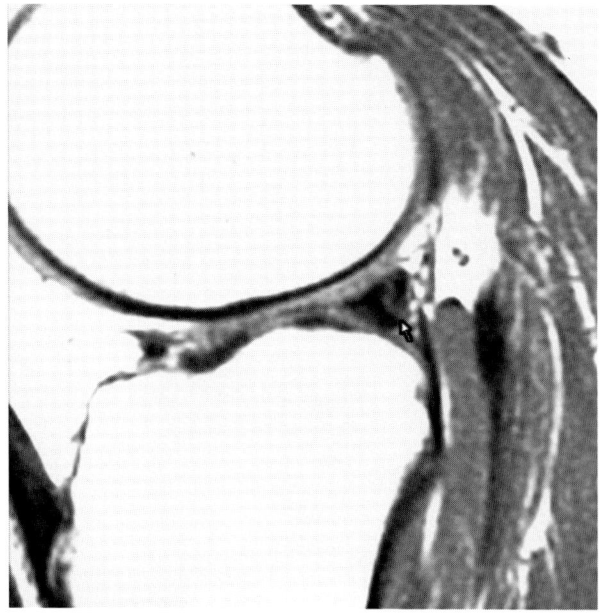

Figure 2–20
Sagittal T1 SE image.
Pseudotear (arrow) *at the insertion site of the meniscofemoral ligament to the posterior horn of the lateral meniscus.*

ness of this sheath can vary significantly and can present as either a thin line or a thick band. True peripheral lateral meniscal tears usually present with an obliquity different from that of the usual course of the popliteus tendon sheath.

The insertion site of a meniscofemoral ligament can mimic the appearance of a vertical tear in the posterior horn of the lateral meniscus (Fig. 2–20). The predominating meniscofemoral ligament can be followed in cross-section on subsequent sagittal images to its confluence with the posterior horn of the lateral meniscus.

Separate portions of the posterior horn may be mistaken for a bucket handle tear because the most posterior coronal images traverse both the body and the posterior horn, especially images of the lateral meniscus (Fig. 2–21). Posterior coronal images through the medial meniscus do not usually appear this way. It should also be noted that a lateral bucket handle tear is much less common than its medial counterpart.

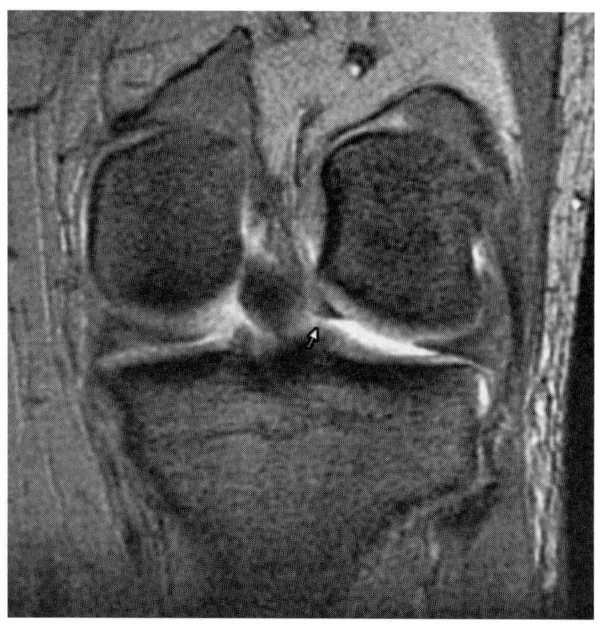

Figure 2–21
Coronal GRE image.
Pseudo–bucket-handle tear of the lateral meniscus (arrow) *due to the coronal plane passing through both the body and the posterior horn of the meniscus.*

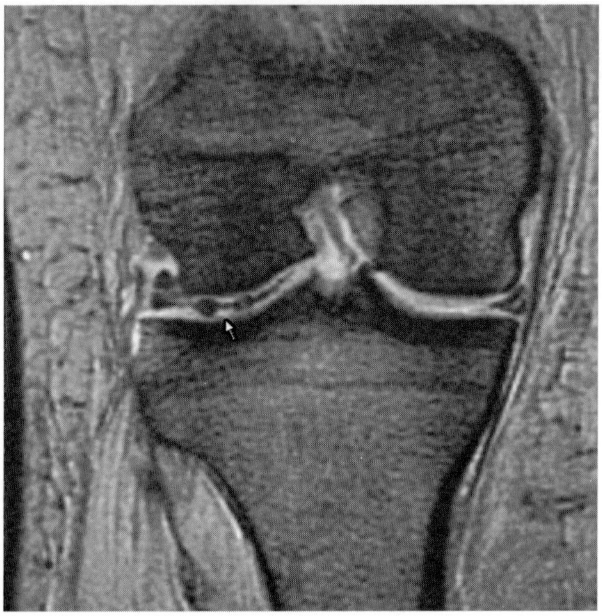

Figure 2–22
Coronal GRE image. *"Blooming" artifact in the lateral compartment of the knee secondary to the magnetic susceptibility of a vacuum phenomenon is manifested by several foci* (arrow) *of dark signal.*

A crescent of air in the joint during imaging can cause a potentially confusing artifact. The "magnetic susceptibility" of intra-articular gas can produce a low-signal-intensity void with an unusual "blooming" artifact on GRE images (Fig. 2–22). This signal void can simulate a tear or even a cartilaginous defect in the meniscus.[25]

The posterior horn of the medial meniscus has a normal superior recess (Fig. 2–23). This recess is smooth and vertically oriented but does not extend below the superior half of the meniscus, a fact that helps distinguish the superior recess from a partial-thickness peripheral tear to the superior articular surface. Lastly, the anterior horn of the medial meniscus can have an unusual cleft-like appearance that can mimic an anterior horn tear (Fig. 2–24).

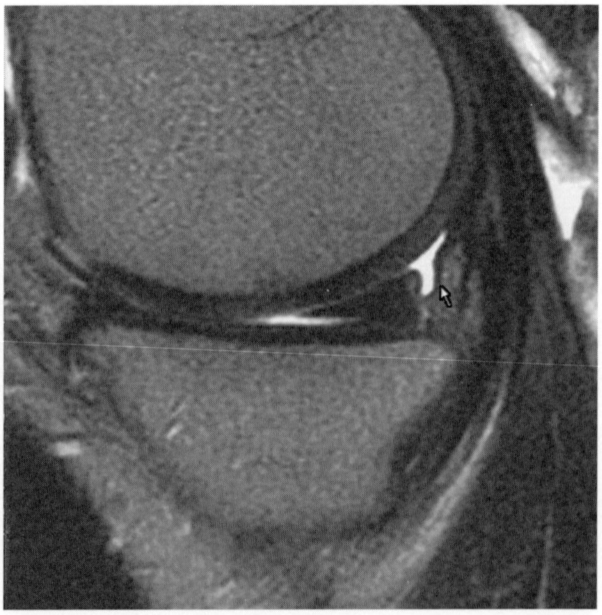

Figure 2–23
Sagittal T2 FSE image, normal superior recess. *Note a vertically oriented line of bright signal* (arrow) *representing fluid in a recess and not a tear of the posterior and peripheral one third of the medial meniscus.*

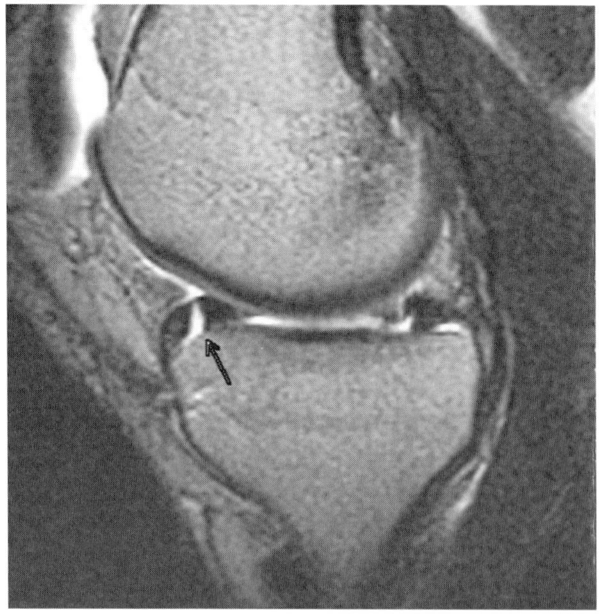

Figure 2–24
Sagittal T2 FSE image. *Pseudotear of the anterior horn of the medial meniscus due to a cleft* (arrow) *in the meniscus. Arthroscopy for other indications incidentally confirmed the absence of any tear at this location.*

Ligamentous Injury

ACL tears appear as a diffuse increase in signal intensity, abnormal angulation, discontinuity, or absence of the ligament. They are more common at their proximal attachment site. A number of secondary signs have been described to increase the accuracy of the MRI diagnosis, which is sometimes difficult because of the partial-volume effect and the oblique course of the ACL. These signs include bone contusions on the lateral femoral condyle and posterior margin of the lateral tibial plateau, anterior displacement of the tibia relative to the condyle, and anterior bowing of the PCL. Chronic tears of the ACL can hinder diagnosis because of the absence of increased signal and the potential fusion of the ACL and PCL.[31] PCL tears are less common but have similar signal characteristics when torn (Fig. 2–25). MRI can be used to evaluate ACL reconstructions, which are best depicted on the

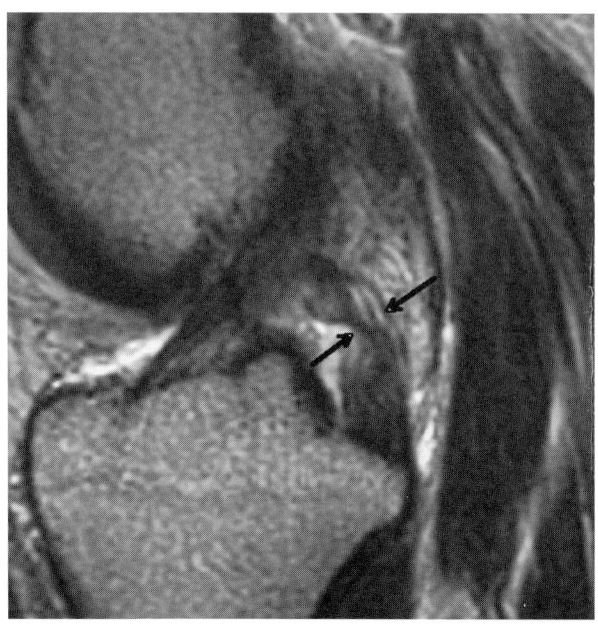

Figure 2–25
Sagittal T2 FSE image, PCL tear. *Note marked attenuation of the midsubstance of the ligament* (arrows) *with minimal increased signal marking the site of injury.*

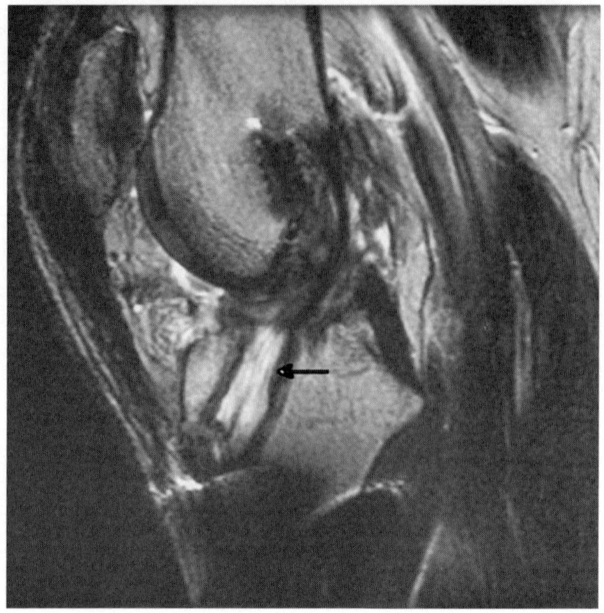

Figure 2–26
Sagittal T2 FSE image, ACL graft impingement. *Note increased signal in the graft* (arrow) *at its distal aspect, secondary to impingement, more proximally in the intercondylar notch.*

sagittal T2 sequence. The graft is normally low-signal and of varying thickness. Localized fluid collections in and around the graft suggest a tear. One should pay attention to the placement of the tibial tunnel. Graft impingement is more likely when the tunnel is anterior to the slope of the intercondylar roof. These same grafts usually reveal increased signal in the graft's distal aspect (Fig. 2–26).[30]

Medial collateral ligament tears are much more common than lateral collateral ligament tears. The spectrum of injury includes minimal periligamentous edema (Grade-1) to partial (Grade-2) or complete (Grade 3) disruption of the ligament. Focal or diffuse bright signal often traverses the ligament, resulting in discontinuity of appearance in both partial and complete tears (Fig. 2–27). This can make it difficult to distinguish them, and such

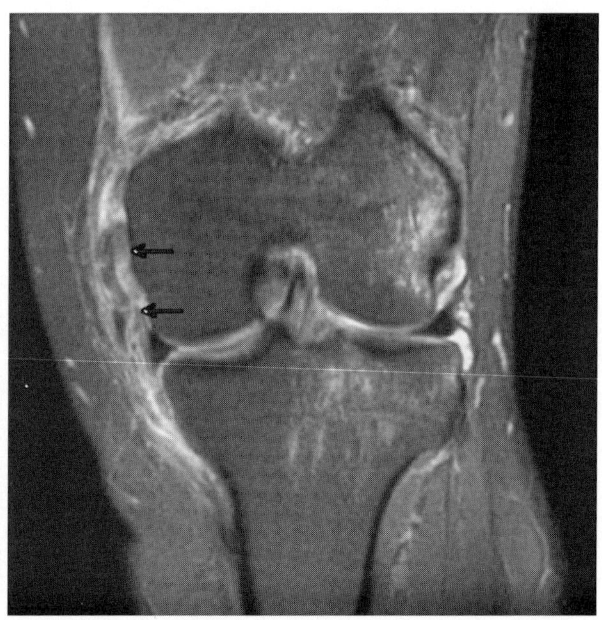

Figure 2–27
Coronal proton-density FSE image with fat suppression, Grade 2/3 MCL injury. *Note proximal altered signal in the MCL* (arrows) *with irregularity of the ligament and surrounding periligamentous edema (bright signal).*

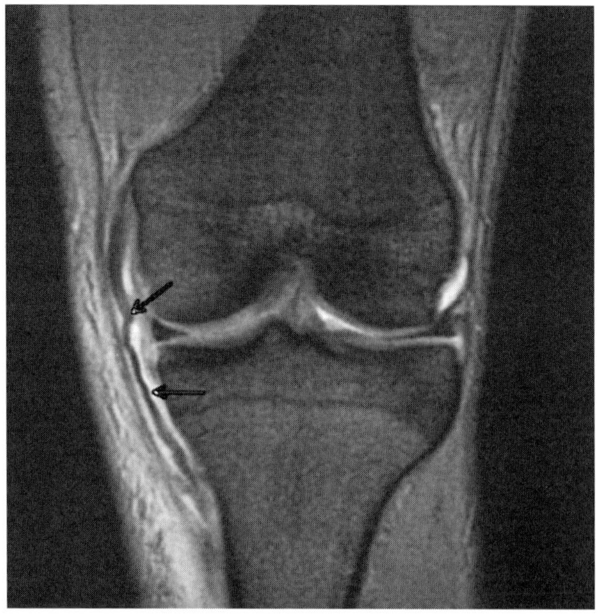

Figure 2–28
Coronal proton-density FSE image with fat suppression. *Note a "wavy" appearance* (arrows) *to the MCL, which was completely torn distally.*

findings are probably best classified as Grade 2 to 3. The MCL usually is torn proximally and can have a wavy appearance when completely torn (Fig. 2–28). Laxity from an MCL injury is evident clinically, but MRI will help demonstrate any associated meniscal tears and bone contusions.[21]

Tendinous Injury

The quadriceps or patellar tendons (Fig. 2–29) can tear with acute trauma. Often, the diagnosis is obvious clinically, but MRI may be useful in partial tears or in spontaneous rupture of the tendon in patients with chronic systemic diseases such as renal failure.[28, 34]

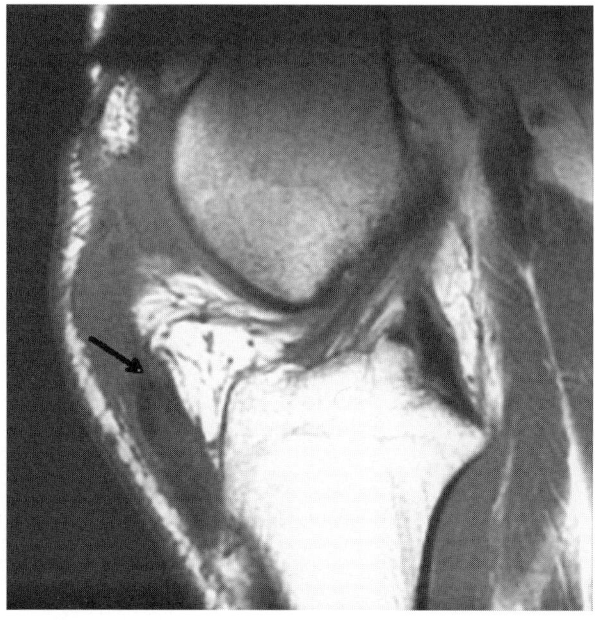

Figure 2–29
Sagittal T1 SE image, patellar tendon tear. *Note abrupt cut-off and thickening of the patellar tendon* (arrow) *as well as surrounding intermediate signal soft tissue edema and hemorrhage.*

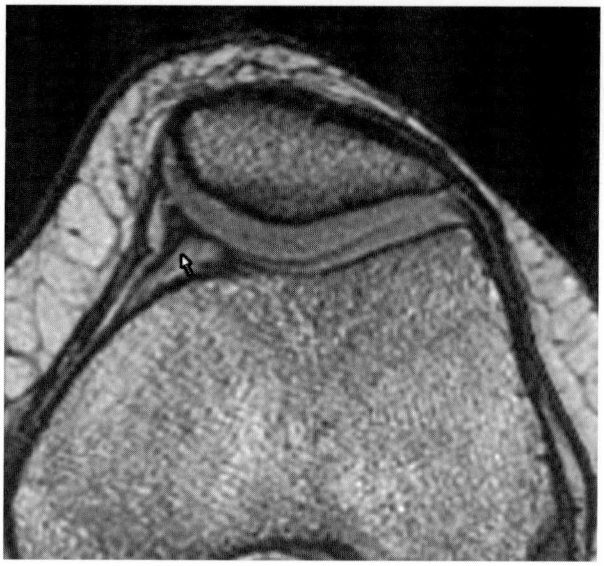

Figure 2–30
Axial GRE image, medial plica. *Note a linear band of dark signal* (arrow) *paralleling the medial retinaculum and inserting on the patella.*

Plicae

Plicae are folds of synovium thought to be embryologic remnants. The most important form is the medial patellar plica that projects into the patellofemoral compartment from the medial aspect of the retropatellar bursa (Fig. 2–30). Trapping of this structure can result in chronic irritation, thickening, and symptoms that may mimic a meniscal tear. These plicae are common and usually are considered incidental and asymptomatic unless thickened.[24]

Osseous and Cartilaginous Injury

Defects in the cartilage appear as focal areas of cartilaginous thinning in which the defect is filled with synovial fluid that demonstrates a characteristic bright signal on T2 images.

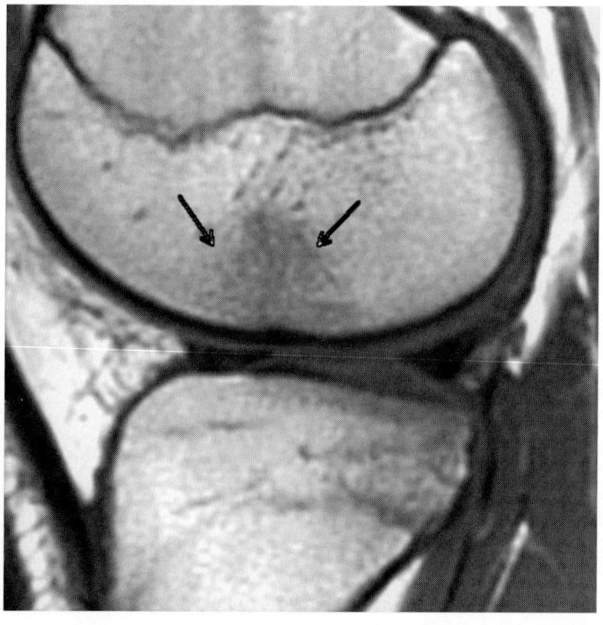

Figure 2–31
Sagittal T1 SE image, bone contusion. *Note an area of decreased signal* (arrows) *in the bone marrow, which is reticular in pattern.*

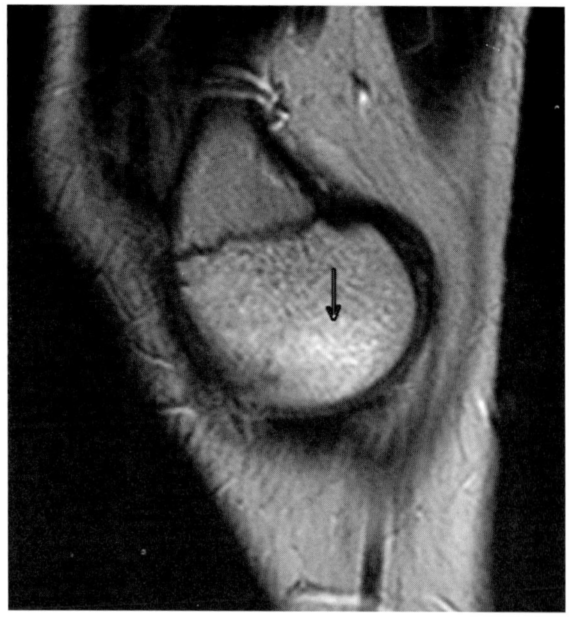

Figure 2–32
Sagittal T2 FSE image, bone contusion. *Note an area of increased signal* (arrow) *in the bone marrow, which is reticular in pattern.*

Diagnosis is often aided by abnormal signal in the underlying bone from associated bone injury. GRE and fat-suppressed proton-density images have proved especially useful.[24]

Bone injury is appreciated as an area of low signal on the T1 sequence (Fig. 2–31) and increased signal on the T2 sequence (Fig. 2–32). Once again, the fat-suppressed proton-density sequence is particularly sensitive to bone injury. A STIR sequence also reveals edema within the bone marrow. Many of these bone injuries resolve spontaneously within a short time. The contusions in the subchondral region of bone (Fig. 2–33), however, are associated with a high incidence of osteochondral abnormalities on follow-up MRI or arthroscopy, such as thinning or loss of cartilage and subchondral sclerosis.[32]

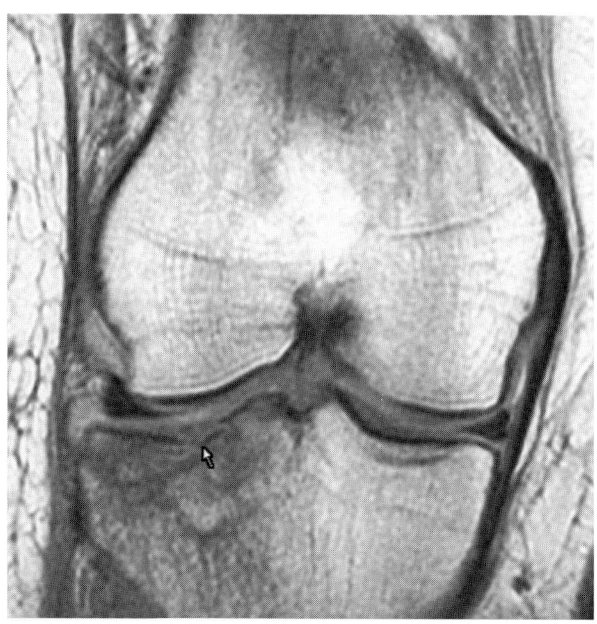

Figure 2–33
Coronal proton-density SE image, osteochondral injury. *Note diffuse subchondral low signal within the bone marrow of the lateral tibial plateau. A smaller focus of intermediate signal disrupts the normally dark signal of the cortical bone* (arrow).

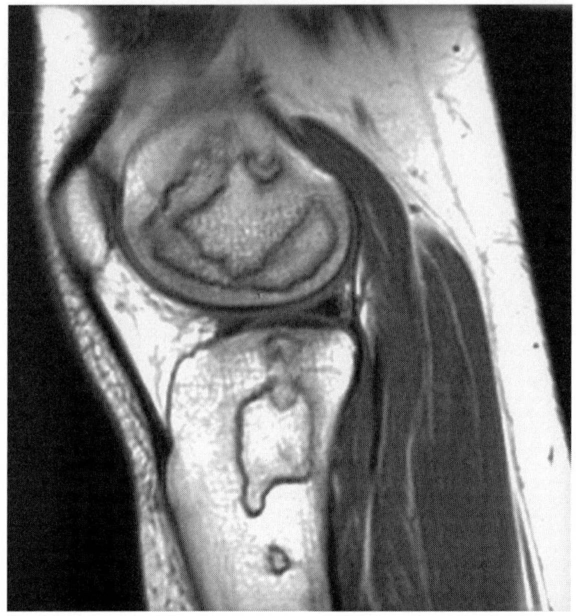

Figure 2–34
Sagittal T1 SE image, medullary infarcts. *Note large areas of infarction on both sides of the joint with central preservation of bone marrow signal outlined by serpentine low-signal margins.*

Medullary bone infarcts (Fig. 2–34) typically occur in the elderly, with collagen vascular disease, and secondary to corticosteroid medication. Although these lesions may be symptomatic, they rarely result in fracture or collapse.

References

1. Applegate GR, Flannigan BD, Tolin BS, et al. MR diagnosis of recurrent tears in the knee: Value of intra-articular contrast material. AJR 1993; 161:821-825.
2. Barnett MJ. MR diagnosis of internal derangements of the knee: Effect of field strength on efficacy. AJR 1993; 161:115-118.
3. Buckwalter KA, Braunstein EM, Janizek DB, et al. MR imaging of meniscal tears: Narrow versus conventional window width photography. Radiology 1993; 187:827-830.
4. Burk DL, Dalinka MK, Kanal E, et al. Meniscal and ganglion cysts of the knee: MR evaluation. AJR 1988; 150:331-336.
5. Chan WP, Rauschning W, Wu CY, et al. Magnetic resonance imaging anatomy and cryomicrotome atlas. *In* Chan WP, Lang P, Genant HK, eds. MRI of the Musculoskeletal System. Philadelphia: WB Saunders, 1994.
6. Crues JV, Mink JH, Levy T, et al. Meniscal tears of the knee. Accuracy of MR imaging. Radiology 1987; 164:445-448.
7. De Smet AA, Graf BK. Meniscal tears missed on MR imaging: Relationship to meniscal tear patterns and anterior cruciate ligament tears. AJR 1994; 162:905-911.
8. De Smet AA, Norris MA, Xandrow DR, et al. MR diagnosis of meniscal tears of the knee: Importance of high signal in the menisci that extends to the surface. AJR 1993; 161:101-107.
9. Deutsch AL, Mink JH, Fox JM, et al. Peripheral meniscal tears: MR findings after conservative therapy or arthroscopic repair. Radiology 1990; 176:485-488.
10. Farley TE, Howell SM, Love KF, et al. Meniscal tears: MR and arthroscopic findings after meniscal repair. Radiology 1991; 180:517-522.
11. Firooznia H, Golimbu C, Rafii M. MR imaging of the menisci: Fundamentals of anatomy and pathology. MRI Clin North Am 1994; 2(3):325-347.
12. Fitzgerald SE. MR imaging of the meniscus: Advanced concepts. MRI Clin North Am 1994; 2(3):349-364.
13. Kaplan PA, Nelson NL, Garvin KI, et al. MR of the knee: The significance of high signal in the meniscus that does not clearly extend to the surface. AJR 1991; 156:333-336.
14. Kornic J, Trefeiner E, McCarthy S, et al. Meniscal abnormalities in the asymtomatic population at MR imaging. Radiology 1990; 177:463-465.
15. Mesgarzadeh M, Moyer R, Leder DS, et al. MR imaging of the knee: Expanded classification and pitfalls in interpretation of meniscal tears. Radiographics 1993; 13:489-500.
16. Mink JH, Deutsch AL. Magnetic resonance imaging of the knee. Clin Orthop Rel Res 1989; 244:29-47.
17. Munk PL, Helms CA, Vellet AD. Technique of magnetic resonance imaging of the knee. *In* Munk PL, Helms CA, eds. MRI of the Knee. Gaithersburg, MD: Aspen, 1992.

18. Munk PL, Helms CA, Vellet A. The menisci. *In* Munk PL, Helms CA, eds. MRI of the Knee. Gaithersburg, MD: Aspen, 1992.
19. Peterfy CG, Janzen DL, Tirman PF, et al. "Magic-Angle" phenomenon: A cause of increased signal in the normal lateral meniscus on short-TE MR images of the knee. AJR 1994; 163:149-154.
20. Reicher MA, Bassett LW, Gold RH. High resolution magnetic resonance imaging of the knee joint: Pathologic correlations. AJR 1985; 145:903-910.
21. Ruiz ME, Erickson SJ. Medial and lateral supporting structures of the knee: Normal MR imaging anatomy and pathologic findings. MRI Clin North Am 1994; 2(3):381-399.
22. Ruwe PA, Wright J, Randall RL, et al. Can MR imaging effectively replace diagnostic arthroscopy? Radiology 1992; 183:335-339.
23. Quinn SF, Brown TF. Meniscal tears diagnosesd with MR imaging vs. arthroscopy: How reliable a standard is arthroscopy? Radiology 1991; 181:843-847.
24. Quinn SF, Rose PM, Brown TR, et al. MR imaging of the patellofemoral compartment. MRI Clin North Am 1994; 2(3):425-440.
25. Shogry ME, Pope TL. Vacuum phenomenon simulating meniscal or cartilaginous injury of the knee at MR imaging. Radiology 1991; 180:513-515.
26. Silverman JM, Mink JH, Deutsch AL. Discoid menisci of the knee: MR imaging appearance. Radiology 1989;173:351-354.
27. Singson RD, Kellet H, Feldman F, et al. MR imaging of medial meniscocapsular separation. Radiology 1989; 173:436.
28. Sonin AH. Magnetic resonance imaging of the extensor mechanism. MRI Clin North Am 1994; 2(3):401-411.
29. Stoller DW, Martin C, Crues JV, et al. Meniscal tears: Pathologic correlation with MR imaging. Radiology 1987; 163:731-735.
30. Stoller DW, Cannon WD, Anderson LJ. The knee. *In* Stoller DW, ed. Magnetic Resonance Imaging in Orthopaedics and Sports Medicine. Philadelphia: JB Lippincott, 1994.
31. Vahey TN, Meyer SF, Shelbourne KD, et al. MR imaging of anterior cruciate ligament injuries. MRI Clin North Am 1994; 2(3):365-380.
32. Vellet AD, Marks P, Fowler P, et al. MRI of occult post-traumatic osteochondral lesions of the knee: Incidence, re-classification and long term sequelae. Radiology 1991; 170:271-276.
33. Weiss KL, Morehouse HT, Levy IM. Sagittal MR images of the knee: A low-signal band parallel to the posterior cruciate ligament caused by a displaced bucket-handle tear. AJR 1991; 156:117-119.
34. Zeiss J, Saddemi SR, Ebraheim NA. MR imaging of the quadriceps tendon: Normal layered configuration and its importance in cases of tendon rupture. AJR 1992; 159:1031-1034.

Knee Arthroscopy

The knee was the first joint in which arthroscopy was applied, and most of the principles and applications of arthroscopy are a direct result of experiences gained from the knee. Professor Kenji Takagi is credited with the first use of endoscopy when he inserted a cystoscope into a cadaver knee in 1918.[8] Since then, endoscopy has been applied to increasing numbers of techniques and surgical procedures.

INDICATIONS

Arthroscopy has diverse application to various forms of knee pathology. Diagnostic arthroscopy helps to confirm suspected knee injuries. Arthroscopy synovectomy can be useful for synovial biopsies to aid the diagnosis of rheumatologic disorders, remove diseased synovium, and resect synovial folds or plicae. A six-portal technique is favored for complete synovectomy (Fig. 2–35).

Treatment of meniscal pathology is perhaps the most common application of arthroscopy. Meniscal tears account for approximately 50% of knee injuries that require surgery.[9] The medial meniscus is most commonly involved. Meniscal tears usually are classified according to their appearance and orientation (Fig. 2–36). Treatment of these injuries includes partial meniscectomy for central or degenerative tears (Fig. 2–37) or meniscal repair for peripheral tears (Fig. 2–38). Meniscal cysts, which are usually associated

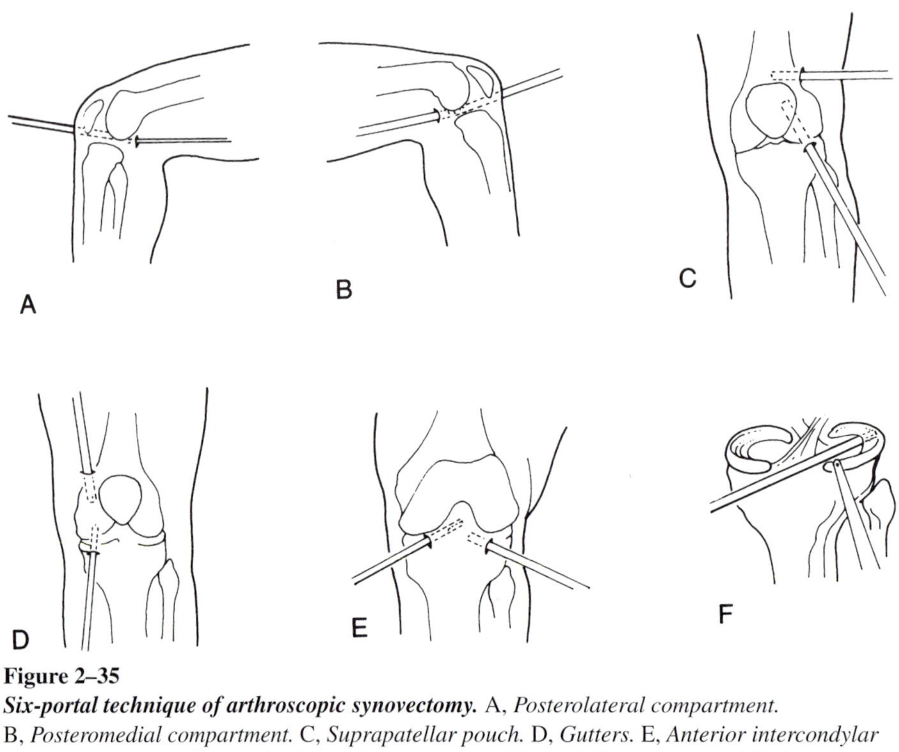

Figure 2–35
Six-portal technique of arthroscopic synovectomy. A, *Posterolateral compartment.* B, *Posteromedial compartment.* C, *Suprapatellar pouch.* D, *Gutters.* E, *Anterior intercondylar area.* F, *Perimeniscal area. (Redrawn from Rosenberg TD et al. Synovectomy of the knee.* In *McGinty JB, ed. Operative Arthroscopy. New York: Raven Press, 1991, p 377.)*

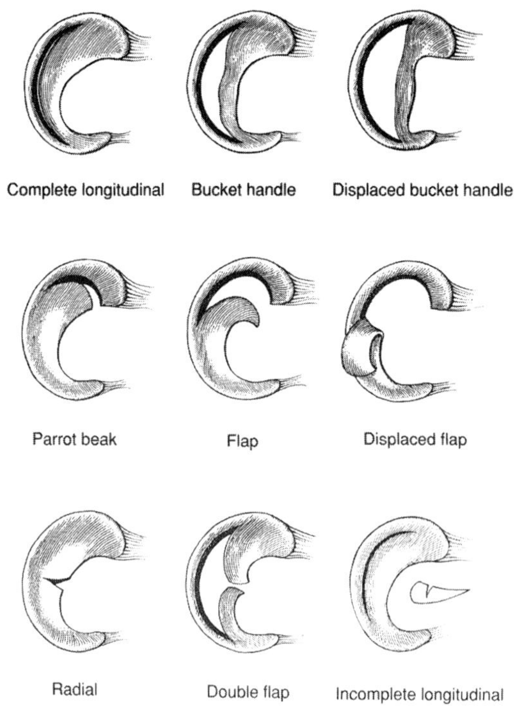

Figure 2–36
Classification of meniscal tears. (From Tria AJ, Klein KS. An Illustrated Guide to the Knee. New York: Churchill Livingstone, 1992.)

with a horizontal meniscal tear of the lateral meniscus, are also treatable arthroscopically by partial meniscectomy and cyst decompression (Fig. 2–39).[3, 13] Arthroscopic techniques also can be used to trim or repair discoid menisci (Fig. 2–40).[12]

Osteochondral lesions are also commonly addressed arthroscopically. Osteochondritis dissecans, classically located at the lateral aspect of the medial femoral condyle, is treated with removal, debridement, or repair of the defect, according to the stage of the lesion (Fig. 2–41). Cartilaginous injuries can occur in older persons, usually involve the medial femoral condyle, and are frequently delaminating injuries (Fig. 2–42) that are less amenable to arthroscopic repair. Treatment includes debridement and some form of chondroplasty. Osteochondral lesions can sometimes be replaced in their original bed and secured with small screws or bioabsorbable pins.

Text continued on page 48

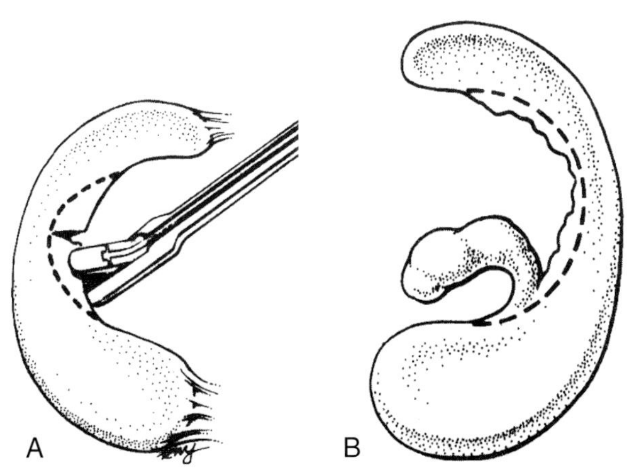

Figure 2–37
Outline of partial meniscectomy necessary for a radial tear (A) *and a degenerative flap tear* (B). *(From Cicotti MG, Shields CL, El Attrach N. Meniscectomy.* In *Fu FH, Harner CD, Vince KG, eds. Knee Surgery. Baltimore: Williams & Wilkins, 1994.)*

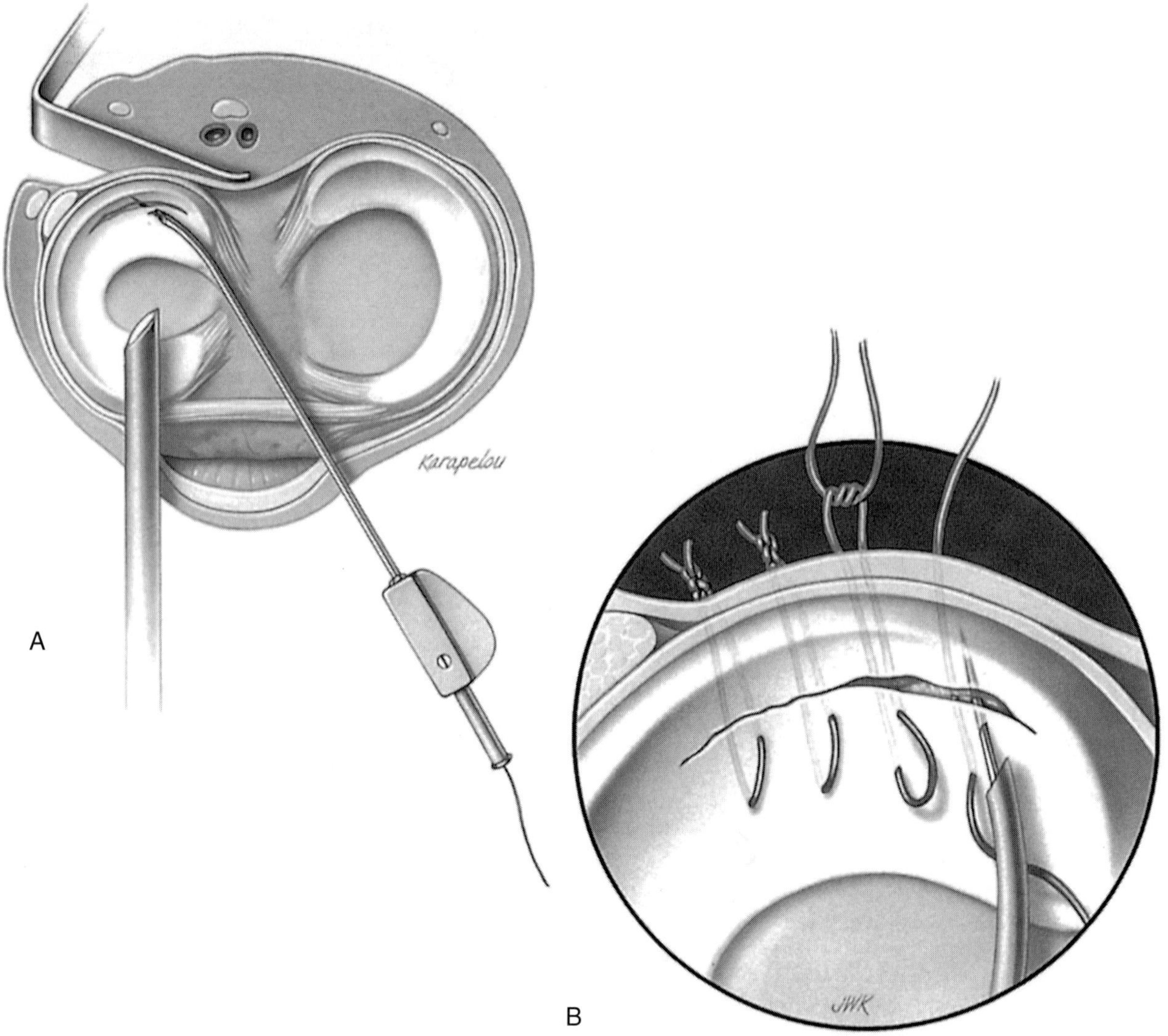

Figure 2–38
Inside-out meniscal repair. A, *Suture placement.* B, *Sutures are tied over the capsule through a small incision. (From Miller MD. Atlas of meniscus repair. Oper Tech Orthop 1995; 5[1]:71.)*

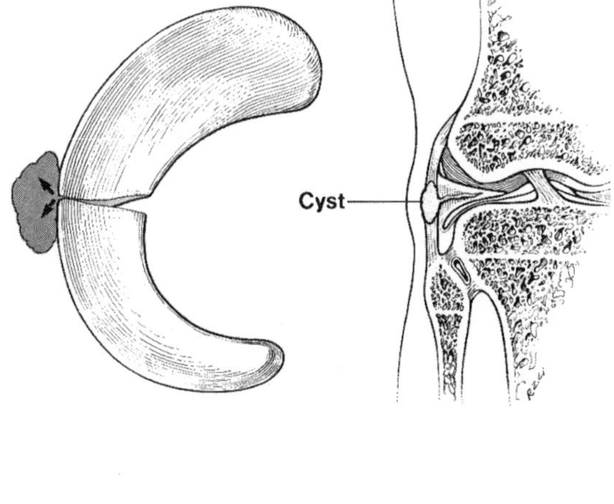

Figure 2–39
Meniscal cyst and associated horizontal meniscal tear. (From Tria AJ, Klein KS. An Illustrated Guide to the Knee. New York: Churchill Livingstone, 1992.)

Figure 2–40
Three types of discoid menisci. A, *Partial (incomplete).* B, *Complete.* C, *Wrisberg variant (deficient peripheral attachment). (From Neuschwander DC. Discoid meniscus.* In *Fu FH, Harner CD, Vince KG, eds. Knee Surgery. Baltimore: Williams & Wilkins, 1994.)*

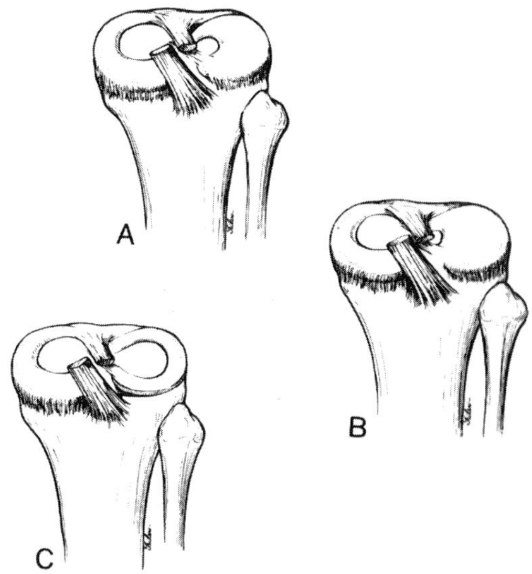

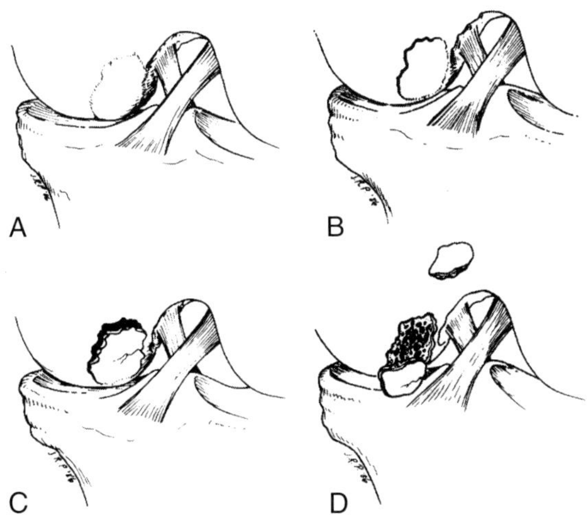

Figure 2–41
Classification of osteochondritis dissecans. A, *In-situ lesion.* B, *Early separation lesion.* C, *Incompletely detached lesion.* D, *Completely detached lesion. (From Rosenberg TD, Paulos LE, Parker RD, Abbott PJ. Arthroscopic surgery of the knee.* In *Chapman MW, ed. Operative Orthopaedics, 2nd ed. Philadelphia: JB Lippincott, 1993.)*

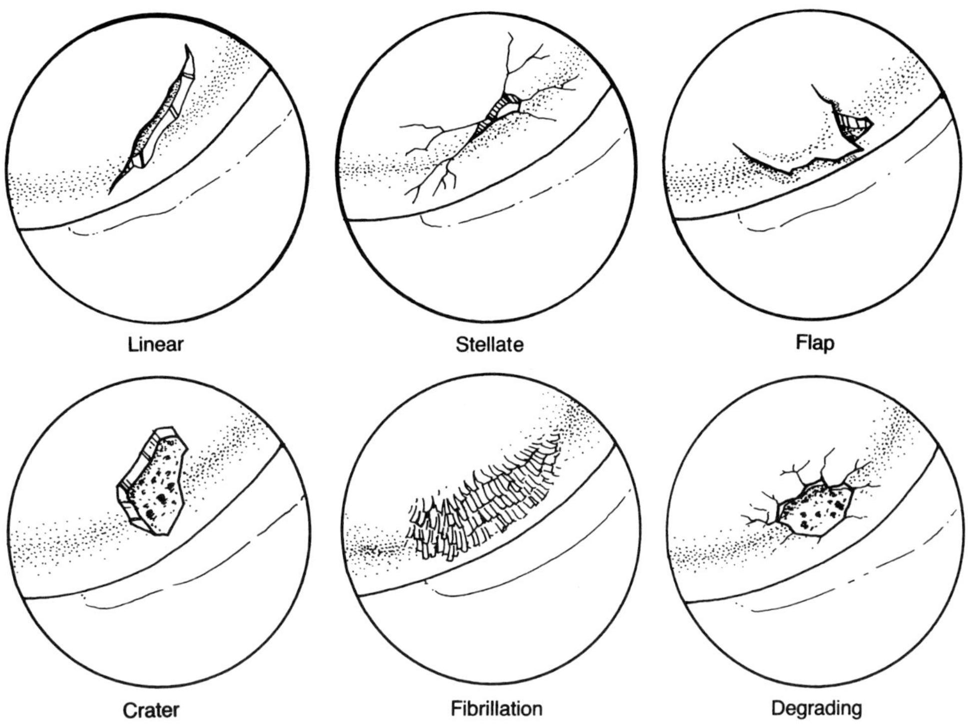

Figure 2–42
Classification of chondral lesions (Bauer and Jackson classification). (Redrawn from Rauer M, Jackson RW. Chondral lesions of the femoral condyles. Arthroscopy 1988; 4:97–102).

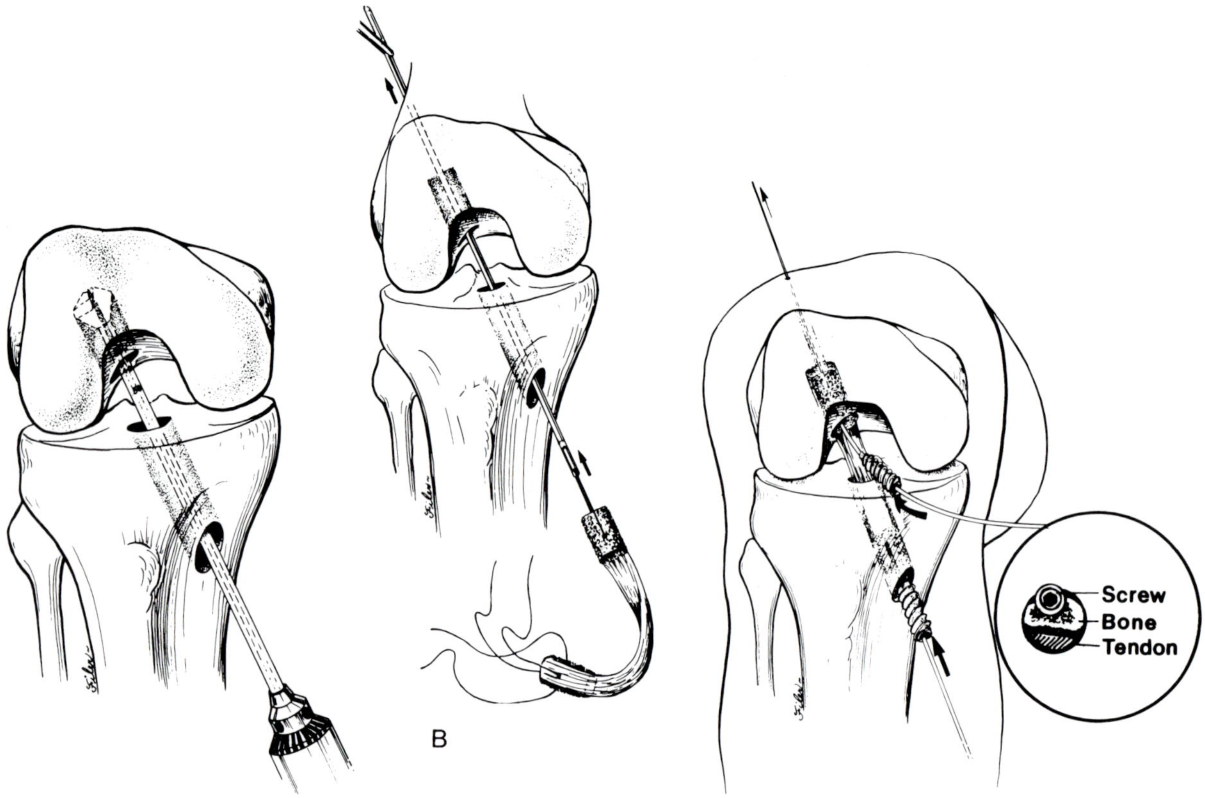

Figure 2–43
Single-incision (endoscopic) technique for ACL reconstruction. A, *Transtibial drilling of the femoral tunnel.* B, *Graft passage.* C, *Graft fixation. (From Miller MD, Fu FH. Arthroscopic allograft ACL Reconstruction. Oper Tech Sports Med 1995; 3[3]:148-156.)*

Injuries to the cruciate ligaments can be easily diagnosed with the arthroscope; endoscopic reconstruction of these ligaments is one of the most common orthopaedic procedures. Techniques for reconstruction of both of these ligaments have been well described elsewhere (Figs. 2–43 and 2–44).[10, 11]

Other procedures that are sometimes aided with arthroscopy include tibial plateau fracture reduction, reduction and fixation of tibial eminence fractures, loose-body removal, anterior fat-pad debridement, lateral release for patellar malalignment, and irrigation and debridement of septic arthritis.

POSITIONING AND PORTAL PLACEMENT

Two different forms of positioning are commonly used for knee arthroscopy. The patient can be placed supine on the operating table, and a lateral post can be used for countertraction. Alternatively, the operative leg can be positioned in a commercially available leg holder (Fig. 2–45). The operative leg is allowed to hang freely over the end of the operating table, and the opposite leg is positioned in a well-padded leg holder with care taken not to compress the peroneal nerve.

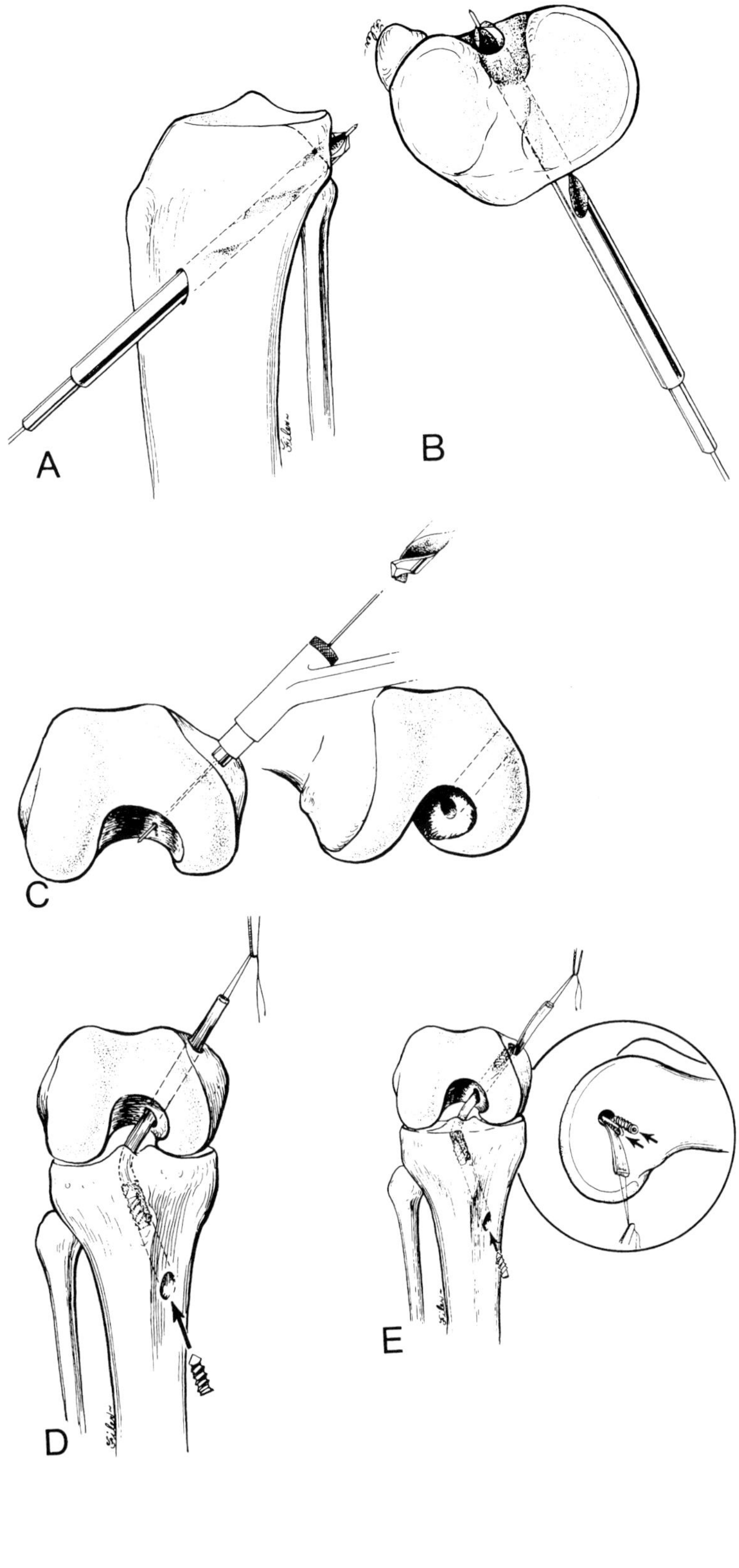

Figure 2–44
Composite drawing of PCL reconstruction technique. A *and* B, *Tibial tunnel preparation.* C, *Femoral tunnel preparation.* D, *Graft passage and tibial fixation.* E, *Femoral fixation. (From Miller MD, Harner CD, Koshiwaguchi S. Acute posterior cruciate ligament injuries.* In *Fu FH, Harner CD, Vince KG, eds. Knee Surgery. Baltimore: Williams & Wilkins, 1994.)*

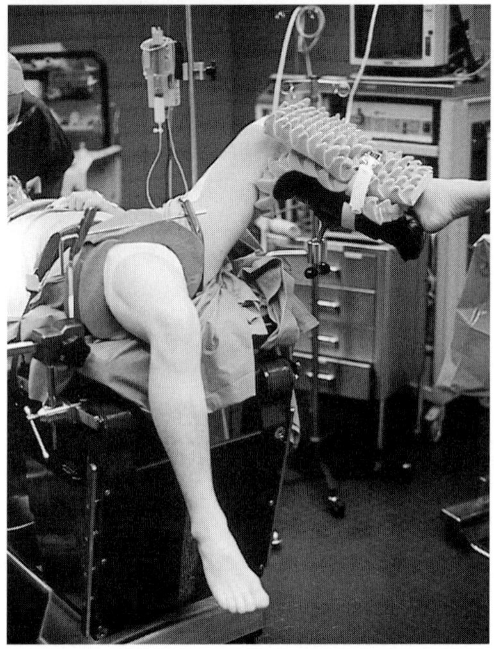

Figure 2–45
Arthroscopic positioning with a commercially available leg holder for the operative leg and a well-padded gynecologic leg holder for the nonoperative extremity.

Standard arthroscopic portals for knee arthroscopy include a superomedial or superolateral portal for fluid inflow and outflow and inferomedial and inferolateral portals positioned just above the joint line on both sides of the patellar tendon for arthroscopy and instrumentation (Fig. 2–46). The inferolateral portal is usually used during diagnostic arthroscopy.

Accessory portals for the knee include the posteromedial, posterolateral, far medial and lateral, and proximal superomedial portals. The posteromedial portal is often helpful for visualizing the PCL[2] and the posterior horn of the medial meniscus.[4] The posterolateral portal, located between the iliotibial band and the biceps tendon, is sometimes helpful, but extreme care should be taken to ensure that the portal is anterior to the biceps tendon to avoid injury to the peroneal nerve. Other portals include the midpatellar portal, far medial and lateral portals (sometimes helpful for instrument placement in hard-to-reach areas), and the proximal superomedial portal, located 4 cm proximal to and in line with the medial edge of the patella (for assessment of patellar tracking).

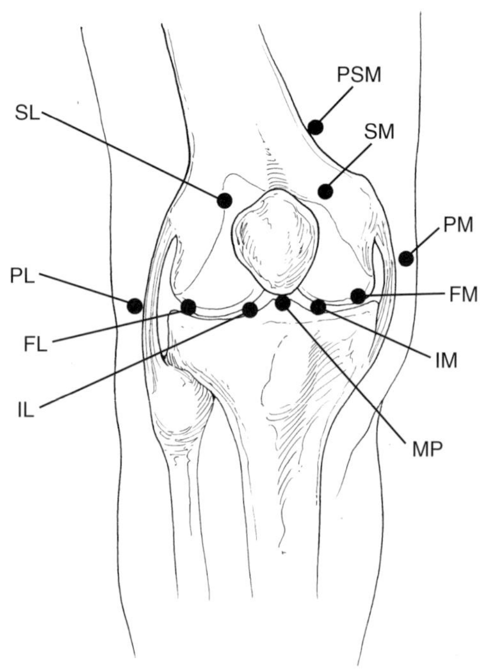

Figure 2–46
Arthroscopic portals. (PSM = proximal superomedial; SM = superomedial; PM = posteromedial; FM = far medial; IM = inferomedial; MP = midpatellar; IL = inferolateral; FL = far lateral; PL = posterolateral; and SL = superolateral.)

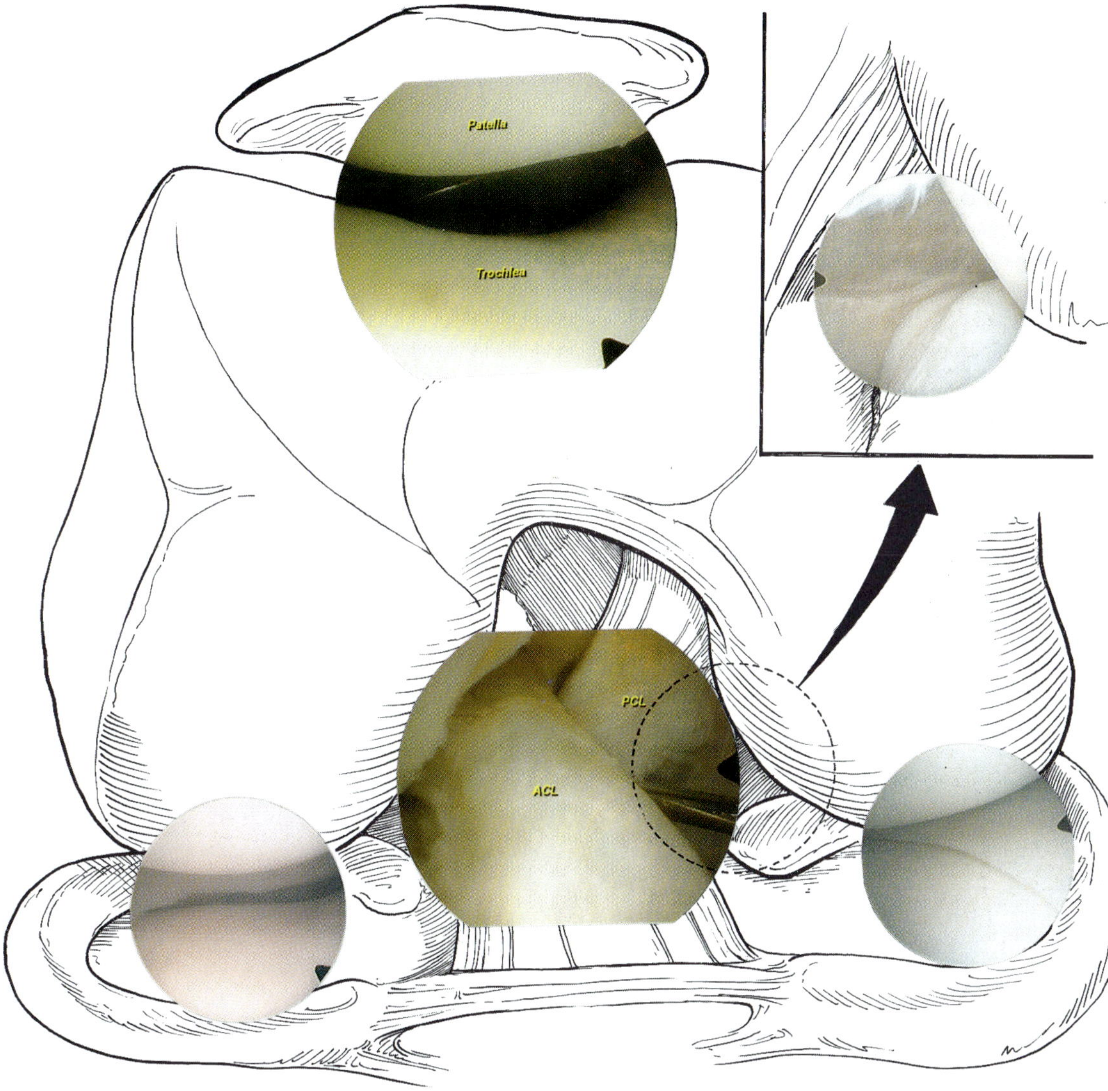

Figure 2–47
Normal arthroscopic anatomy. (Inset shows posteromedial aspect of the knee as seen through the notch.)

ARTHROSCOPIC ANATOMY

As with any joint, systematic examination of the knee is appropriate. Prior to positioning the patient, a complete examination under anesthesia is conducted to assess instability in all planes. An arthroscopic cannula is placed in the superomedial or superolateral portal for inflow and outflow, and the arthroscope is introduced into the inferolateral portal. Although many examination sequences are possible, it is important to visualize the suprapatellar pouch, patellofemoral joint, medial and lateral gutters, medial and lateral compartments (meniscus and articular cartilage), and intercondylar notch (cruciate ligaments) in all patients. Accessory viewing portals are established as necessary if other areas need to be evaluated. After a complete evaluation of the joint (Fig. 2–47), all surgical pathology is addressed.

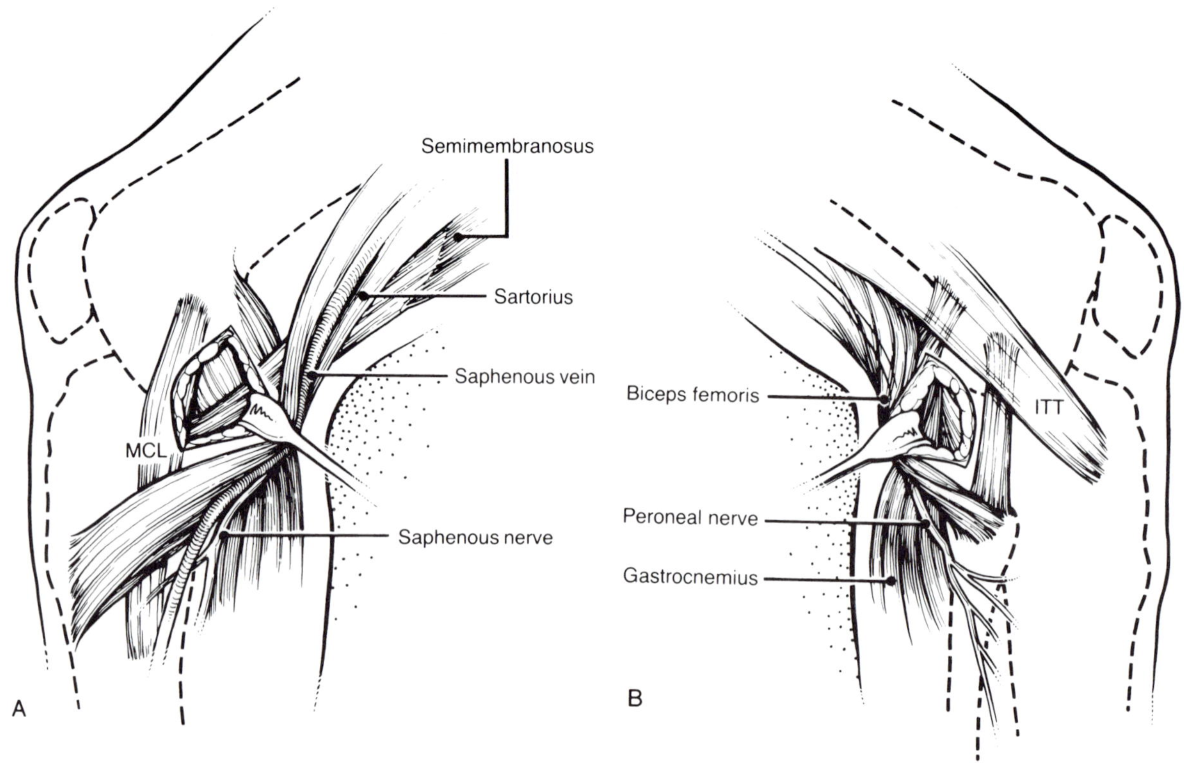

Figure 2–48
Meniscal repair incisions and their relationship to important structures medially (A) *and laterally* (B). *MCL, medial collateral ligament; ITT, iliotibial band. (From Scott WN, ed. Arthroscopy of the Knee. Philadelphia: WB Saunders, 1990.)*

COMPLICATIONS

In addition to the general arthroscopic complications discussed in Chapter 1, several potential complications peculiar to arthroscopic procedures of the knee should be emphasized. The branches of the saphenous nerve (medially) and the common peroneal nerve (laterally) must be carefully protected during meniscus repair (Fig. 2–48). It is also important to use extreme care when working in the posterior aspect of the knee (such as during PCL tibial tunnel preparation) to avoid injury to the popliteal artery. The arthroscopist should also be acutely aware of the unusual complications, including deep vein thrombosis,[14] reflex sympathetic dystrophy,[1] postoperative adhesions and fibrosis,[6, 7] and loss of motion.[5]

References

1. Cooper DE, DeLee JC, Ramamurthy S. Reflex sympathetic dystrophy of the knee. J Bone Joint Surg [Am] 1989; 71:365-369.
2. Fanelli GC, Giannetti BF, Edson CJ. The posterior cruciate ligament: Evaluation and treatment. Curr Concepts Rev Arthrosc 1994; 10:673-688.
3. Glasgow MMS, Allen PW, Blakeway C. Arthroscopic treatment of cysts of the lateral meniscus. J Bone Joint Surg [Br] 1993; 75:299-302.
4. Gold DL, Schaner PJ, Sapega AA. The posteromedial portal in knee arthroscopy: An analysis of diagnostic and surgical utility. Arthroscopy 1995; 11(2):139-145.
5. Harner CD, Irrgang JJ, Paul J, Dearwater S, Fu FH. Loss of motion after anterior cruciate ligament reconstruction. Am J Sports Med 1992; 20:499-506.
6. Hoffa A. The influence of the adipose tissue with regard to the pathology of the knee joint. JAMA 1904; 43:795.
7. Jackson DW, Schaefer RK. Cyclops syndrome: Loss of extension following intraarticular anterior cruciate ligament reconstruction. Arthroscopy 1990; 6:171-178.

8. Jackson RW. History of arthroscopy. *In* McGinty JB, ed. Operative Arthroscopy. New York: Raven Press, 1991, pp 1-4.
9. Jensen JE, Conn RR, Hazelrigg G, Hewell JE. Symptomatic evaluation of acute knee injuries. Clin Sports Med 1985; 4:295.
10. Miller MD, Fu FH. Arthroscopic allograft anterior cruciate ligament reconstruction. Op Tech Sports Med 1995; 3(3):148-156.
11. Miller MD, Harner CD, Koshiwaguchi S. Acute posterior cruciate ligament injuries. *In* Fu FH, Harner CD, Vince KG, eds. Knee Surgery. Baltimore: Williams & Wilkins, 1994, pp 749-767.
12. Neuschwander DC. Discoid lateral meniscus. *In* Fu FH, Harner CD, Vince KG, eds. Knee Surgery. Baltimore: Williams & Wilkins, 1994, pp 393-403.
13. Parisien JS. Arthroscopic treatment of cysts of the menisci. A preliminary report. Clin Orthop 1990; 257:154-158.
14. Walker RH, Dillingham M. Thrombophlebitis following arthroscopic surgery of the knee. Contemp Orthop 1983; 6:29-33.

Illustrative Cases—Knee

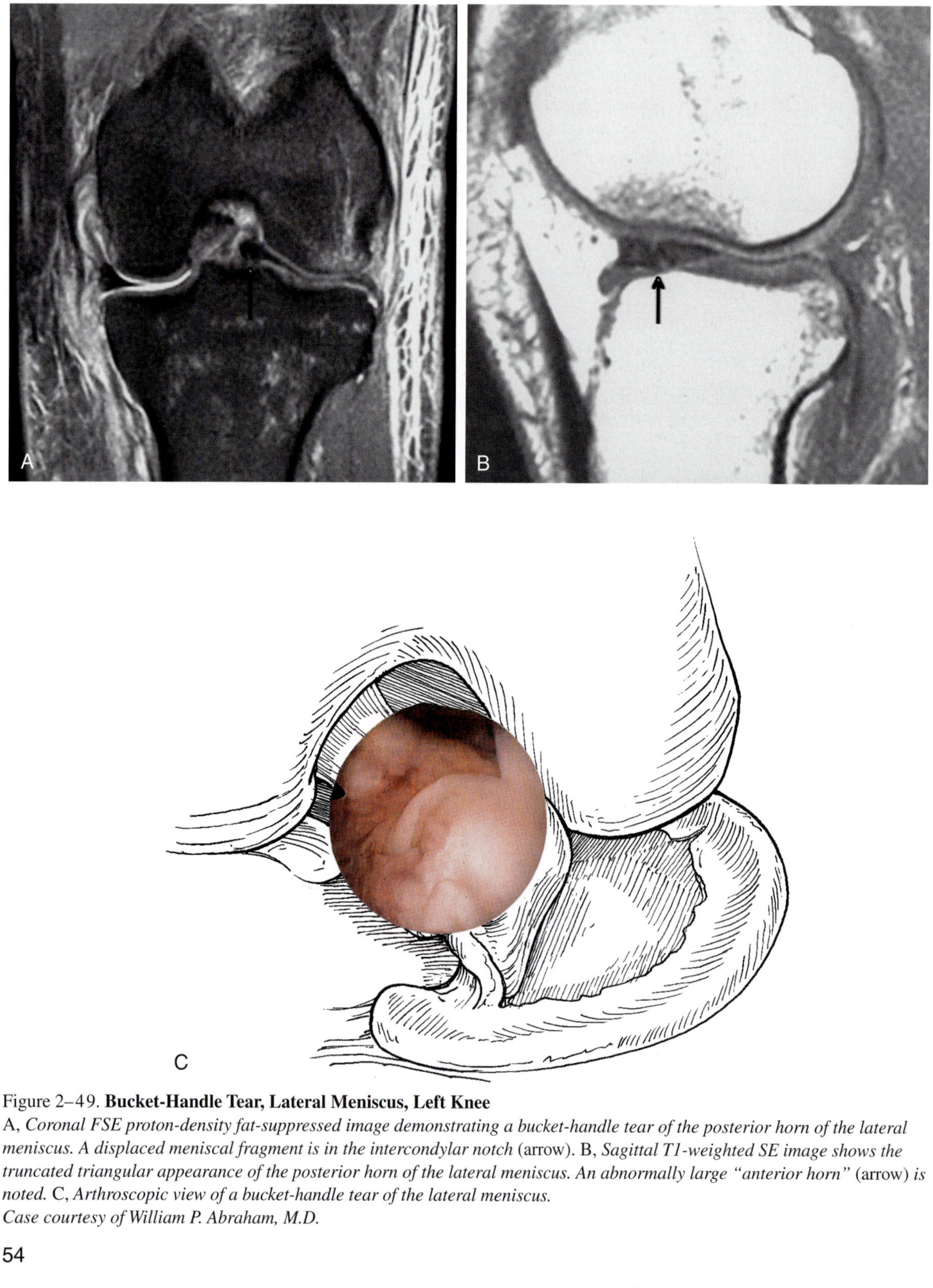

Figure 2–49. **Bucket-Handle Tear, Lateral Meniscus, Left Knee**

A, *Coronal FSE proton-density fat-suppressed image demonstrating a bucket-handle tear of the posterior horn of the lateral meniscus. A displaced meniscal fragment is in the intercondylar notch* (arrow). B, *Sagittal T1-weighted SE image shows the truncated triangular appearance of the posterior horn of the lateral meniscus. An abnormally large "anterior horn"* (arrow) *is noted.* C, *Arthroscopic view of a bucket-handle tear of the lateral meniscus.*

Case courtesy of William P. Abraham, M.D.

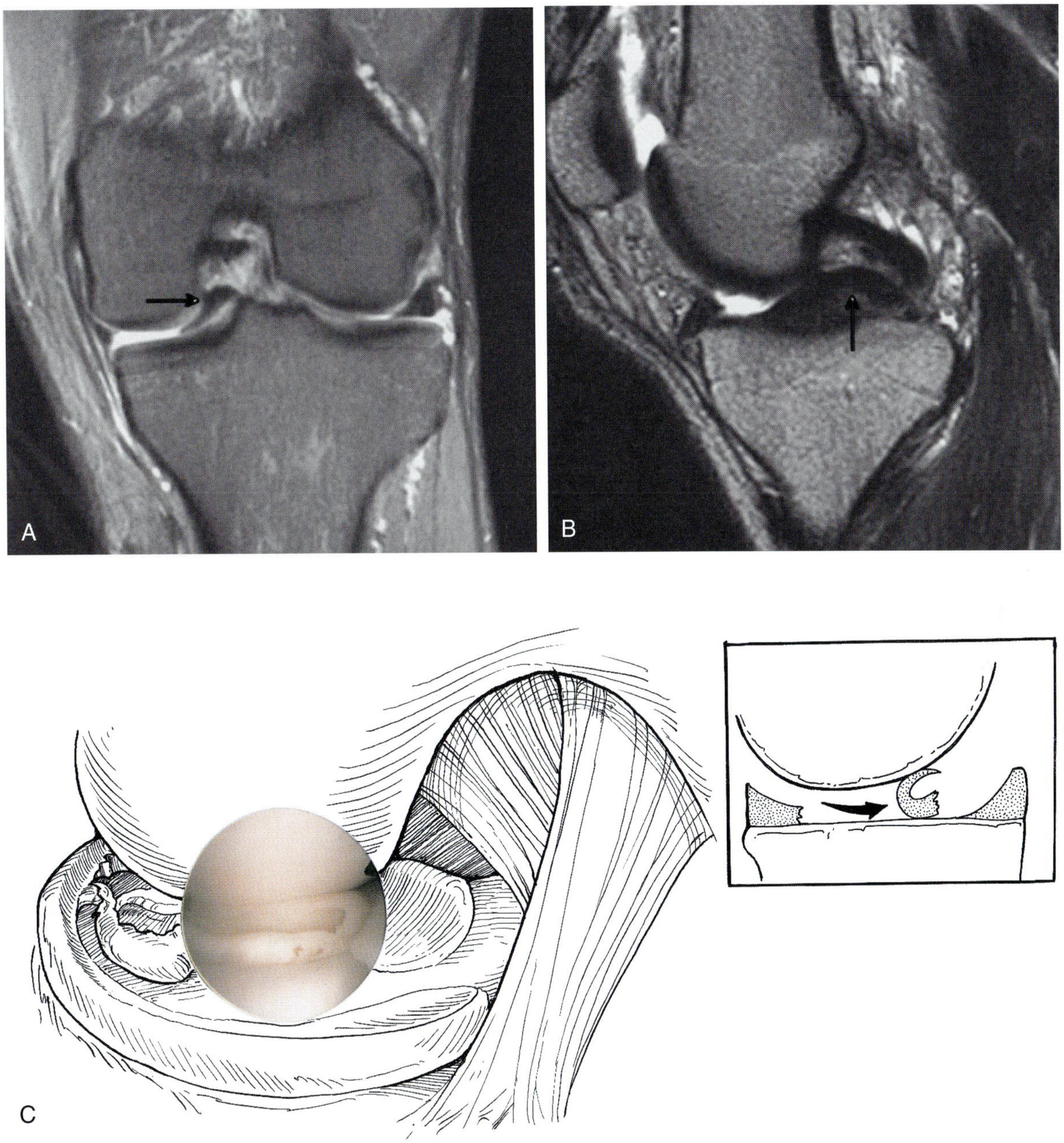

Figure 2–50. **Bucket-Handle Tear, Medial Meniscus, Left Knee**

A, *Coronal FSE proton-density fat-suppressed image demonstrating a bucket-handle tear of the posterior horn of the medial meniscus. A displaced meniscal fragment is in the intercondylar notch* (arrow) *below the posterior cruciate ligament.* B, *Sagittal FSE T2-weighted image shows the displaced fragment* (arrow) *in the intercondylar notch immediately below the posterior cruciate ligament ("double PCL sign").* C, *Arthroscopic view of a bucket-handle tear of the medial meniscus.*

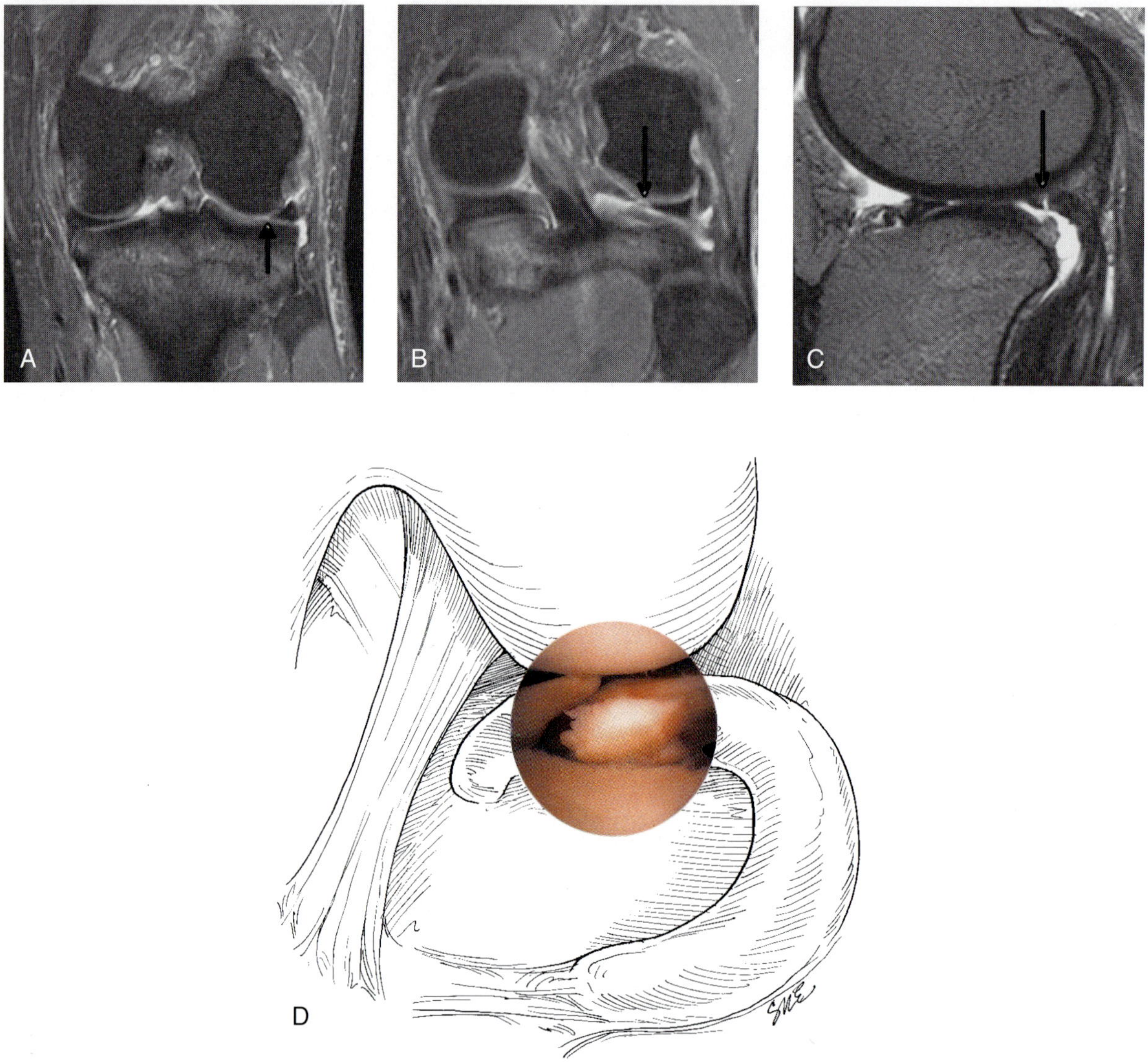

Figure 2–51. **Double Flap Tear, Posterior Horn Lateral Meniscus, Left Knee**
A, *Coronal FSE proton-density fat-suppressed image demonstrating truncation of the posterior horn lateral meniscus* (arrow). B, *Coronal FSE proton-density fat-suppressed image posterior to A showing a focus of bright signal* (arrow) *within the posterior horn lateral meniscus.* C, *Sagittal FSE T2-weighted image reveals a vertical tear pattern* (arrow) *confirming a flap tear of the posterior horn lateral meniscus.* D, *Arthroscopic view demonstrating a double-flap tear of the lateral meniscus with an interposed meniscal fragment.*

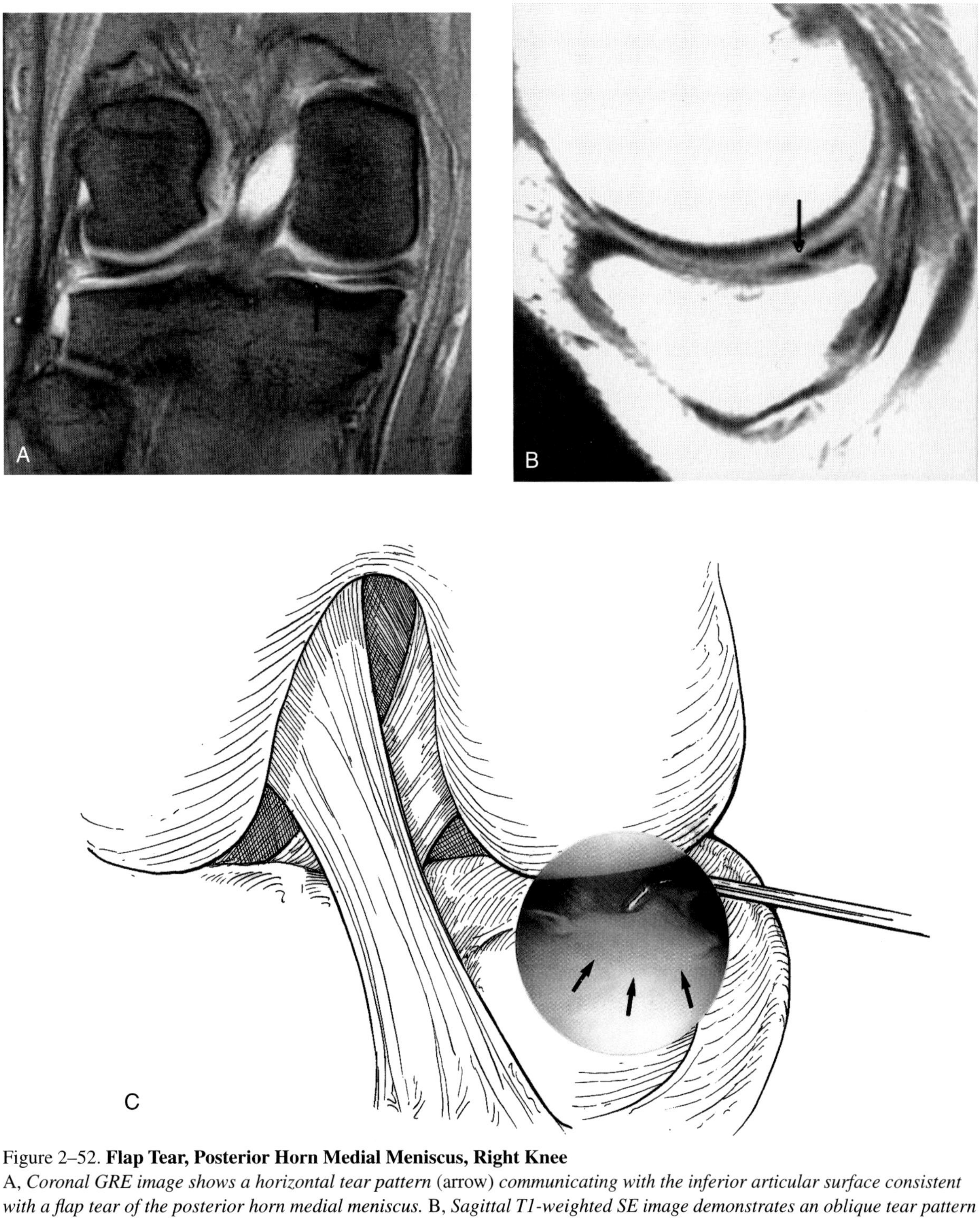

Figure 2–52. **Flap Tear, Posterior Horn Medial Meniscus, Right Knee**
A, *Coronal GRE image shows a horizontal tear pattern* (arrow) *communicating with the inferior articular surface consistent with a flap tear of the posterior horn medial meniscus.* B, *Sagittal T1-weighted SE image demonstrates an oblique tear pattern* (arrow) *communicating with the superior articular surface, confirming a flap tear.* C, *Arthroscopic view demonstrating a flap tear (displaced centrally with a probe) of the posterior horn of the medial meniscus.*

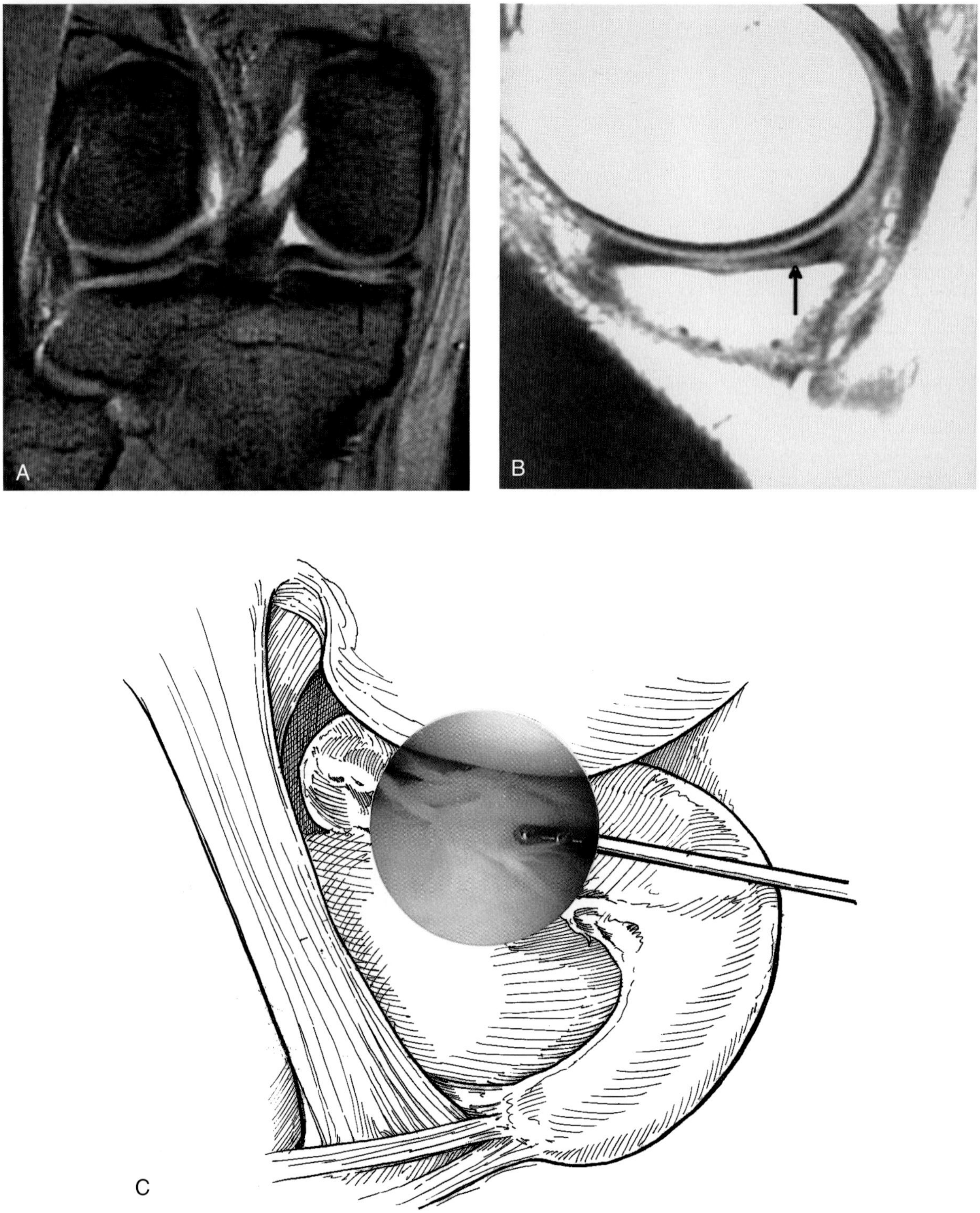

Figure 2–53. **Flap Tear, Posterior Horn Medial Meniscus, Right Knee**
A, *Coronal GRE image reveals an oblique tear pattern within the posterior horn medial meniscus* (arrow) *that communicates with the inferior articular surface.* B, *Sagittal T1-weighted SE image shows similar findings* (arrow). C, *Arthroscopic view demonstrates displacement of the flap tear (displaced by a probe) into the center of the medial compartment.*

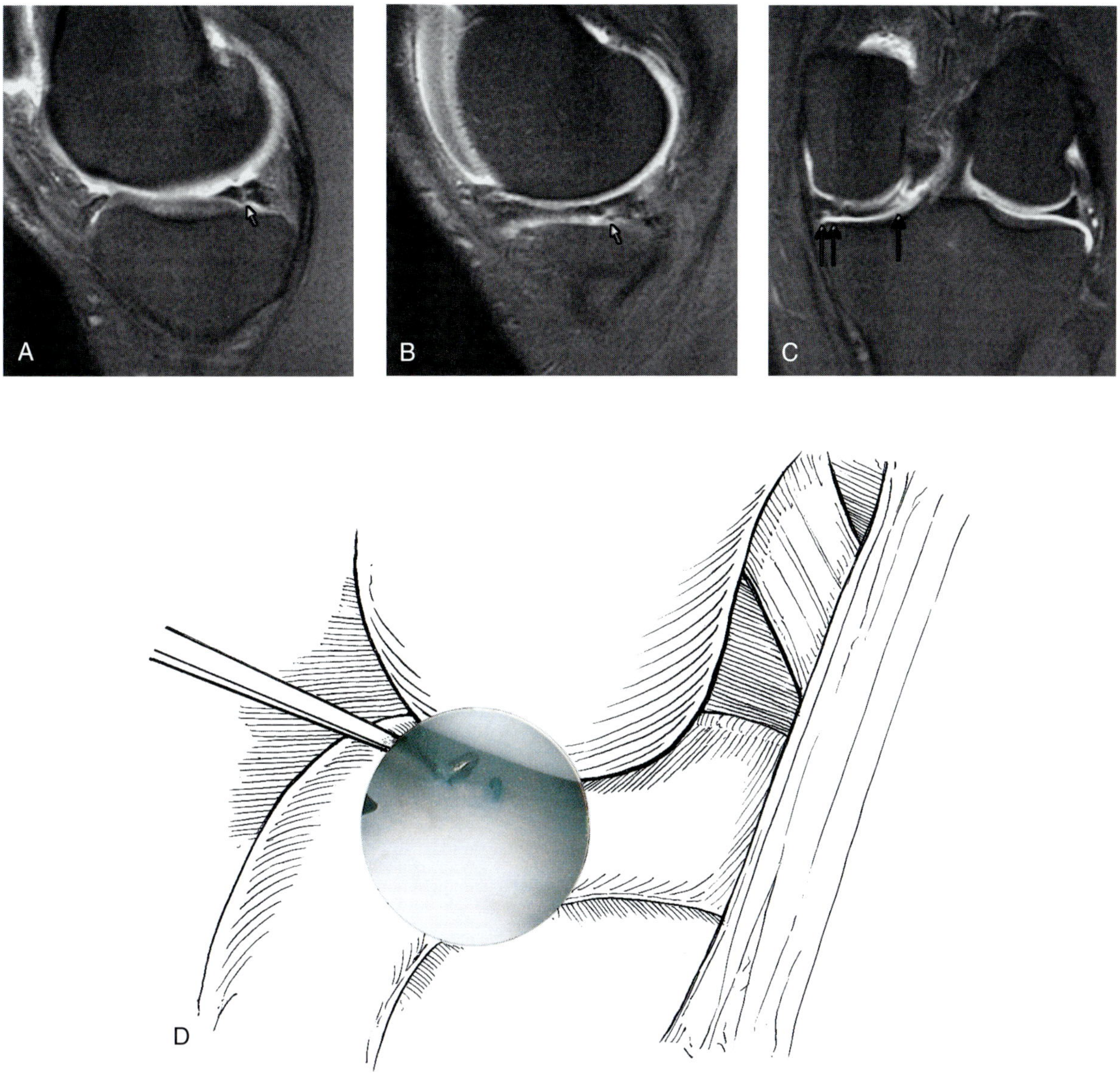

Figure 2–54. **Recurrent Medial Meniscal Tear, Left Knee**
A, *Sagittal T1-weighted SE fat-suppressed image reveals a stellate area of bright signal in the posterior horn medial meniscus* (arrow) *following administration of intra-articular gadolinium contrast.* B, *Sagittal T1 weighted SE fat-suppressed image reveals a peripheral focus of bright signal* (arrow) *at the inferior surface of the posterior horn medial meniscus.* C, *Coronal T1-weighted SE fat-suppressed image shows a focus of bright signal* (arrow) *in the posterior horn medial meniscus toward the intercondylar notch and a smaller, peripheral focus of bright signal* (double arrow) *at the inferior meniscal surface.* D, *Arthroscopic image demonstrating recurrent tear and sutures from a previously attempted repair (probe).*

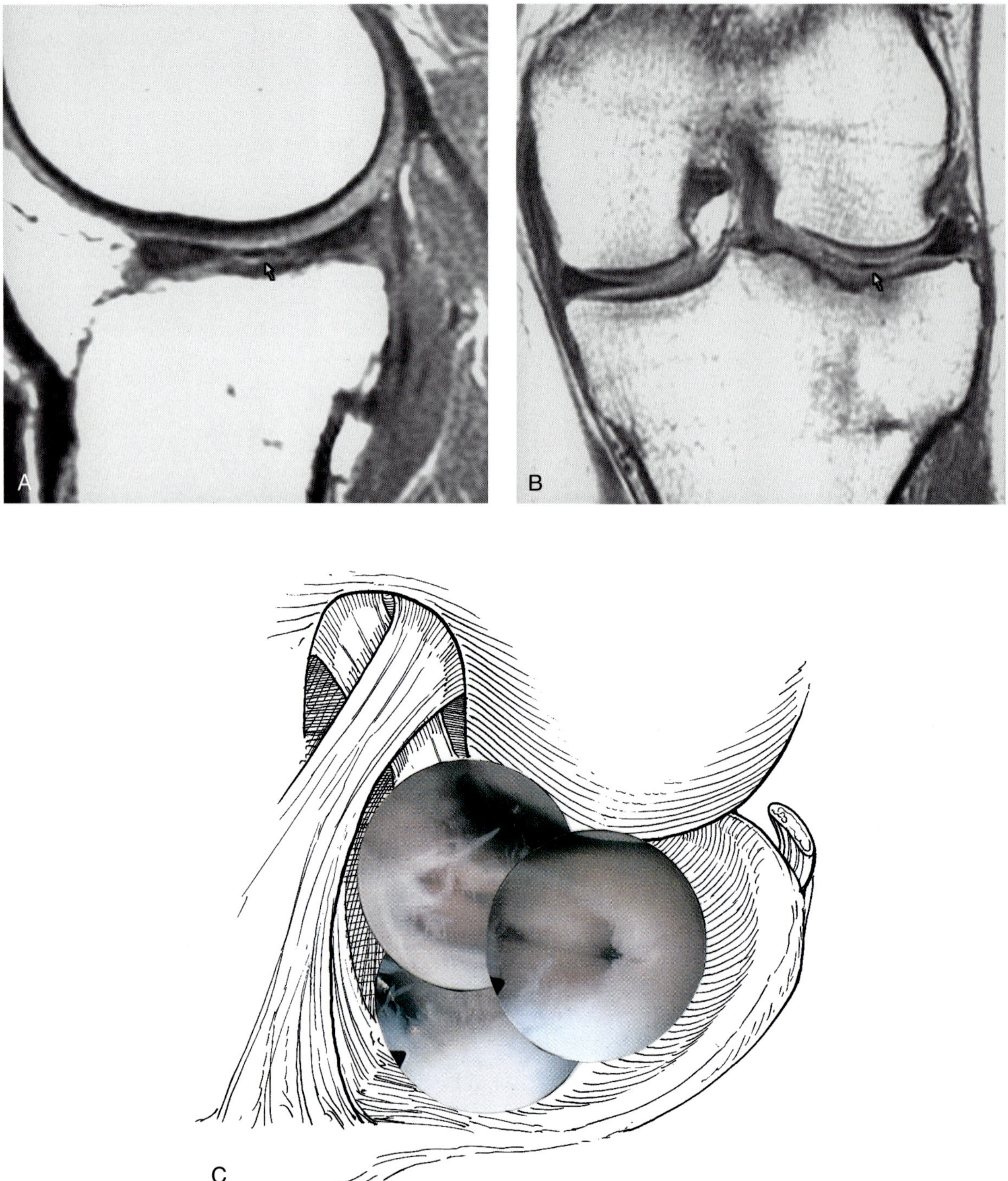

Figure 2–55. **Degenerative Lateral Meniscal Tear, Left Knee**
A, *Sagittal T1-weighted SE image shows irregularity of the free margin, lateral meniscus* (arrow). B, *Coronal T1-weighted SE image yields similar findings* (arrow). C, *Arthroscopic image shows degenerative fraying of the lateral meniscus.*

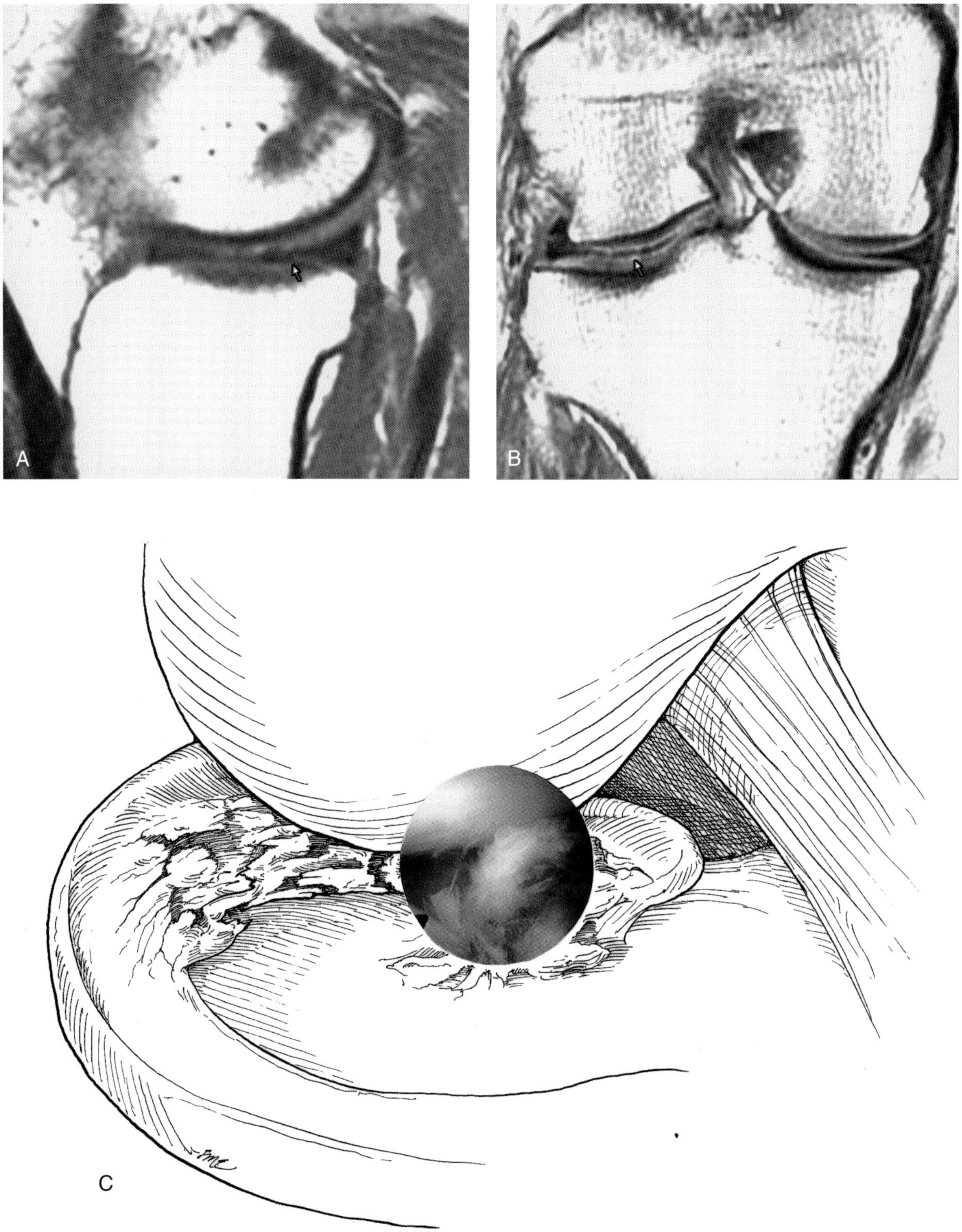

Figure 2–56. **Degenerative Lateral Meniscal Tear, Right Knee**
A, *Sagittal T1-weighted SE image shows irregularity of the free margin, lateral meniscus* (arrow). B, *Coronal T1-weighted SE image yields similar findings* (arrow). C, *Arthroscopic image shows degenerative fraying of the lateral meniscus.*

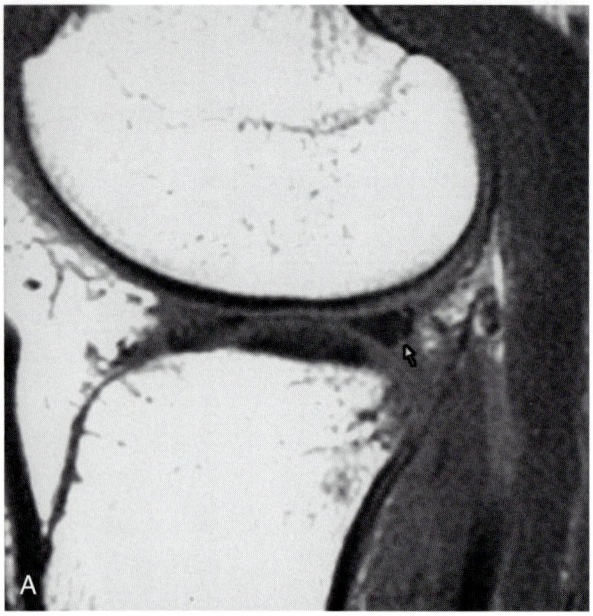

Figure 2–57. **Incomplete Tear, Superior Surface, Posterior Horn Lateral Meniscus, Right Knee**
A, *Sagittal T1-weighted SE image demonstrating a vertical tear pattern of the peripheral one third of the posterior horn lateral meniscus communicating with the superior articular surface* (arrow). B, *Arthroscopic image, viewed through the notch, demonstrating a peripheral tear behind the lateral femoral condyle.*

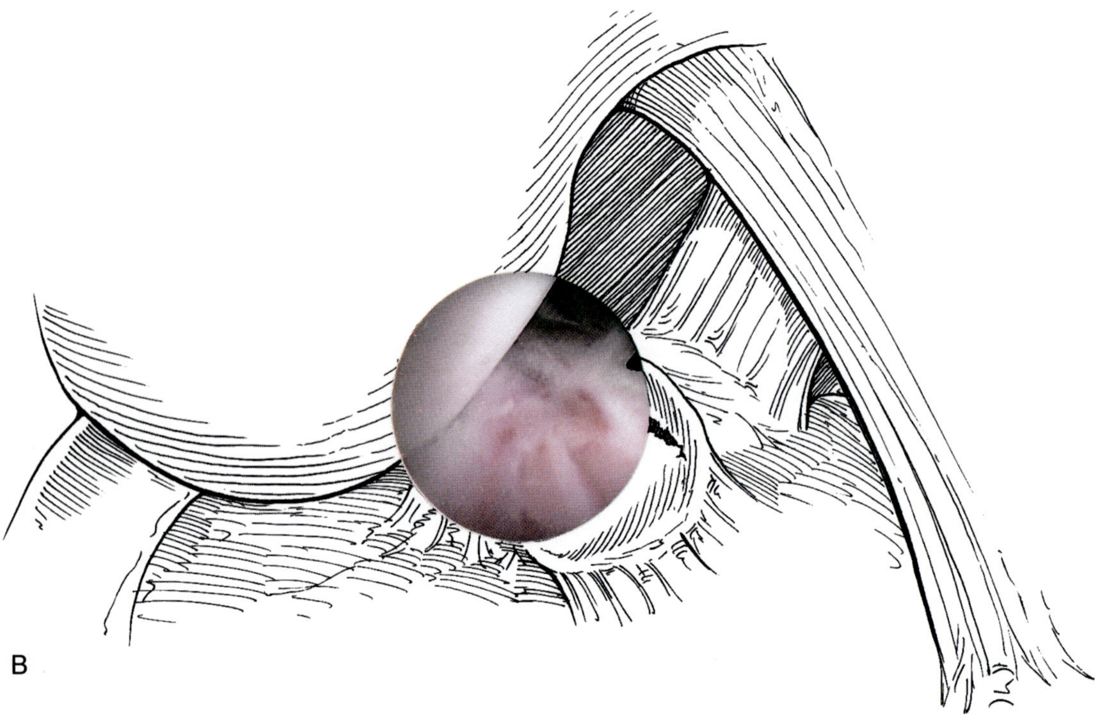

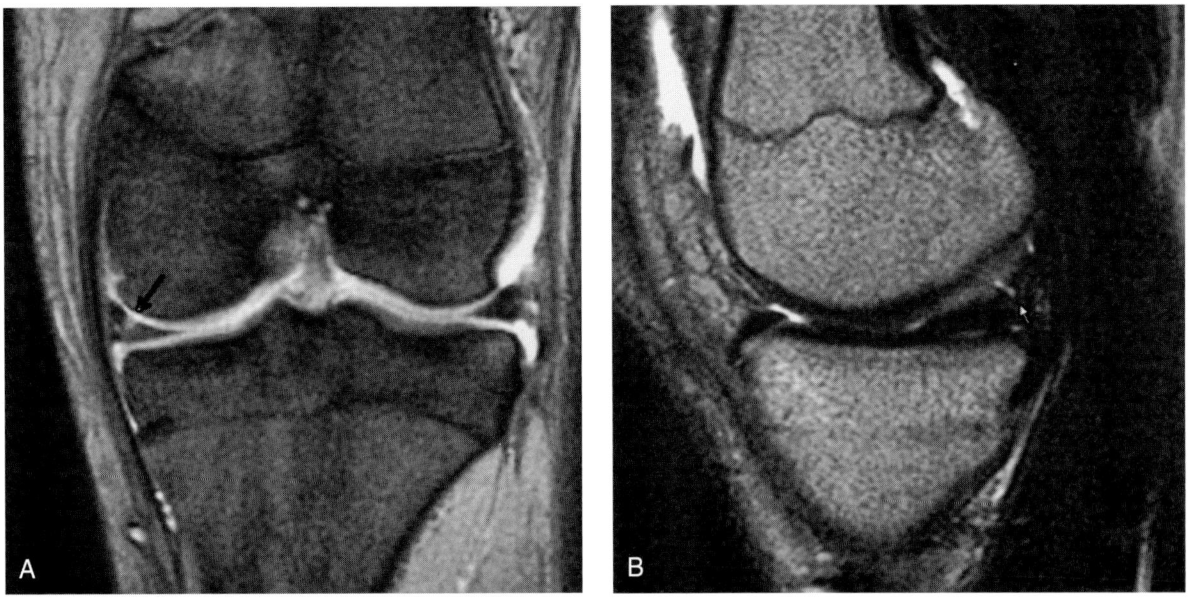

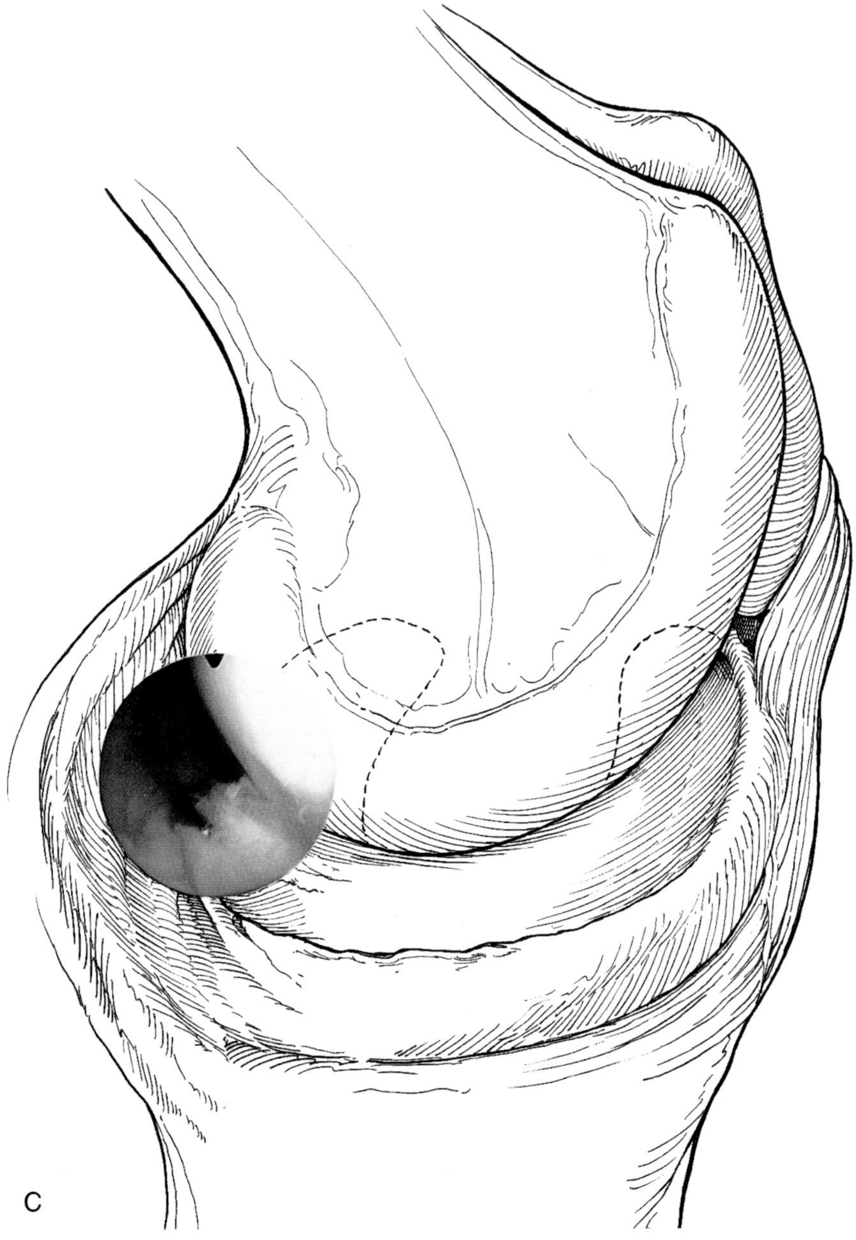

Figure 2–58. **Incomplete Tear, Superior Surface, Posterior Horn Medial Meniscus, Left Knee**
A, *Coronal GRE image reveals an incomplete vertical tear pattern communicating to the superior articular surface of the posterior horn medial meniscus* (arrow). B, *Sagittal FSE T2-weighted image shows a focus of bright signal at the superior surface of the posterior horn* (arrow). C, *Arthroscopic photo, viewed through the notch, demonstrating the peripheral tear behind the medial femoral condyle.*

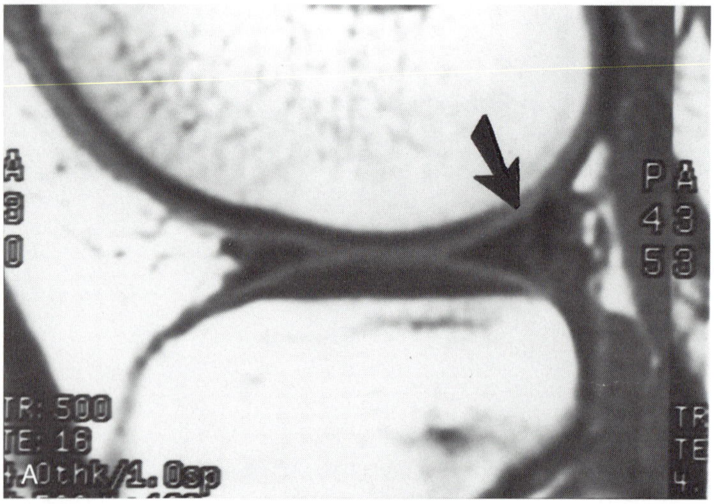

Figure 2–59. **Complete Vertical Tear, Posterior Horn Lateral Meniscus, Right Knee**

A, *Sagittal T1-weighted SE image shows a complete vertical tear pattern* (arrow) *communicating with superior and inferior articular surfaces within the peripheral one third of the posterior horn lateral meniscus.* B, *Arthroscopic view demonstrating a complete vertical (longitudinal) tear (probe).*

Case courtesy of Ronald Jones, M.D.

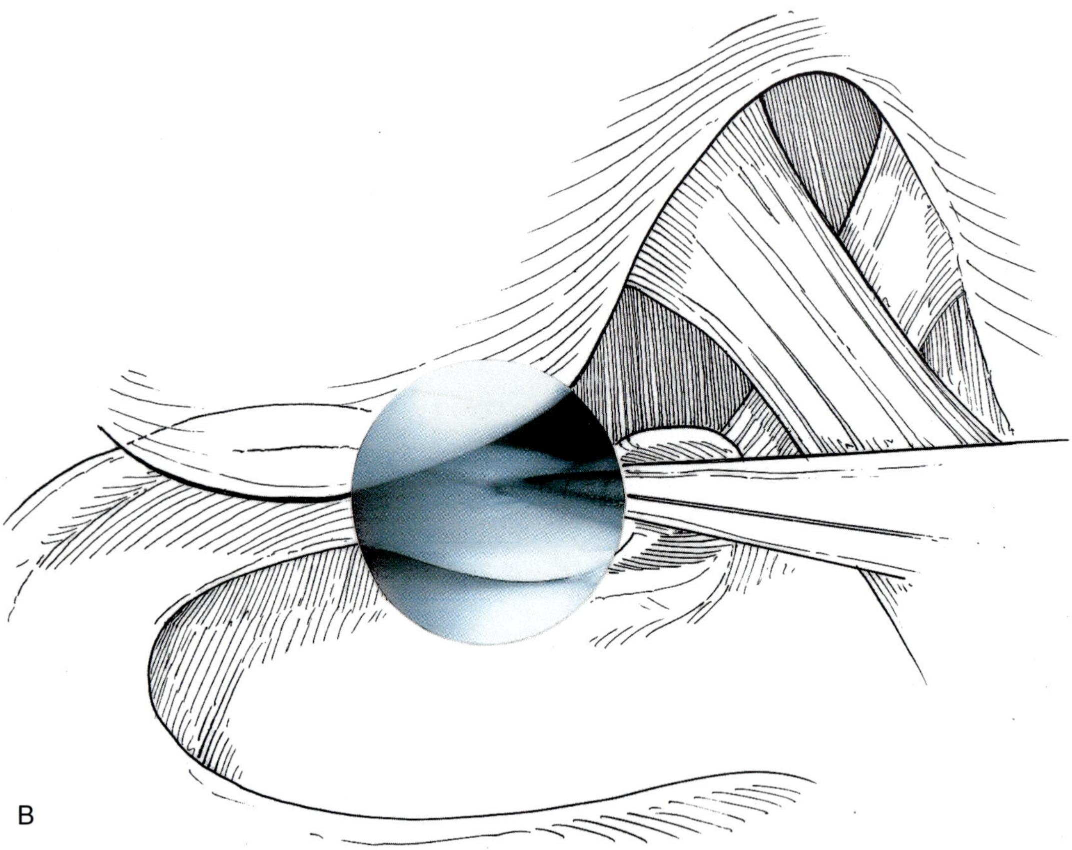

B

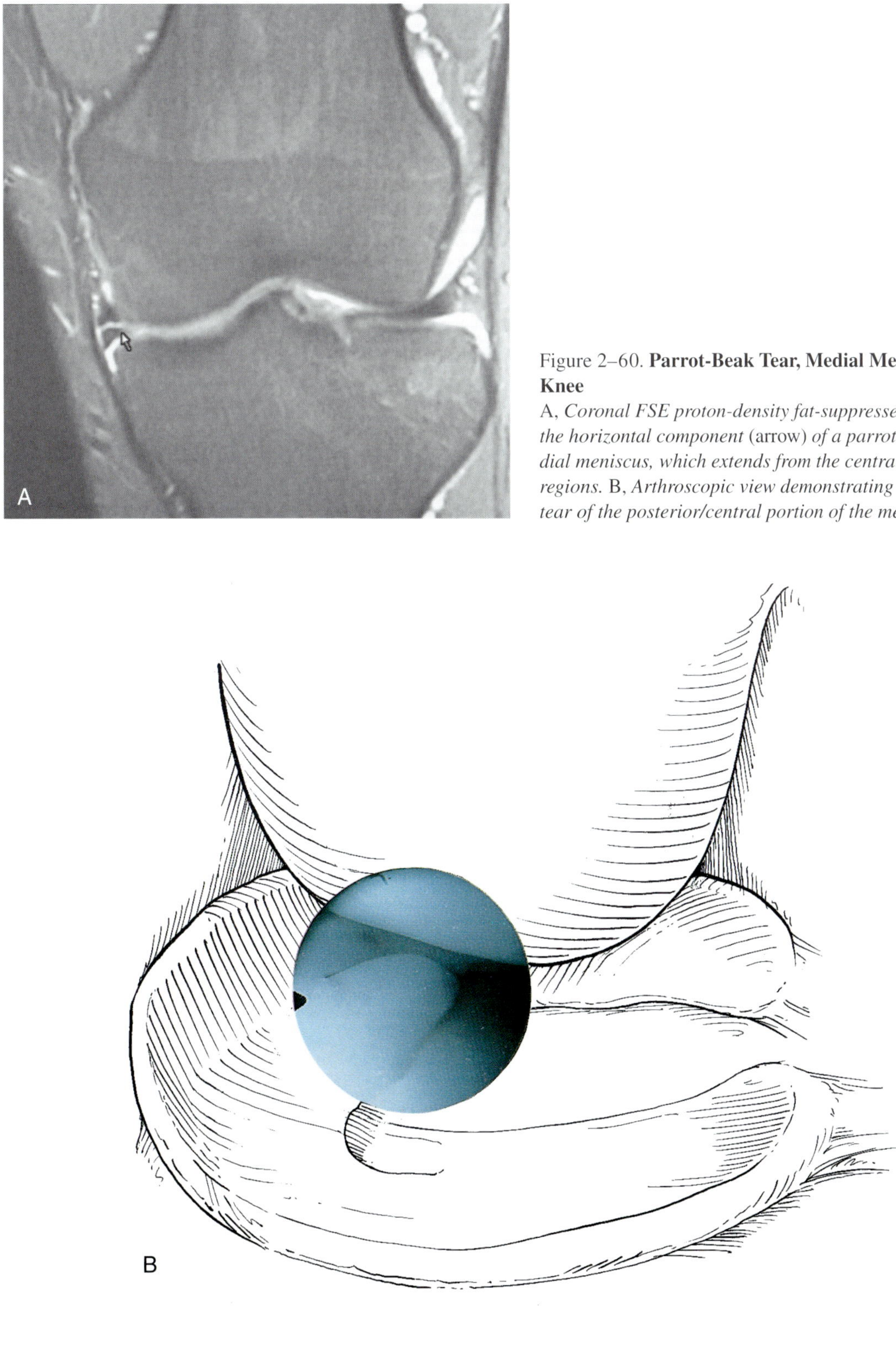

Figure 2–60. **Parrot-Beak Tear, Medial Meniscus, Left Knee**

A, *Coronal FSE proton-density fat-suppressed image shows the horizontal component* (arrow) *of a parrot-beak tear, medial meniscus, which extends from the central to peripheral regions.* B, *Arthroscopic view demonstrating a parrot-beak tear of the posterior/central portion of the medial meniscus.*

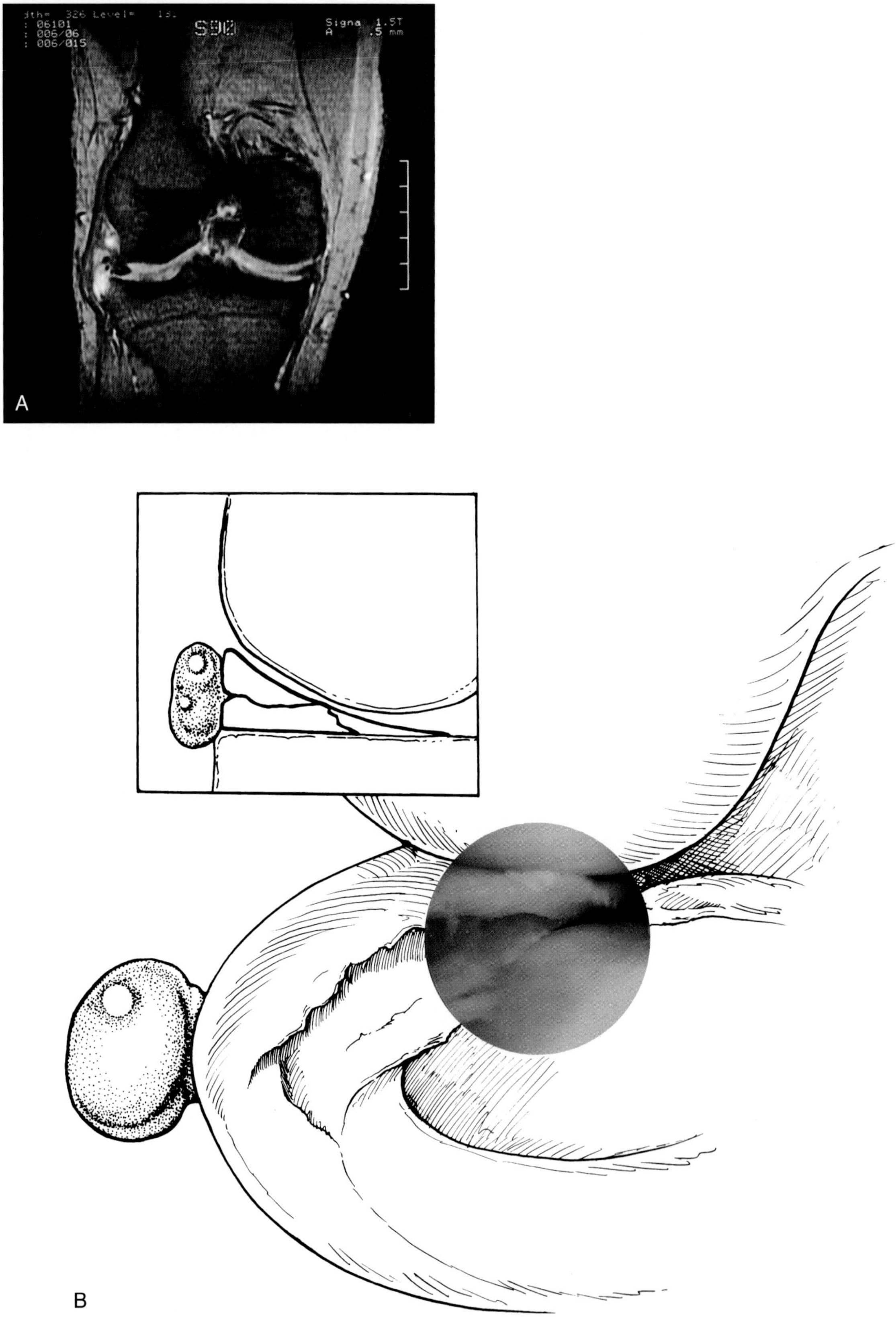

Figure 2–61. **Horizontal Lateral Meniscal Tear and Meniscal Cyst, Right Knee**
A, *Coronal GRE image shows a horizontal cleavage tear of the lateral meniscal tear with direct communication with a meniscal cyst in the peripheral region.* B, *Arthroscopic view demonstrates a complex meniscal tear that communicates with the tear. Case courtesy of J. Serge Parisien, M.D.*

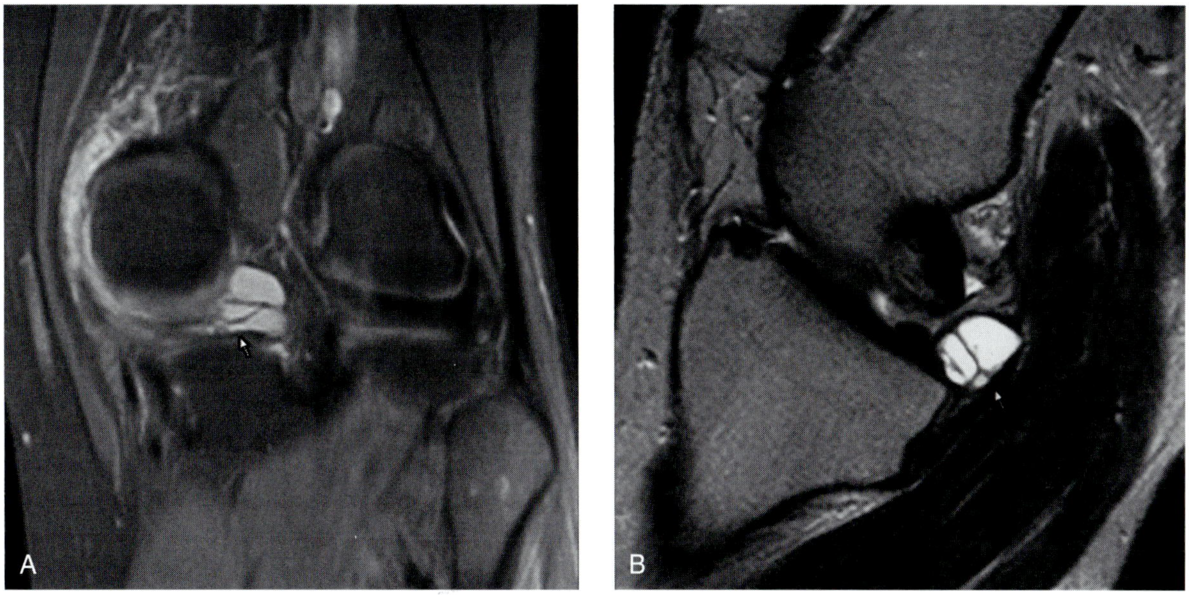

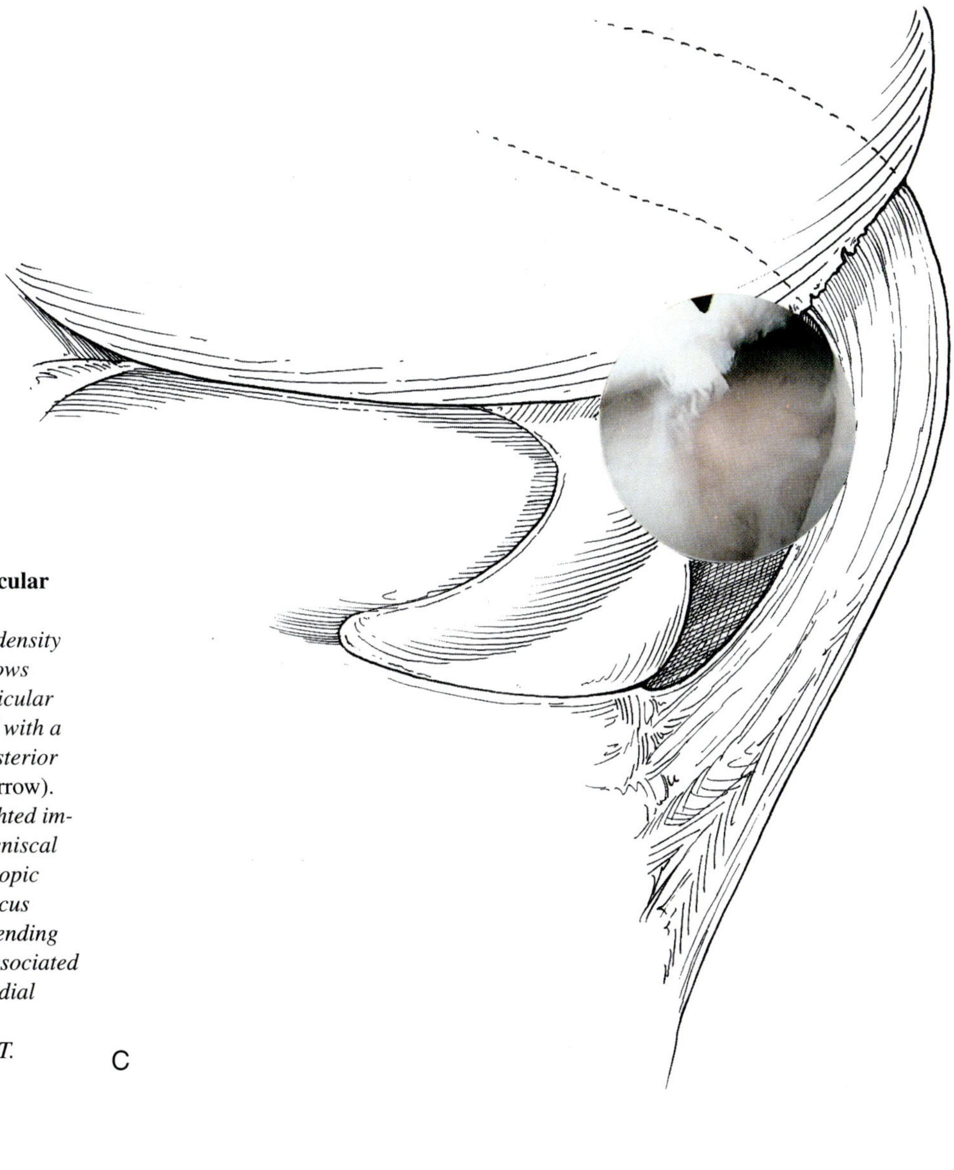

C

Figure 2–62. **Intra-Articular Meniscal Cyst**
A, *Coronal FSE proton-density fat-suppressed image shows multi-loculated intra-articular meniscal cyst associated with a horizontal tear in the posterior horn medial meniscus* (arrow). B, *Sagittal FSE T2-weighted images demonstrating a meniscal cyst* (arrow). C, *Arthroscopic view of the medial meniscus demonstrating a cyst extending into the notch from an associated horizontal tear of the medial meniscus.*
Case courtesy of Daniel T. Hinkin, M.D.

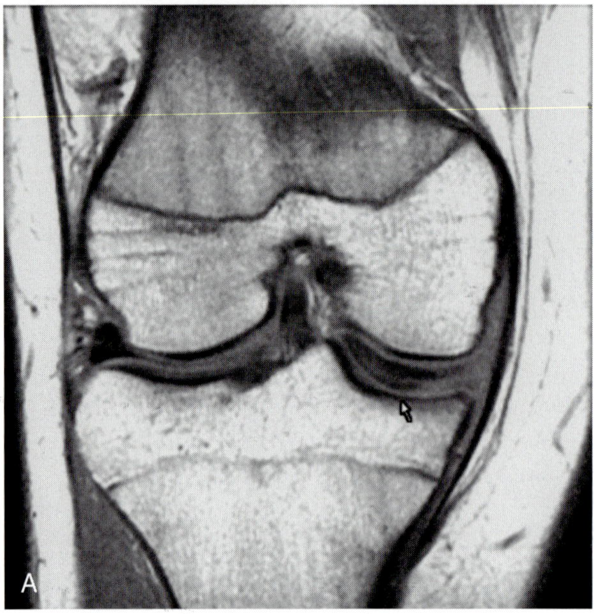

Figure 2–63. **Discoid Medial Meniscus, Right Knee**
A, *Coronal proton-density SE image of the medial compartment. The meniscus is unusually large and extends into the intercondylar notch* (arrow), *consistent with a discoid meniscus. Linear inter-substance signal did not represent a tear at the time of arthroscopy.* B, *Arthroscopic view demonstrating the medial tibial plateau completely covered by meniscal tissue.*
Case courtesy of Daniel T. Hinkin, M.D.

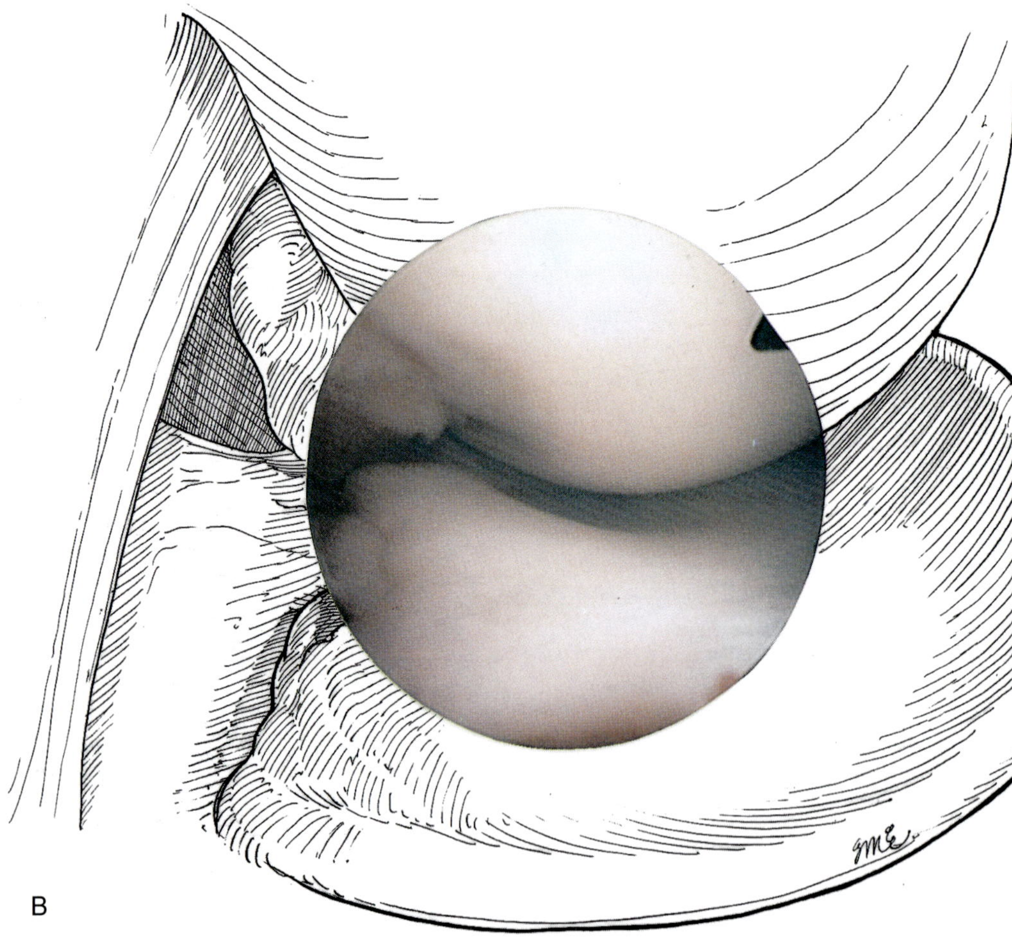

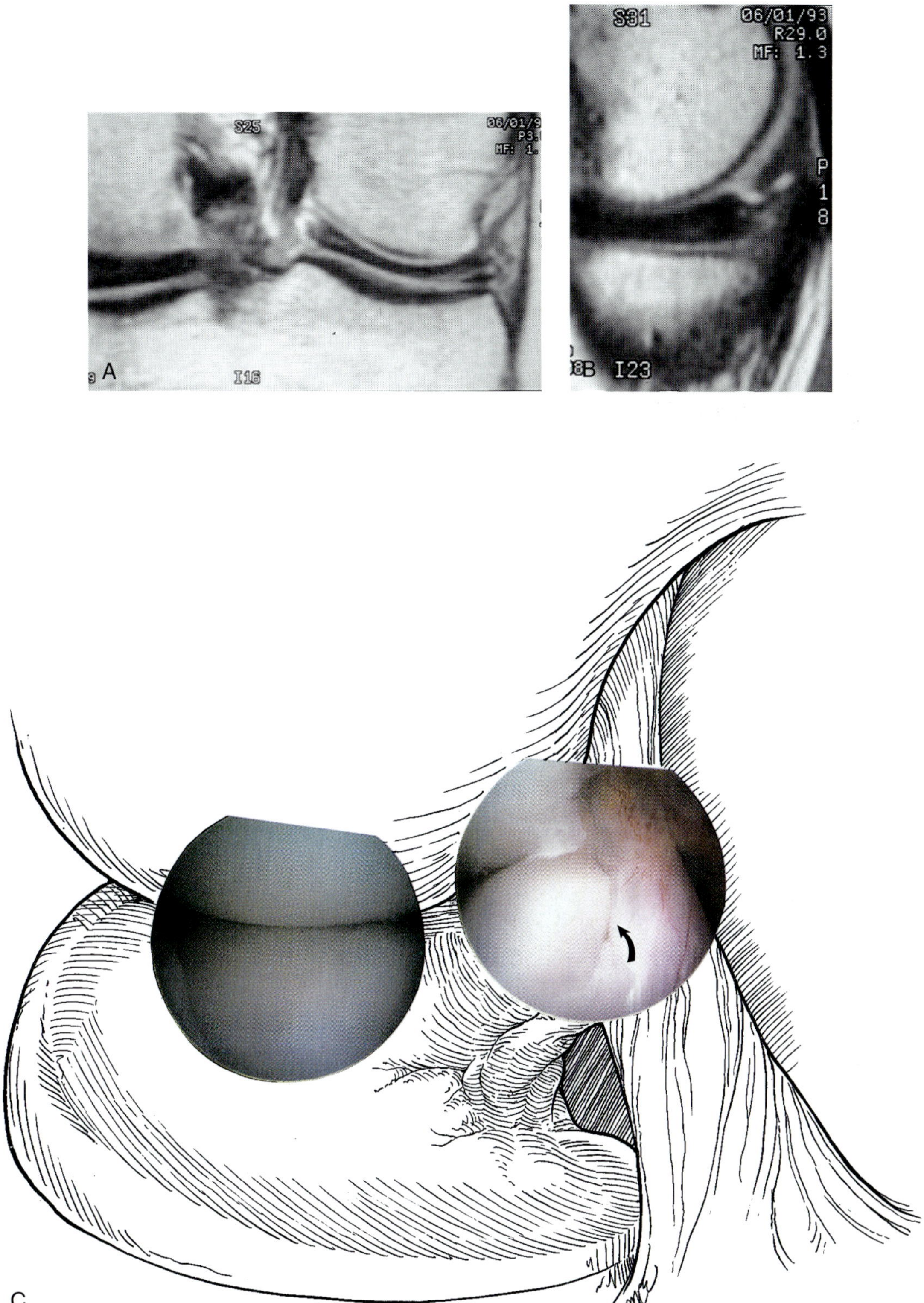

Figure 2–64. **Discoid Lateral Meniscus, Right Knee**
A, *Coronal proton-density SE image shows an abnormally large lateral meniscus at mid-body extending into the intercondylar notch.* B, *Sagittal proton-density SE image shows thickened lateral discoid meniscus.* C, *Arthroscopic view demonstrates thick meniscus that extends into the notch* (arrow).
Case courtesy of Christopher D. Harner, M.D.

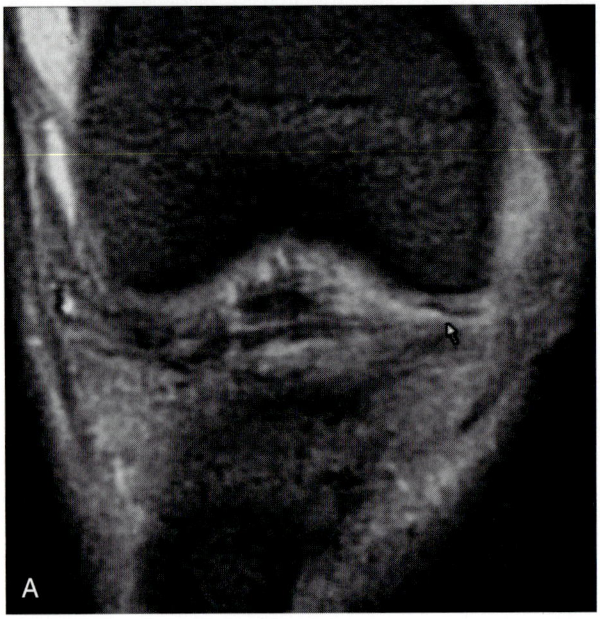

Figure 2–65. **Chondrocalcinosis, Right Knee**
A, *Coronal GRE image reveals a linear signal void within the articular cartilage of the anterior aspect of the medial femoral condyle* (arrow), *consistent with calcium pyrophosphate dihydrate deposits.* B, *Arthroscopic image demonstrating diffuse deposition of crystalline deposits.*

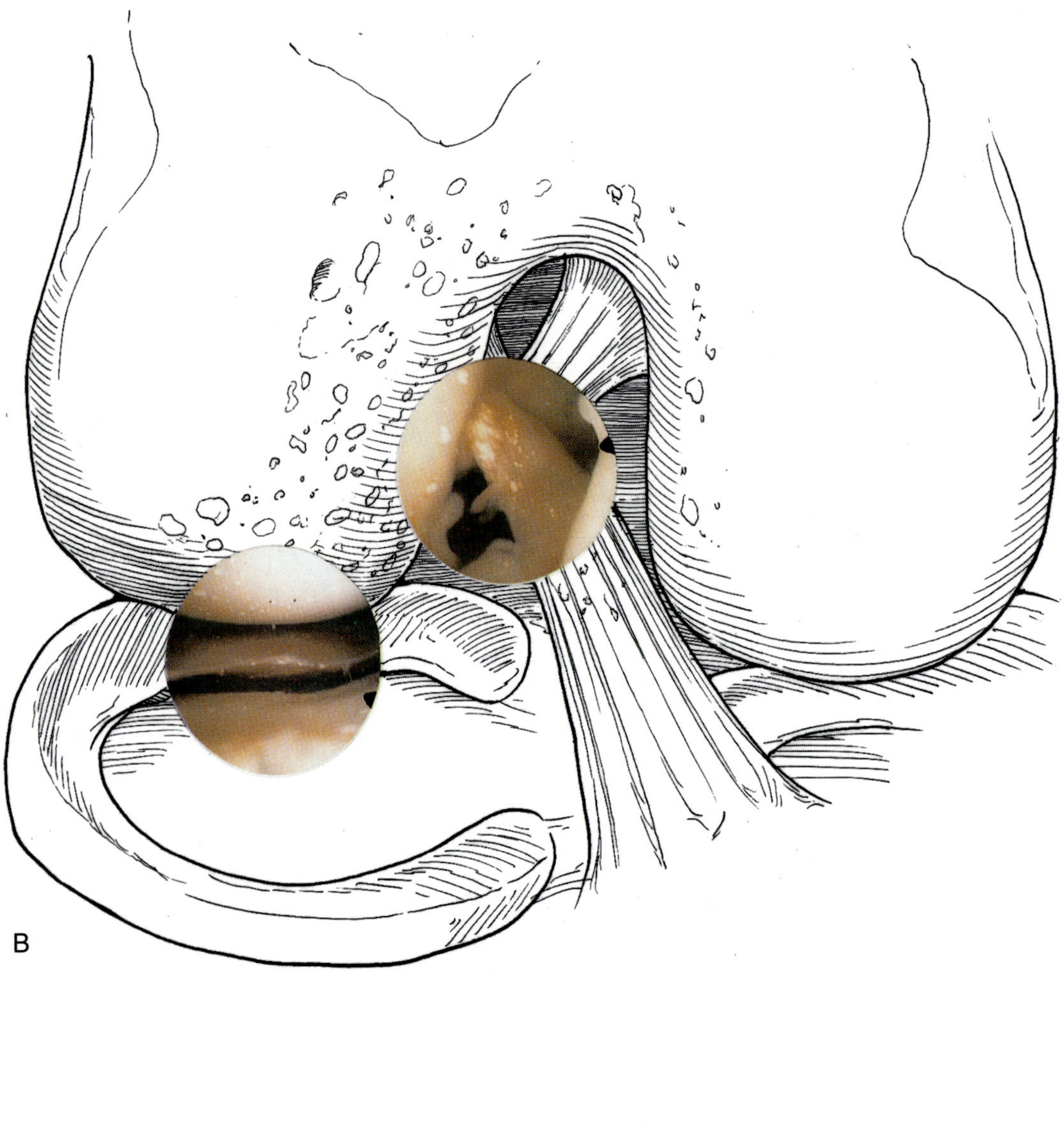

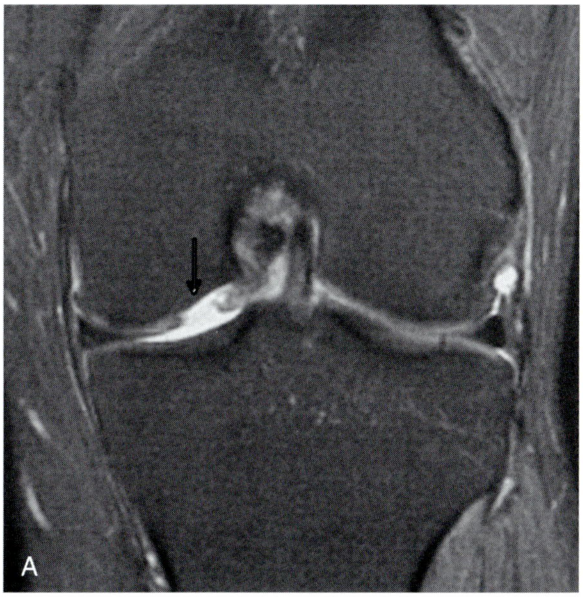

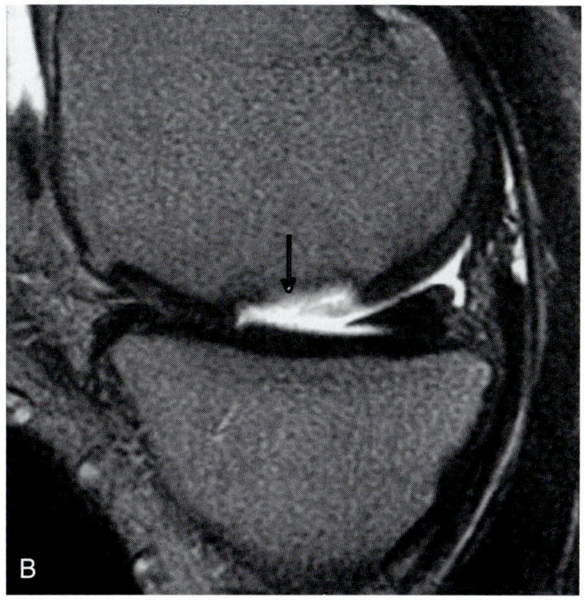

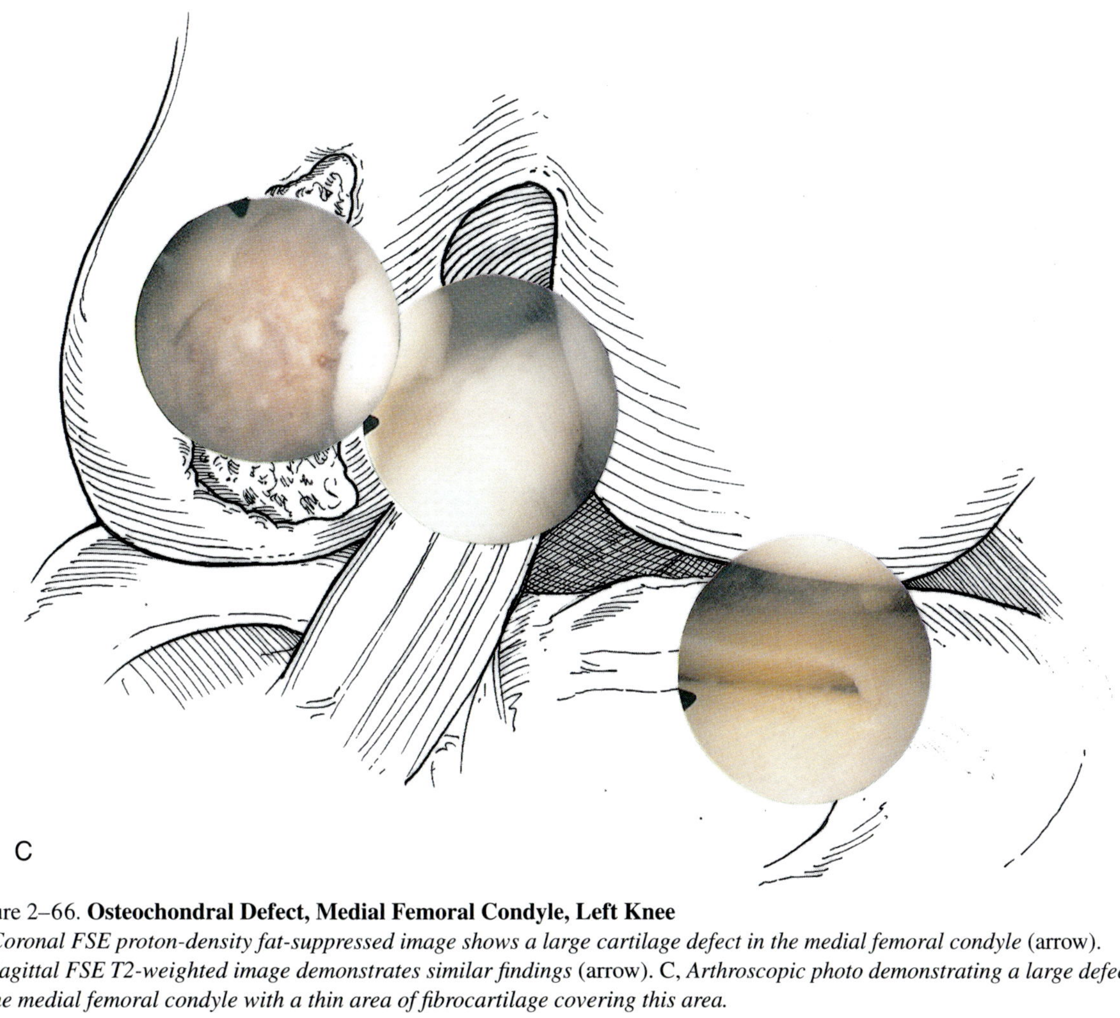

Figure 2–66. **Osteochondral Defect, Medial Femoral Condyle, Left Knee**
A, *Coronal FSE proton-density fat-suppressed image shows a large cartilage defect in the medial femoral condyle* (arrow). B, *Sagittal FSE T2-weighted image demonstrates similar findings* (arrow). C, *Arthroscopic photo demonstrating a large defect in the medial femoral condyle with a thin area of fibrocartilage covering this area.*

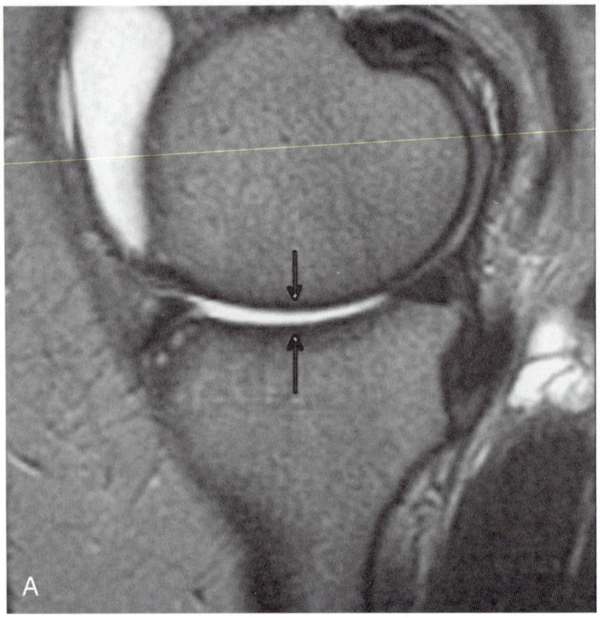

Figure 2–67. **Advanced Chondrosis, Medial Compartment, Left Knee**

A, *Sagittal FSE T2-weighted image reveals bare cortical bone surfaces of the medial femoral condyle and medial tibial plateau* (arrows). *Bright signal between the femur and tibia represents fluid.* B, *Arthroscopic view demonstrating a "kissing lesion" or exposed bone on both the medial femoral condyle and the medial tibial plateau.*

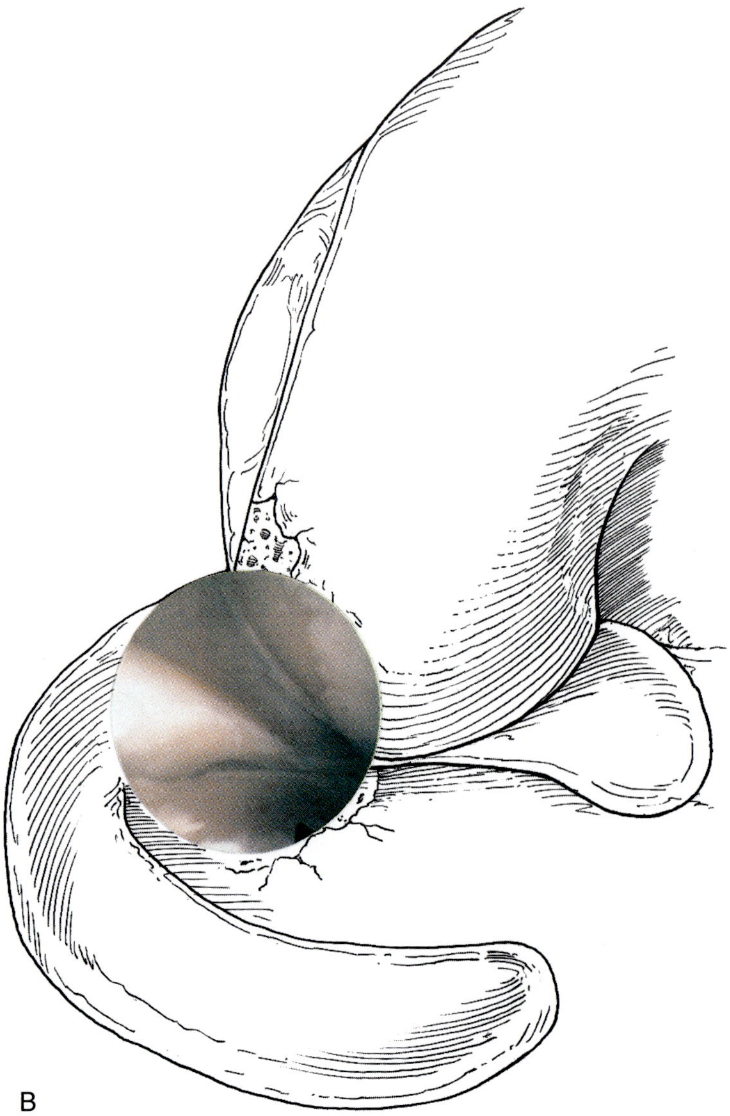

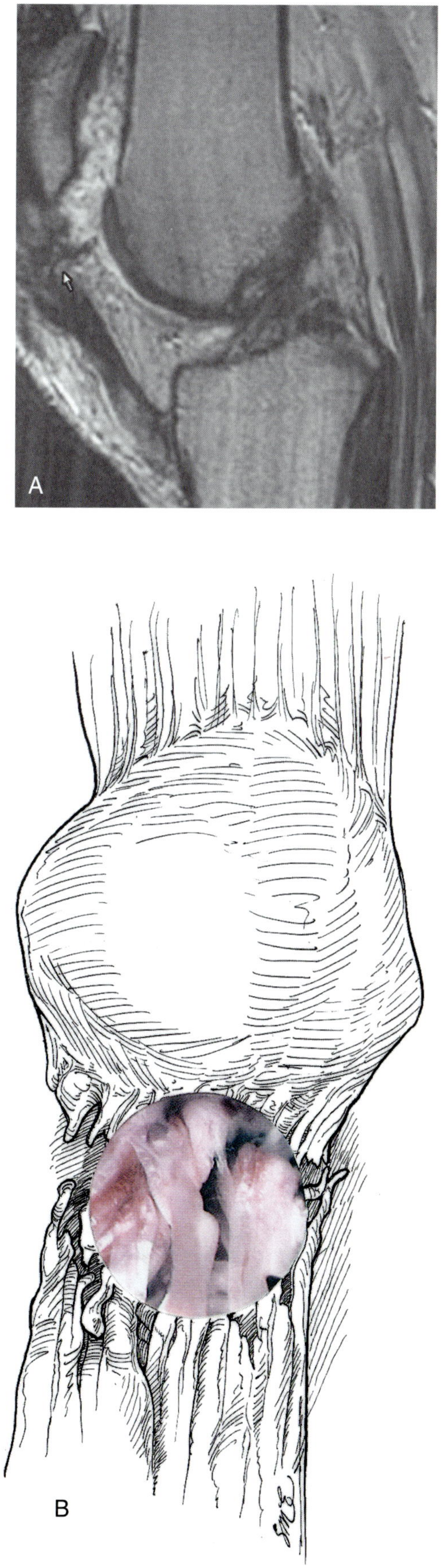

Figure 2–68. **Patellar Tendon Rupture, Right Knee**

A, *Sagittal FSE T2-weighted image shows disruption of the proximal patellar tendon* (arrow) *with associated high-riding patella.* B, *Arthroscopic view through the defect demonstrating a shredded "mop-end" patellar tendon.*

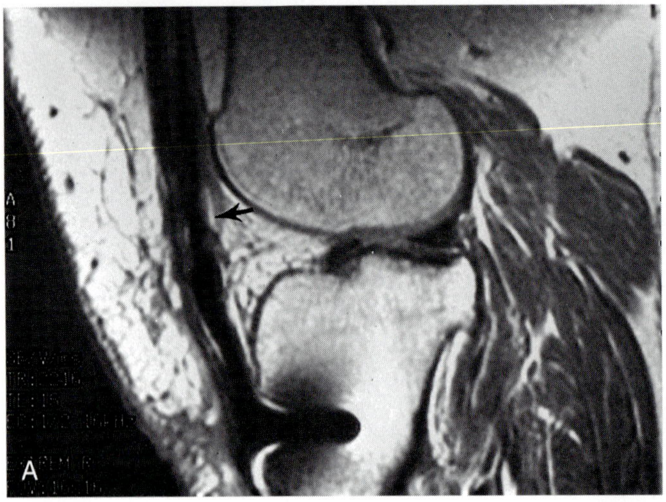

Figure 2–69. **Extensor Mechanism Defect, Status Following Patellectomy, Right Knee**
A, *Sagittal proton-density SE image shows marked attenuation of the extensor mechanism in the area of the previous patellectomy* (arrow). B, *Arthroscopic view demonstrating significant thinning of the extensor mechanism.*

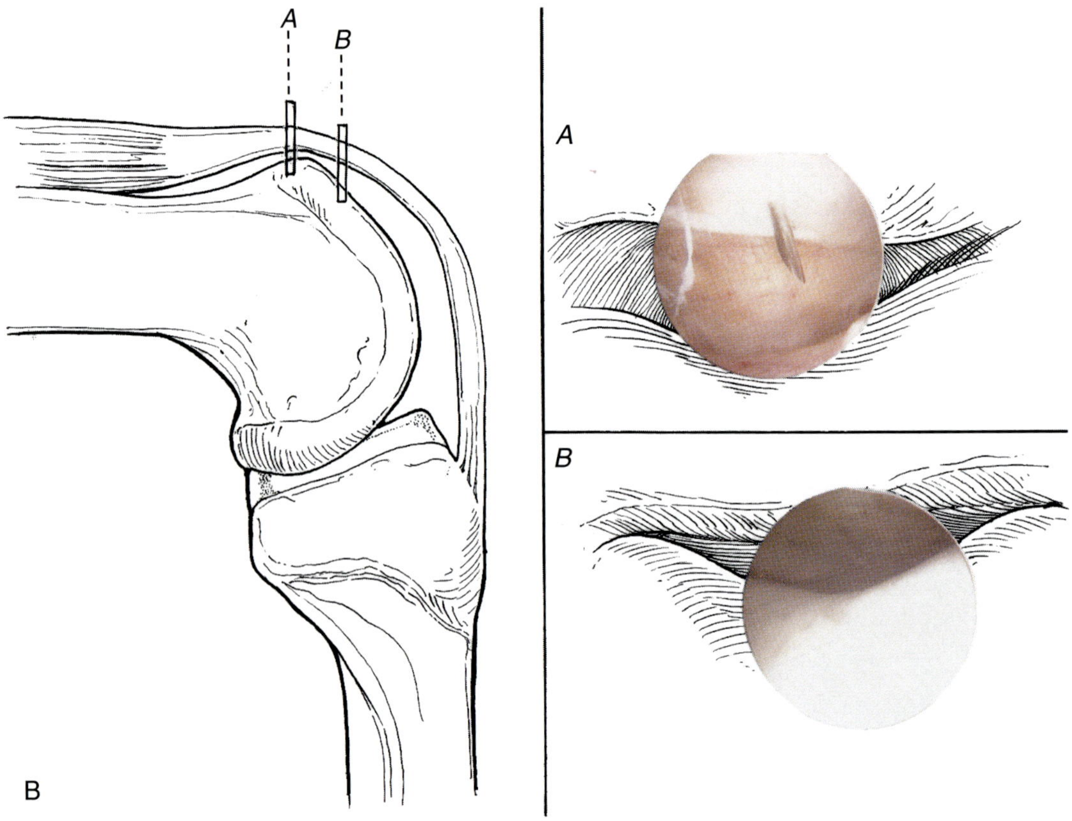

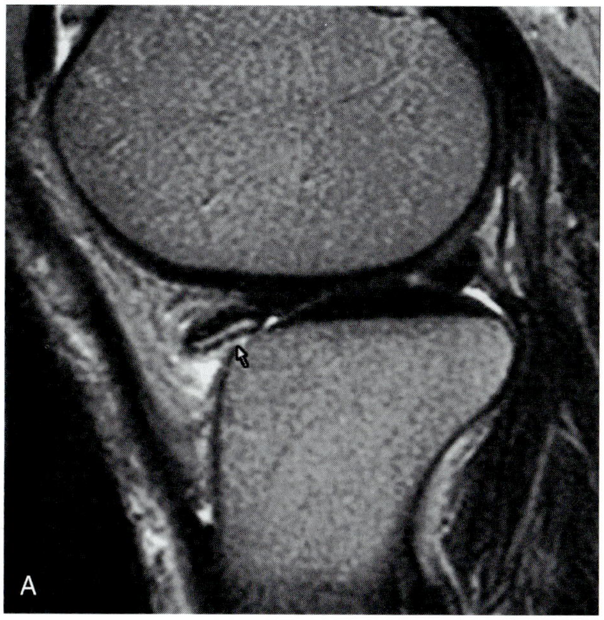

Figure 2–70. **Loose Body, Lateral Compartment, Right Knee**

A, *Sagittal FSE T2-weighted image shows an ovoid loose body* (arrow) *beneath the anterior horn lateral meniscus.*
B, *Arthroscopic view of an osteochondral loose body under the lateral meniscus.*

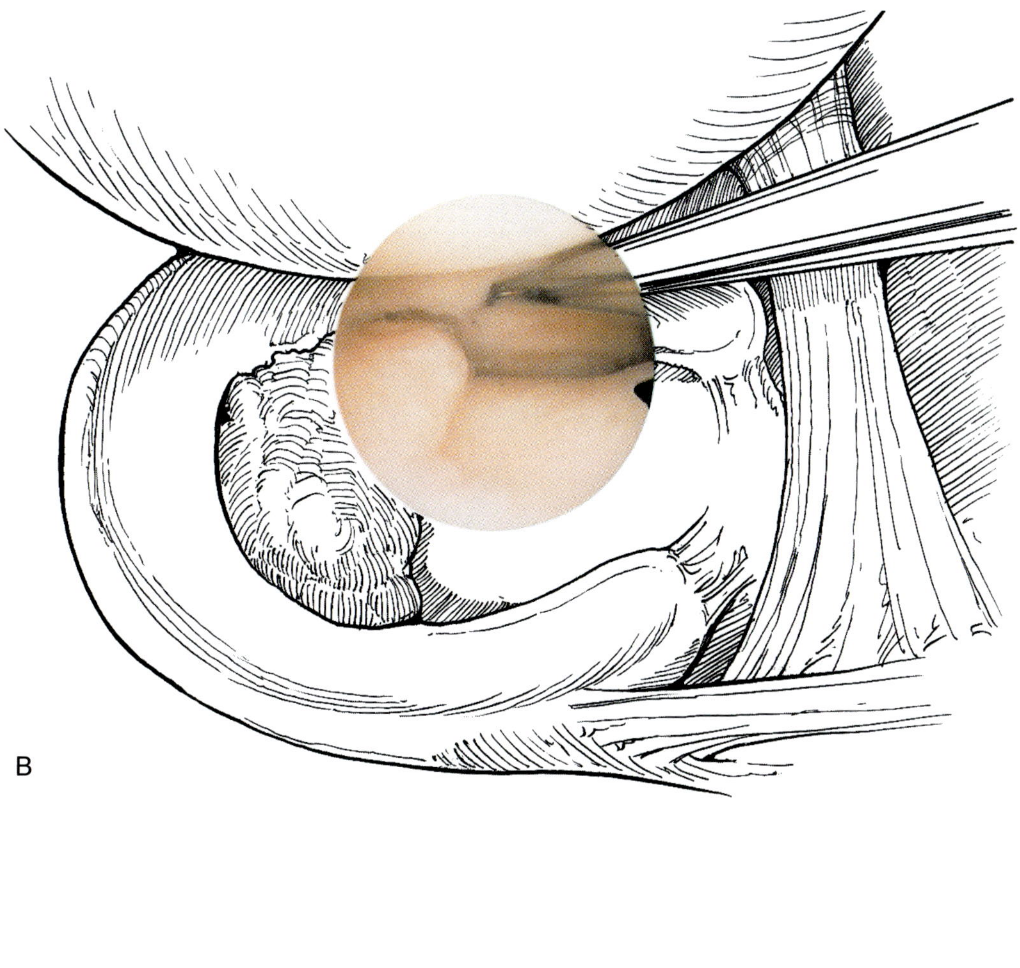

B

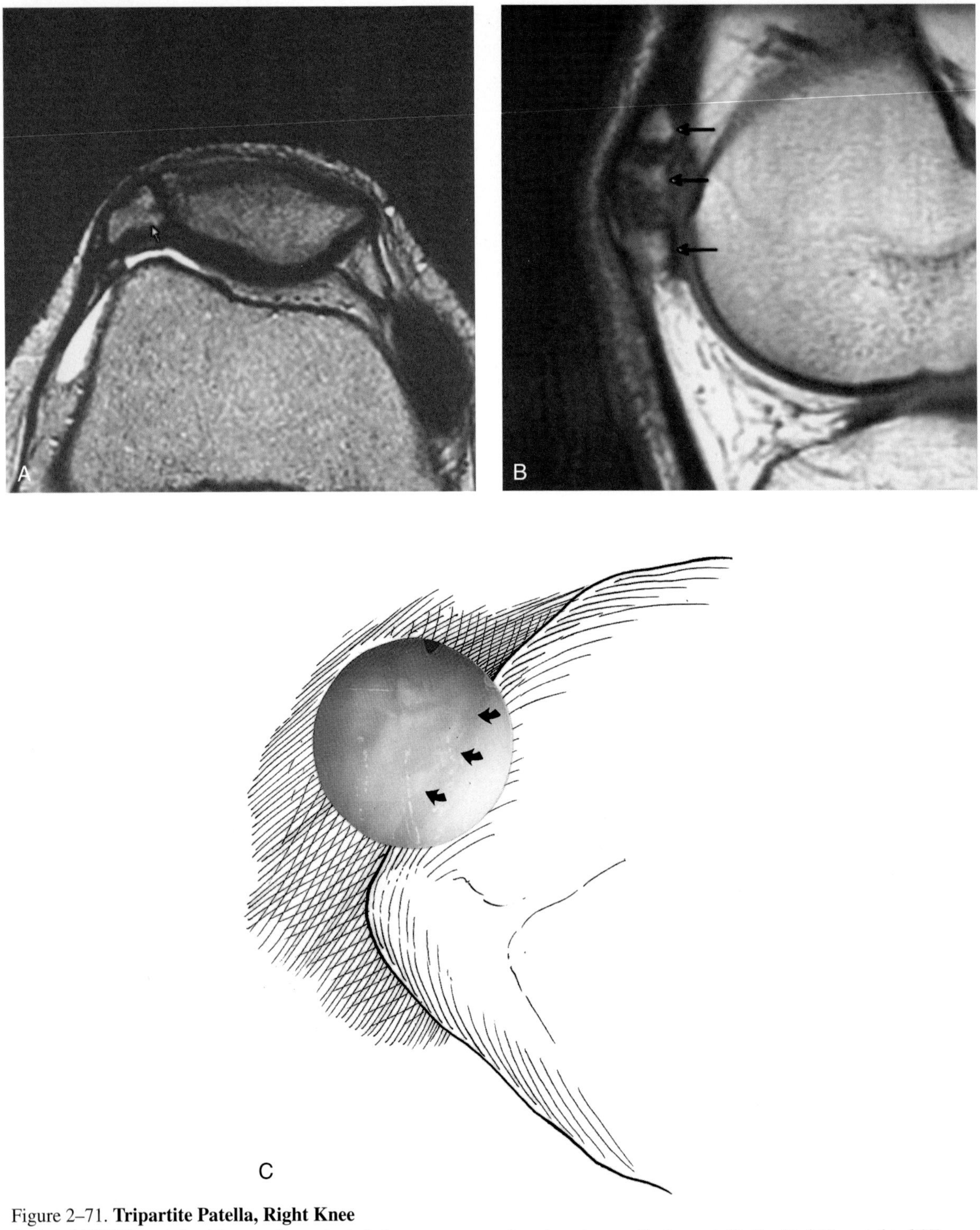

Figure 2–71. **Tripartite Patella, Right Knee**
A, *Axial FSE T2-weighted image shows the inferior component of a tripartite patella* (arrow). B, *Sagittal T1-weighted SE image shows all three components of a tripartite patella* (arrows). C, *Arthroscopic view demonstrates the separation of the symptomatic lateral fragments* (arrows).

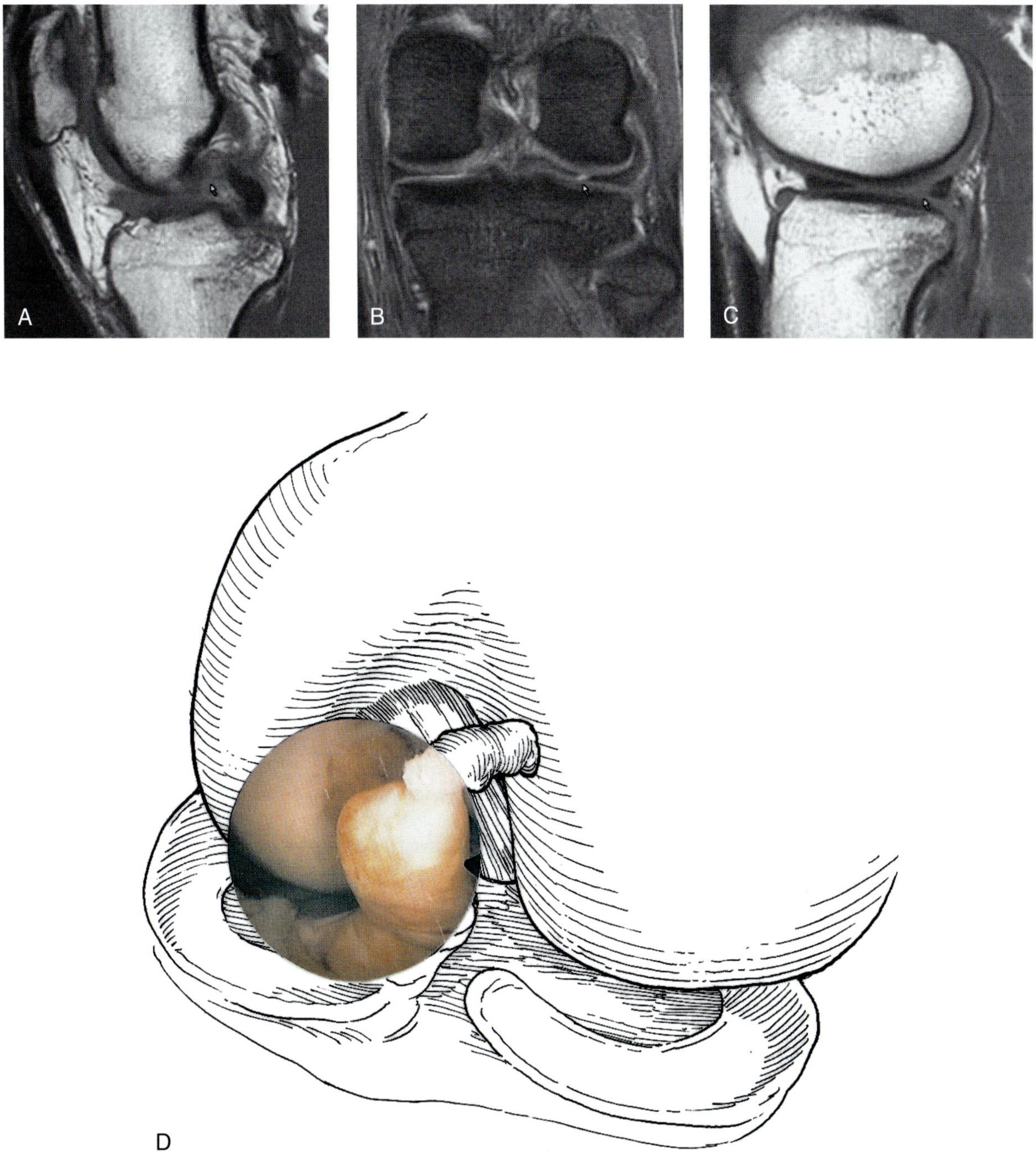

Figure 2–72. **Subacute Tear, Anterior Cruciate Ligament, and Lateral Meniscal Tear, Left Knee**
A, *Sagittal T1-weighted SE image shows discontinuity of the anterior cruciate ligament* (arrow) *consistent with complete disruption.* B, *Coronal GRE image demonstrating a focus of bright signal in the posterior horn lateral meniscus* (arrow) *consistent with a parrot-beak tear.* C, *Sagittal T1-weighted SE image reveals blunting of the free margin of the posterior horn lateral meniscus* (arrow). D, *Arthroscopic view of the ACL stump and a parrot-beak tear of the lateral meniscus.*

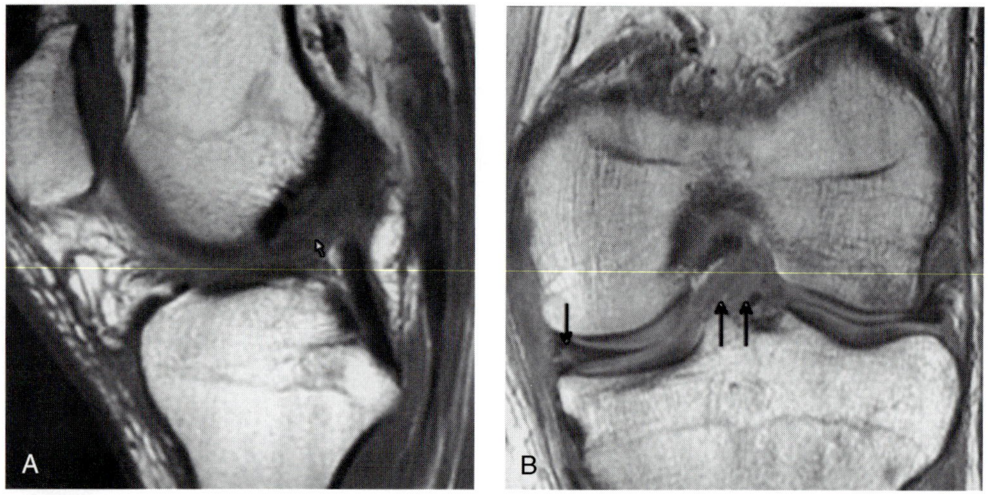

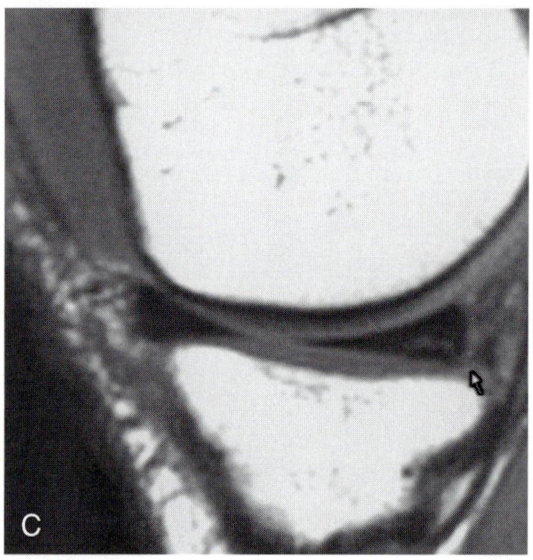

Figure 2–73. **Two-Bundle Tear, ACL, and Inferior Surface Medial Meniscal Tear, Left Knee**
A, *Sagittal T1-weighted SE image demonstrates mass effect, increased signal, and loss of continuity of the ACL* (arrow). B, *Coronal proton density SE image shows a peripheral stellate pattern of bright signal within the medial meniscus* (arrow) *and disruption of the ACL at the tibial eminence manifested by mass effect and increased signal intensity* (double arrow). C, *Sagittal T1-weighted SE image shows a stellate pattern of increased signal in the posterior horn medial meniscus with communication to the inferior articular surface* (arrow). D, *Arthroscopic view demonstrating a double-bundle ACL tear and a medial meniscal tear (probe).*

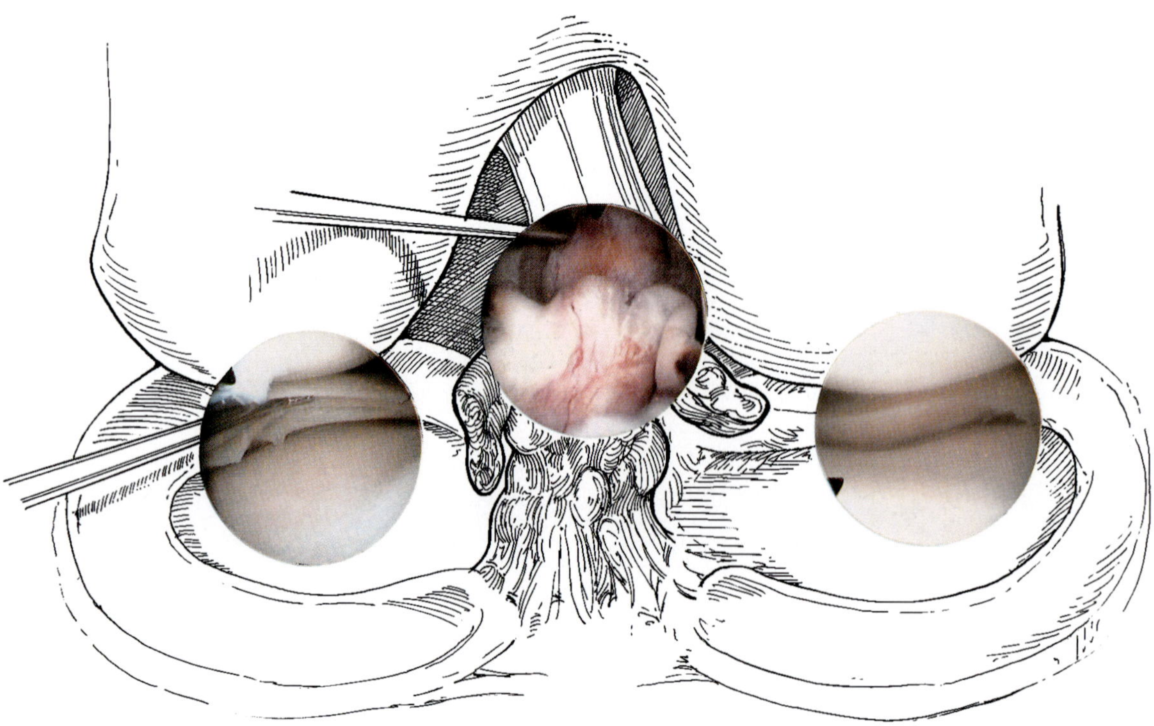

D

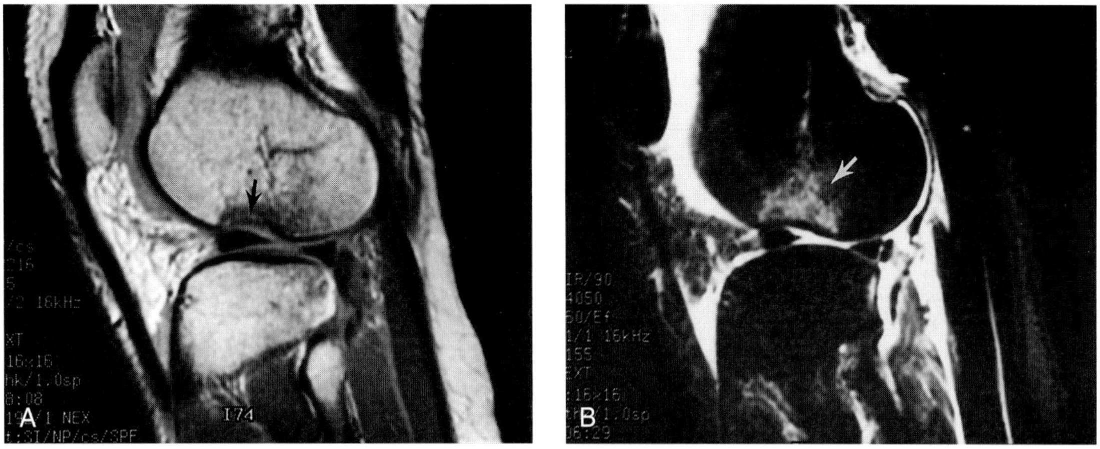

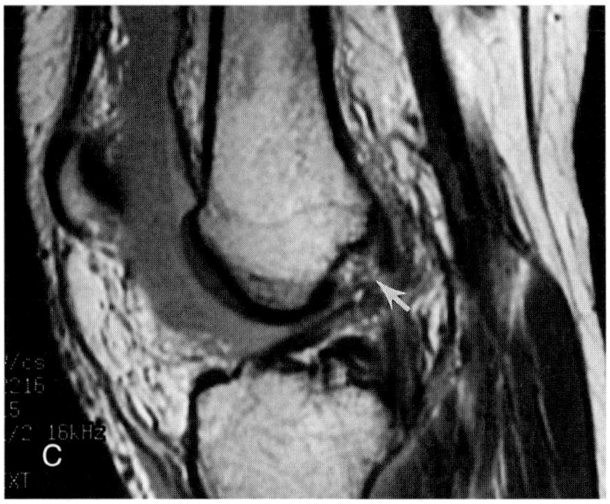

Figure 2–74. **Osteochondral Impaction Fracture (Bone Bruise) with ACL Tear, Right Knee**
A, *Sagittal proton-density SE image shows geographic osteochondral injury with impaction of the articular surface of the lateral femoral condyle* (arrow). B, *Sagittal STIR image shows an associated bright signal within the subchondral bone marrow consistent with a "bone bruise"* (arrow). C, *Sagittal proton-density SE image demonstrates complete disruption of the proximal ACL.* D, *Arthroscopic figure demonstrating an impaction fracture (severe bone bruise) in lateral femoral condyle.*
Case courtesy of Christopher D. Harner, M.D.

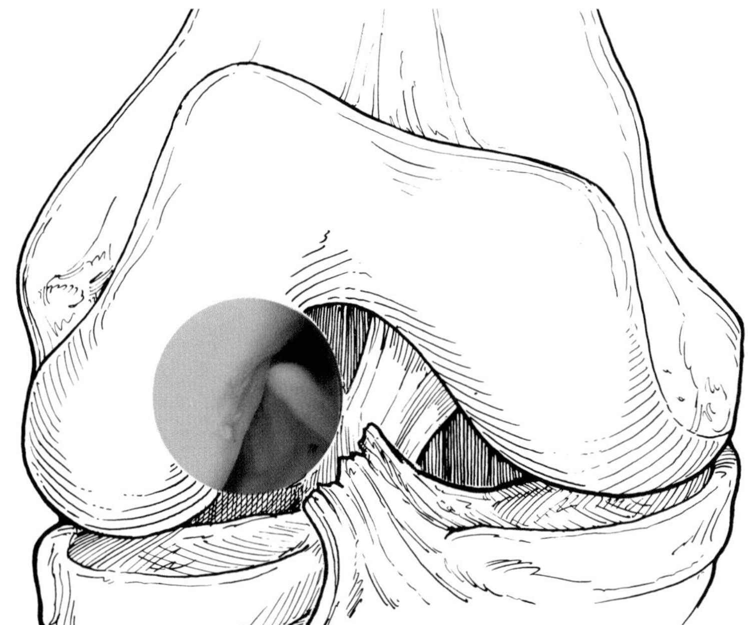

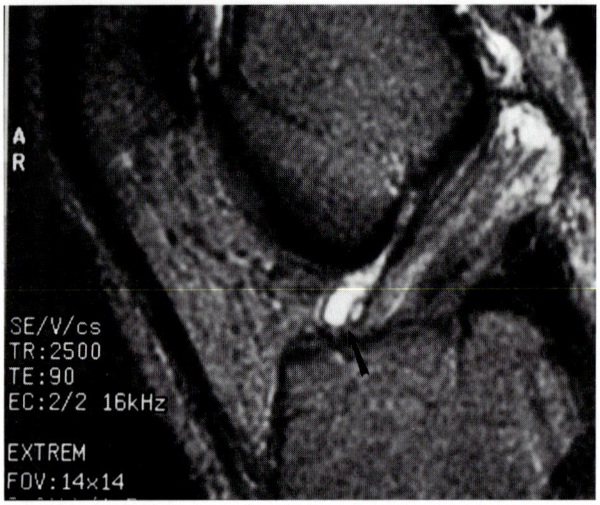

A

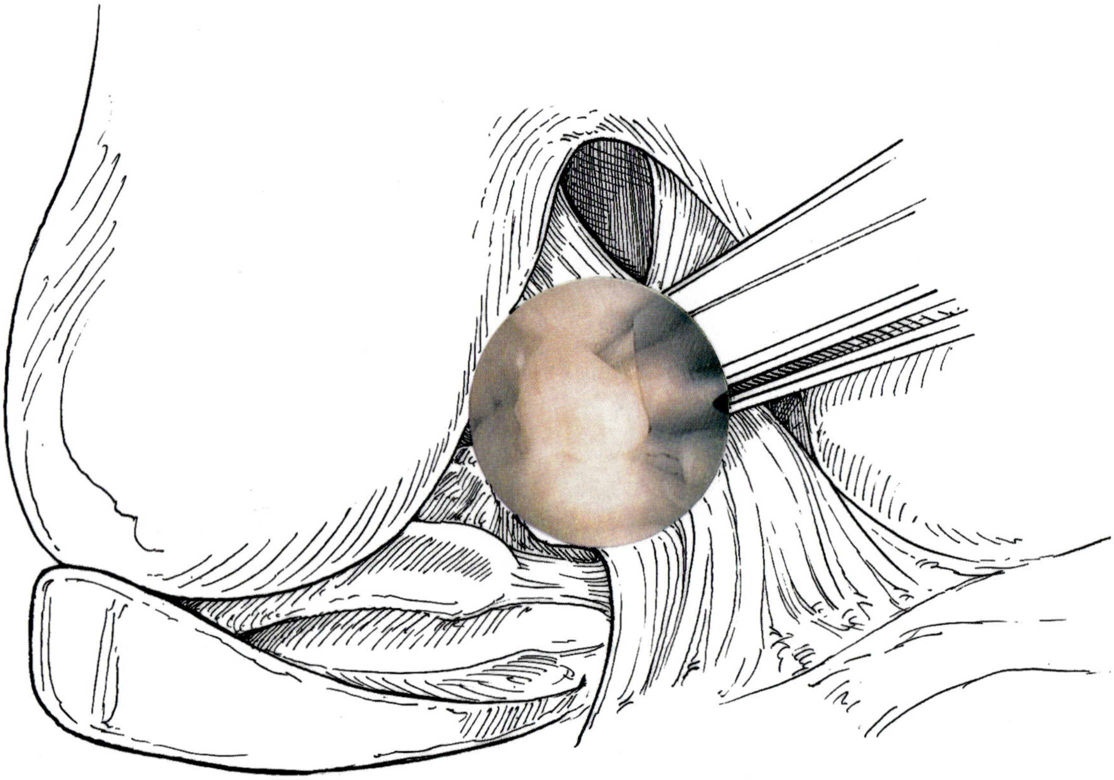

B

Figure 2–75. **ACL Ganglion, Right Knee**
A, *Sagittal SE T2-weighted image reveals a small (< 1 cm), loculated fluid collection* (arrow) *associated with the ACL near its tibial attachment.* B, *Arthroscopic image demonstrating a ganglion (shaver) intimately associated with the ACL.*

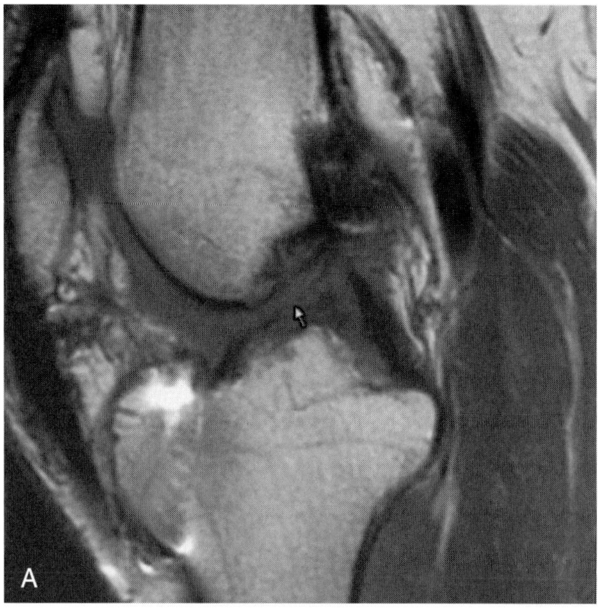

Figure 2–76. **ACL Graft Failure, Right Knee**
A, *Sagittal T1-weighted SE image showing marked attenuation of an ACL graft* (arrow) *in the intercondylar notch.*
B, *Arthroscopic image shows attenuation and laxity of the graft. Note the lack of vascularization with the "shiny" appearance of residual graft tissue.*

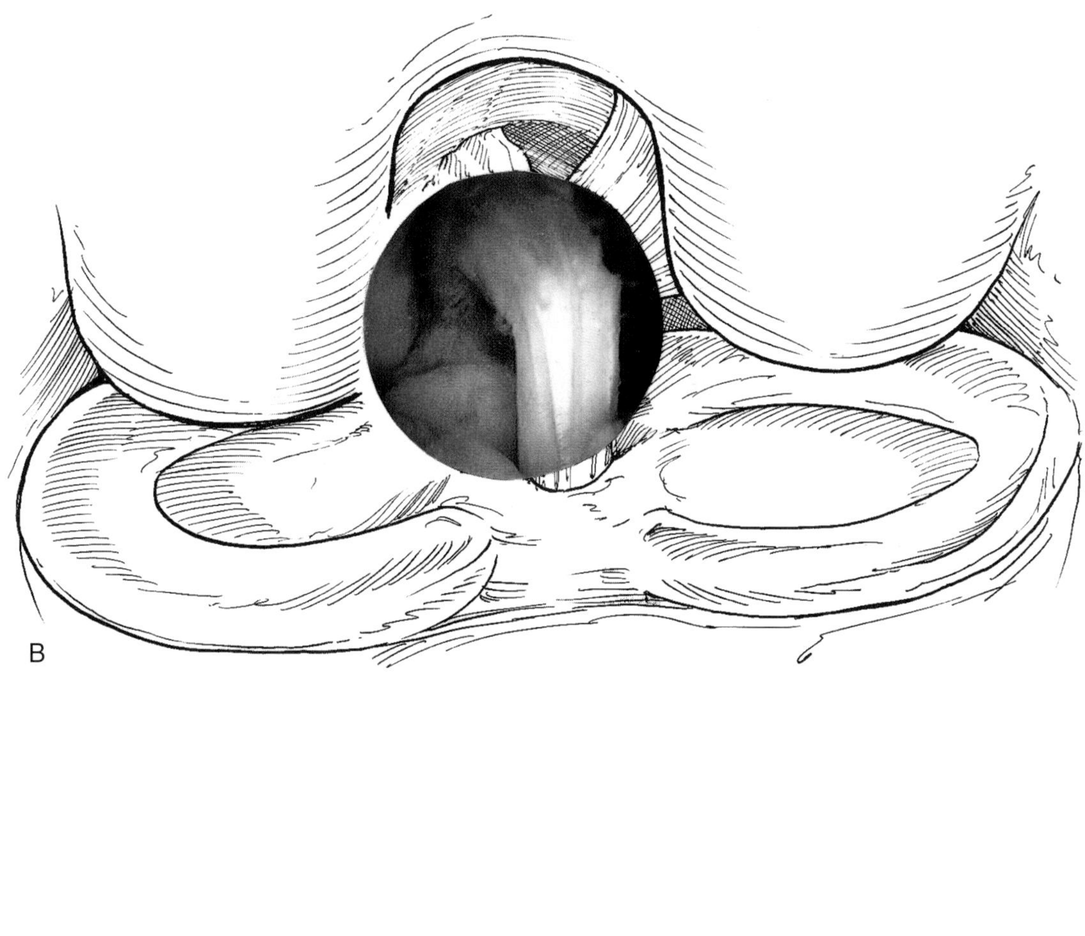

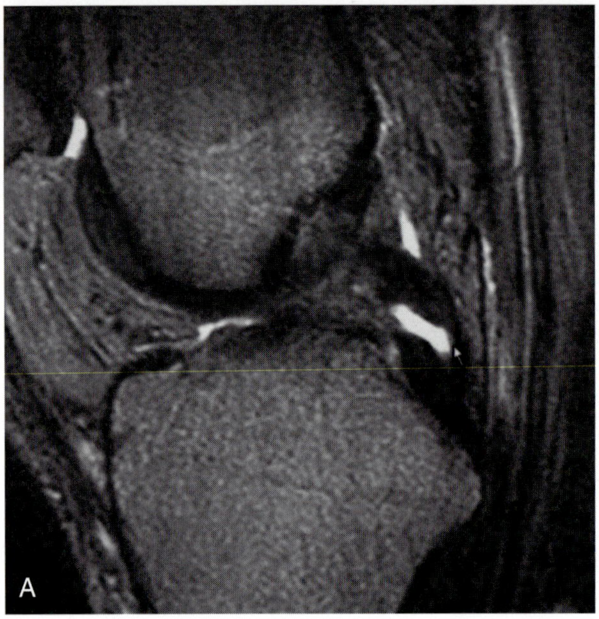

Figure 2–77. **PCL Injury, Left Knee**
A, *Sagittal FSE T2-weighted image shows bright signal intensity from fluid surrounding the tibial stump of the torn PCL* (arrow). B, *Arthroscopic view of the PCL stump as viewed through the notch.*

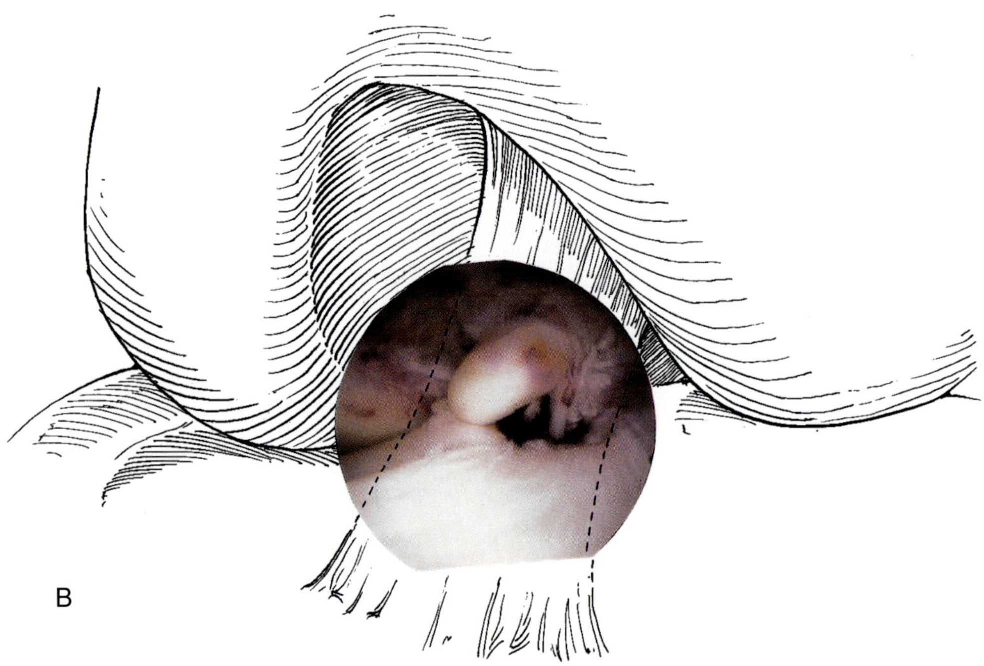

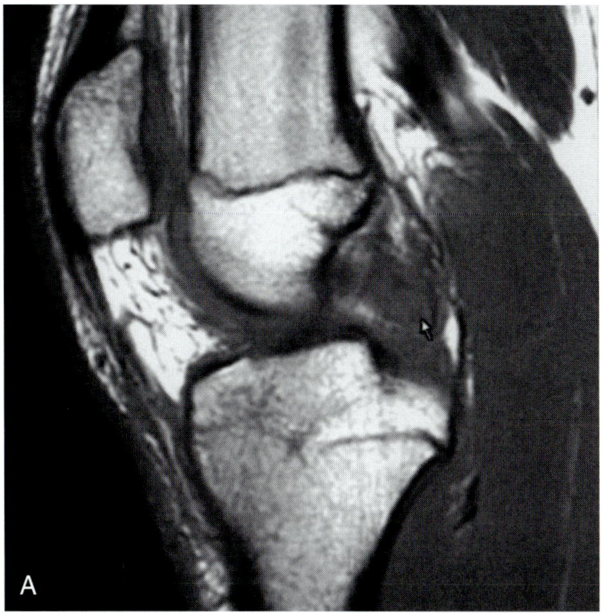

A

Figure 2–78. **PCL Contusion, Left Knee**
A, *Sagittal T1-weighted image demonstrates intermediate signal within the body of the posterior cruciate ligament* (arrow). B, *Arthroscopic view through the notch demonstrating a contusion in the posterior cruciate ligament.*

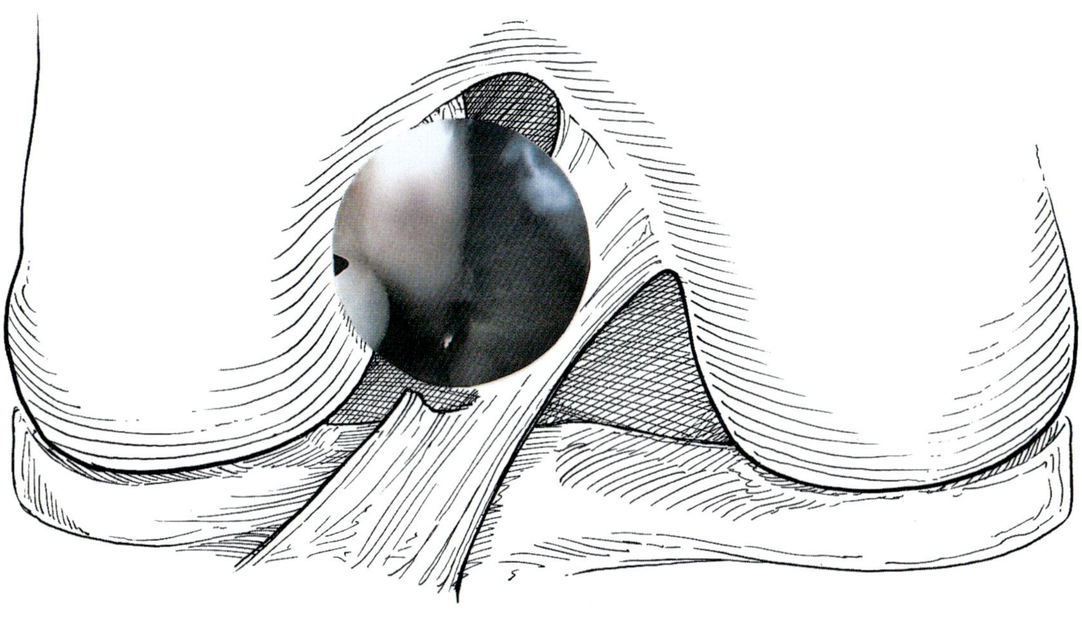

B

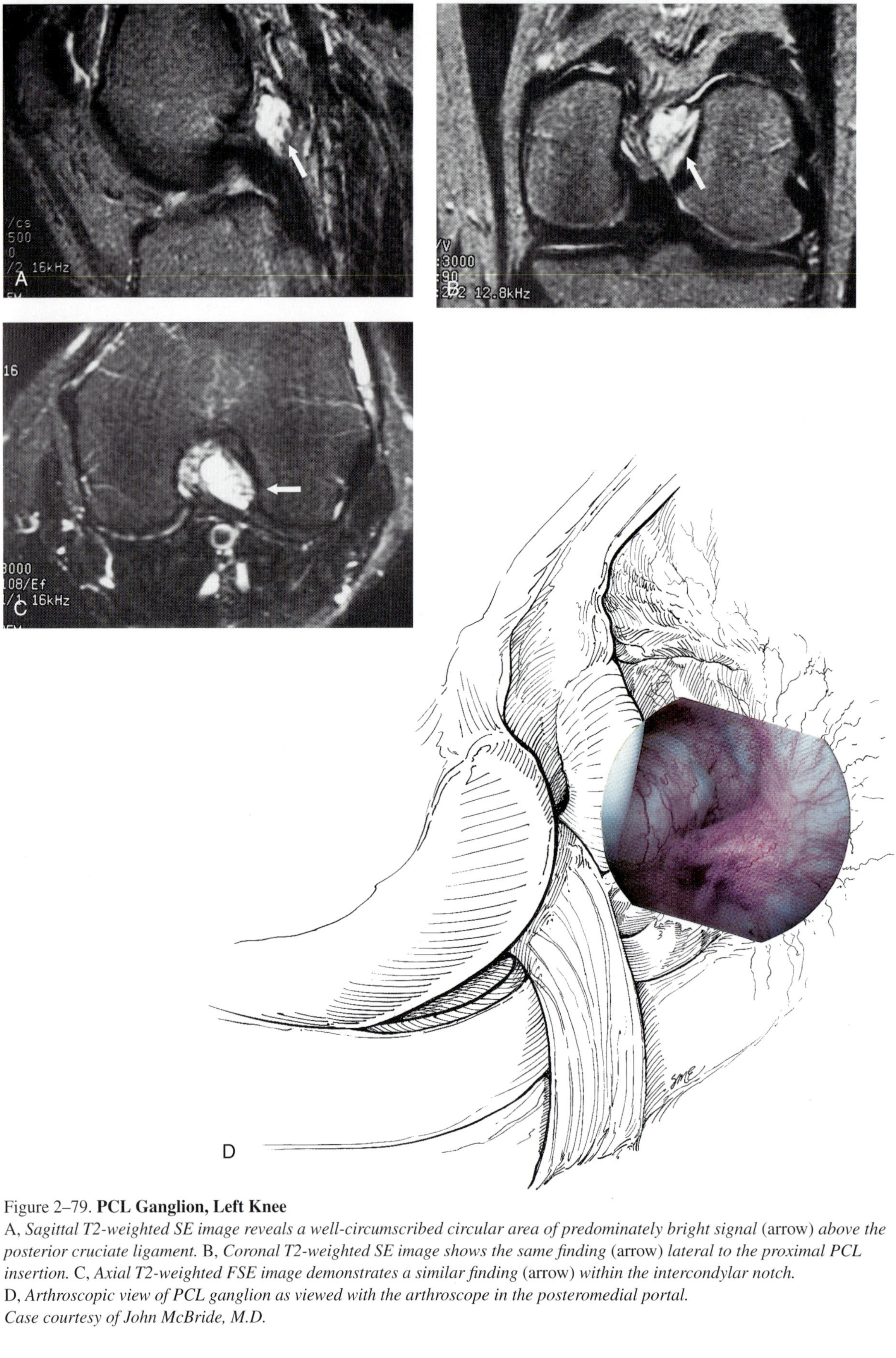

Figure 2–79. **PCL Ganglion, Left Knee**

A, *Sagittal T2-weighted SE image reveals a well-circumscribed circular area of predominately bright signal* (arrow) *above the posterior cruciate ligament.* B, *Coronal T2-weighted SE image shows the same finding* (arrow) *lateral to the proximal PCL insertion.* C, *Axial T2-weighted FSE image demonstrates a similar finding* (arrow) *within the intercondylar notch.*
D, *Arthroscopic view of PCL ganglion as viewed with the arthroscope in the posteromedial portal.*
Case courtesy of John McBride, M.D.

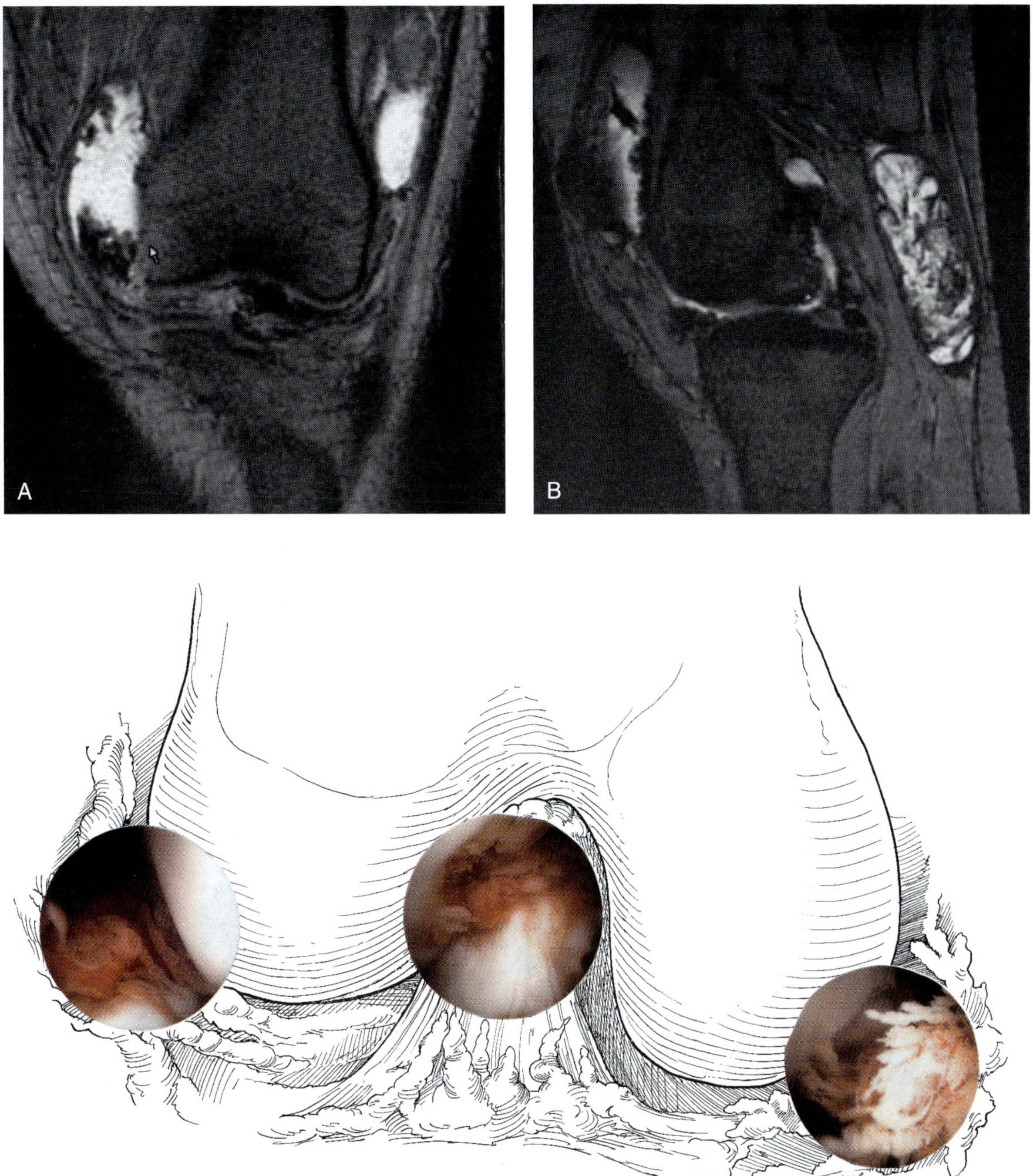

C

Figure 2–80. **Pigmented Villonodular Synovitis (PVNS), Left Knee**

A, *Coronal GRE image demonstrates multiple synovial deposits of diffuse dark signal intensity* (arrow) *throughout the knee.* B, *Sagittal GRE image shows similar findings.* C, *Arthroscopic view showing proliferative PVNS throughout the knee.*

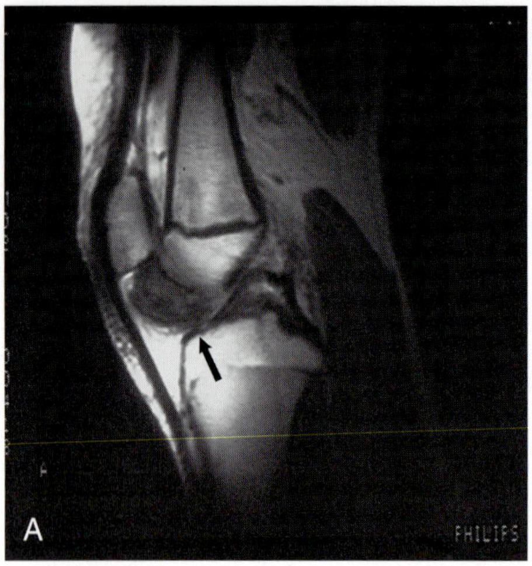

Figure 2–81. **Localized PVNS, Left Knee**
A, *Sagittal proton-density image reveals a focal area of heterogenous signal intensity* (arrow) *consistent with localized PVNS.* B, *Arthroscopic photograph demonstrates localized PVNS in the anterior notch of the left knee.*
Case courtesy of J. Serge Parisien, M.D.

B

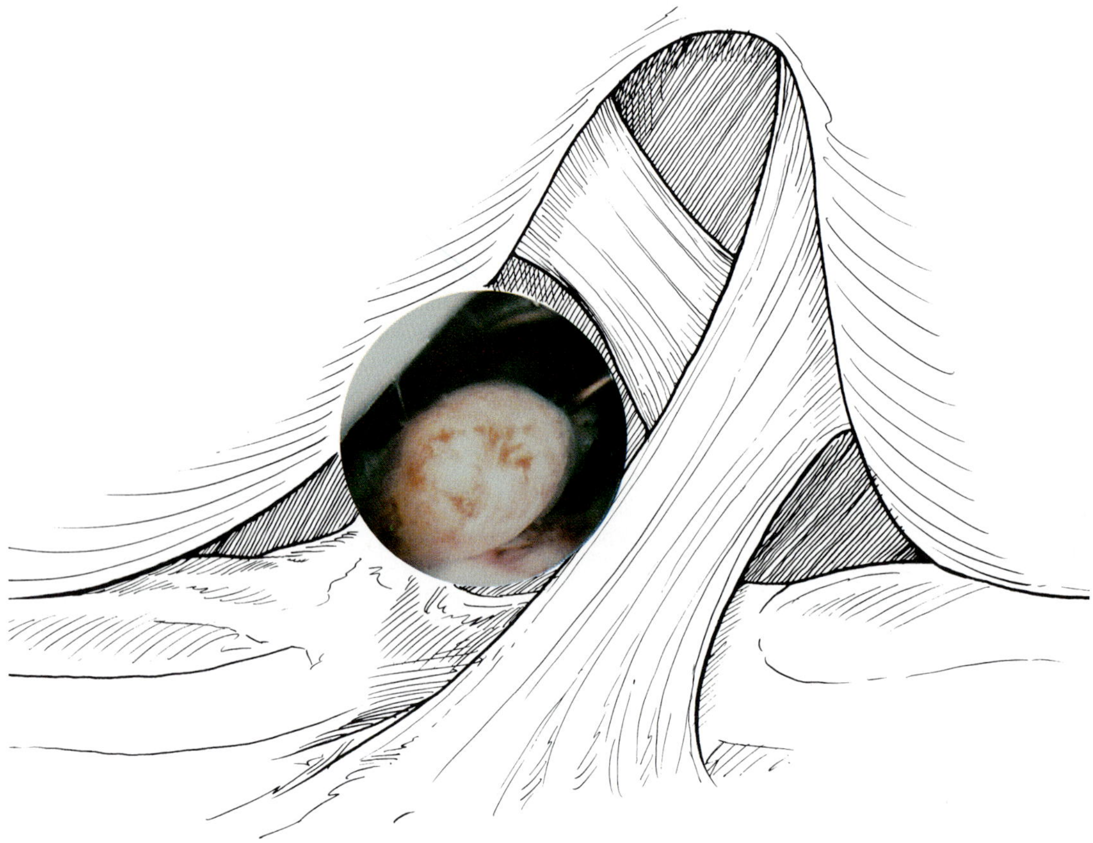

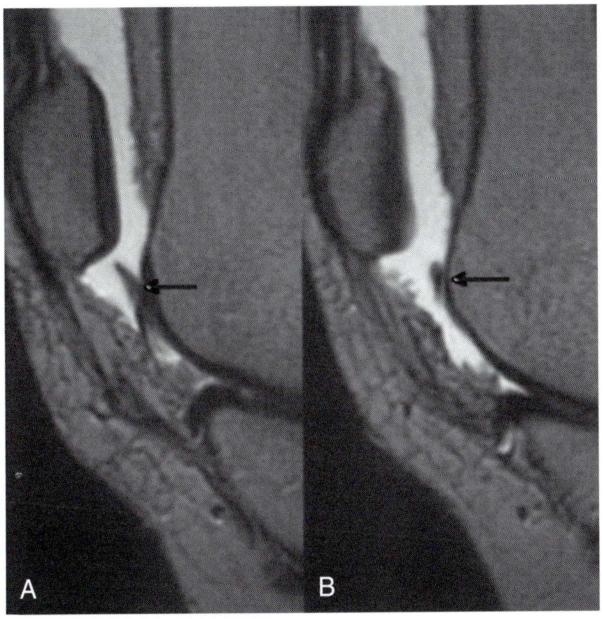

Figure 2–82. **Medial Patellar Plica, "Shelf," Left knee**
A, *Sagittal FSE T2-weighted image shows medial patellar plica* (arrows) *contacting the medial femoral condyle.* B, *Sagittal FSE T2-weighted image immediately lateral to A demonstrating thickening of the same plica* (arrow).
C, *Arthroscopic view demonstrating a medial patellar plica contacting the condyle and associated chondral abrasion. Case courtesy of Scott Smith, M.D.*

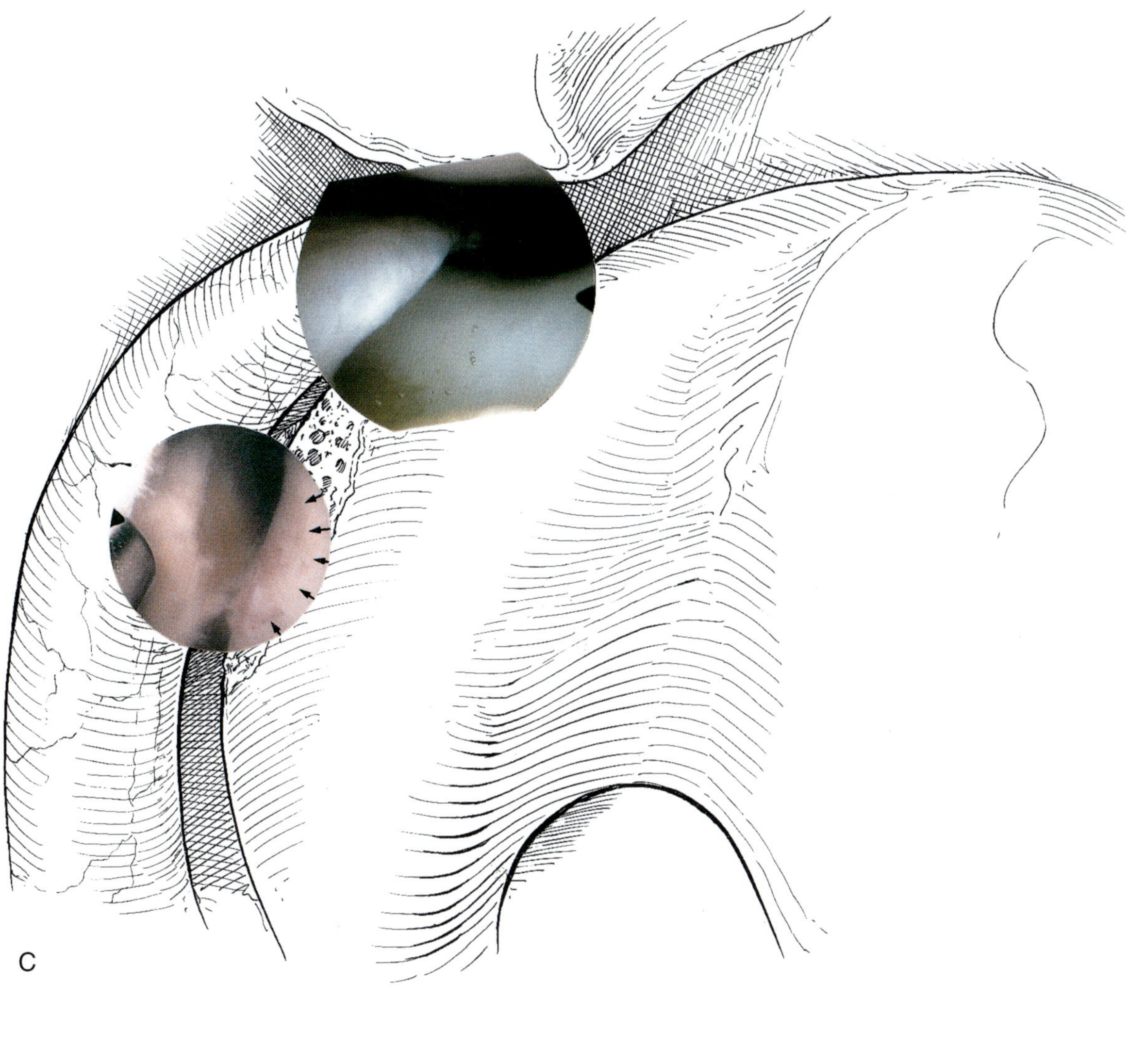

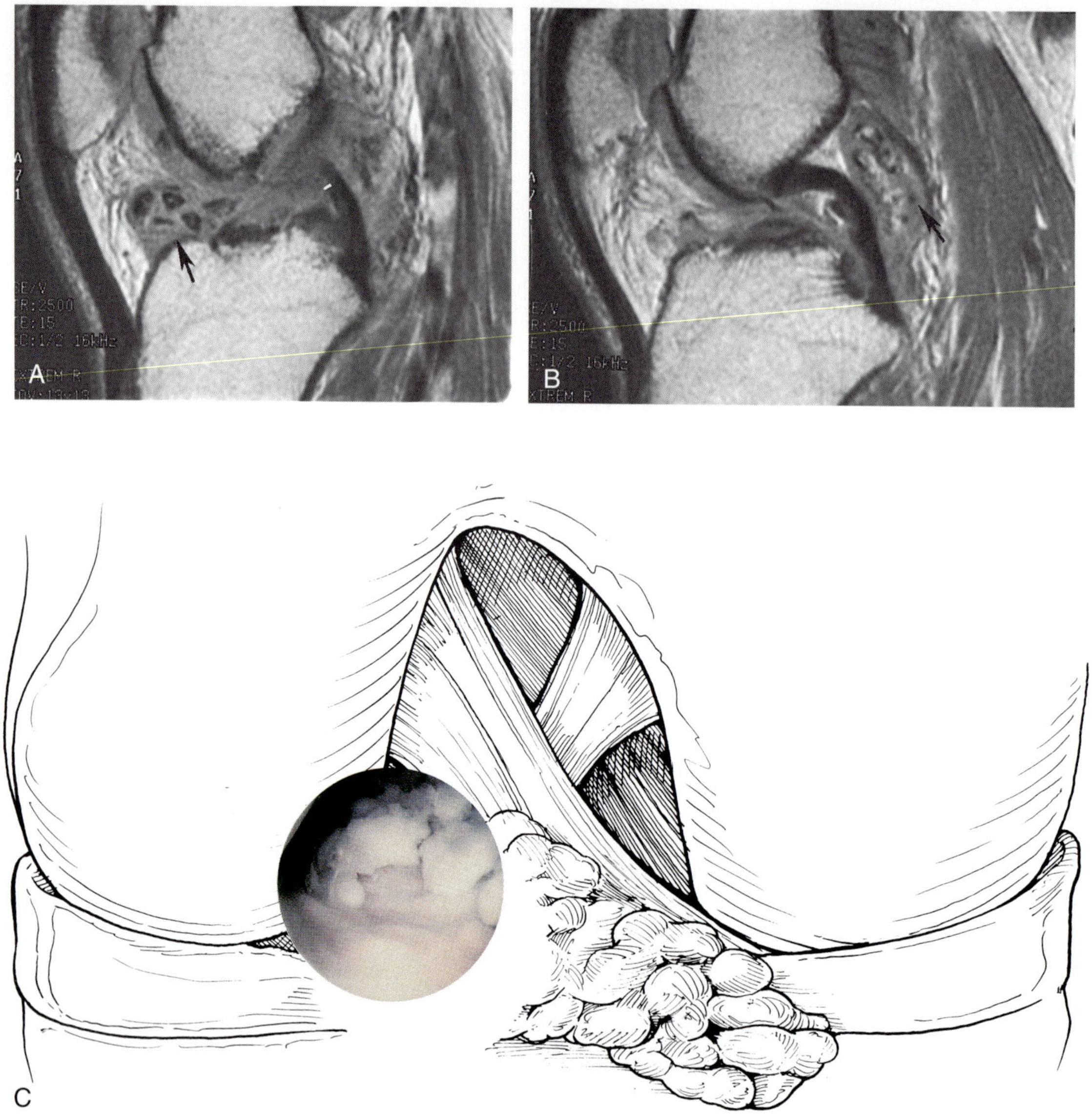

Figure 2–83. **Synovial Osteochondromatosis, Right knee**

A, *Sagittal proton-density SE image shows multiple osteochondral loose bodies* (arrow) *within the anterior recess of the knee joint.* B, *Sagittal proton-density SE image, slightly medial to A, demonstrates similar findings* (arrow) *posterior to the PCL.* C, *Arthroscopic view demonstrating osteochondral loose bodies anterior to the cruciate ligaments.*
Case courtesy of J Serge Parisien, M.D.

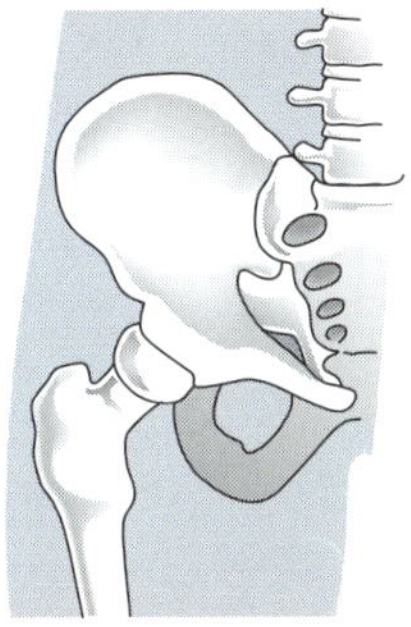

CHAPTER

3 Hip

MRI of the Hip

MRI of the hip is widely accepted as the primary modality for the early detection of avascular necrosis (AVN) in the femoral head. This was one of the earliest musculoskeletal applications of MRI. Wider applications have since emerged to include Legg-Calvé-Perthes disease, transient osteoporosis, articular and periarticular trauma, and congenital dysplasia of the hip. Hip pain remains a common problem. Preliminary evaluation almost always begins with plain radiography. If the plain radiographic information does not direct patient management or remains equivocal, bone scintigraphy, computed tomography, or MRI may be indicated.

TECHNIQUE

Numerous techniques have been described for the evaluation of hip disorders. Coronal images obtained in the body coil adequately display the acetabular and proximal femoral bone marrow, primarily for detection of AVN. These images, however, do not provide adequate spatial resolution for articular cartilage or labral pathology. Application, then, of surface coil imaging (Fig. 3–1) yields the necessary resolution for intra-articular pathology. Spin-echo (SE) sequences have generally been the standard in hip imaging; however, appreciation is growing for inversion recovery sequences for bone-marrow pathology and gradient-echo sequences for articular cartilage. The choice of technique, then, depends on the clinical indications, although most cases include coronal T1, T2, short tau inversion recovery (STIR), and axial T2 sequences. Typical body-coil parameters include 40-cm field of view, 4- to 5-mm slice thickness, and 192×256 matrix.[10]

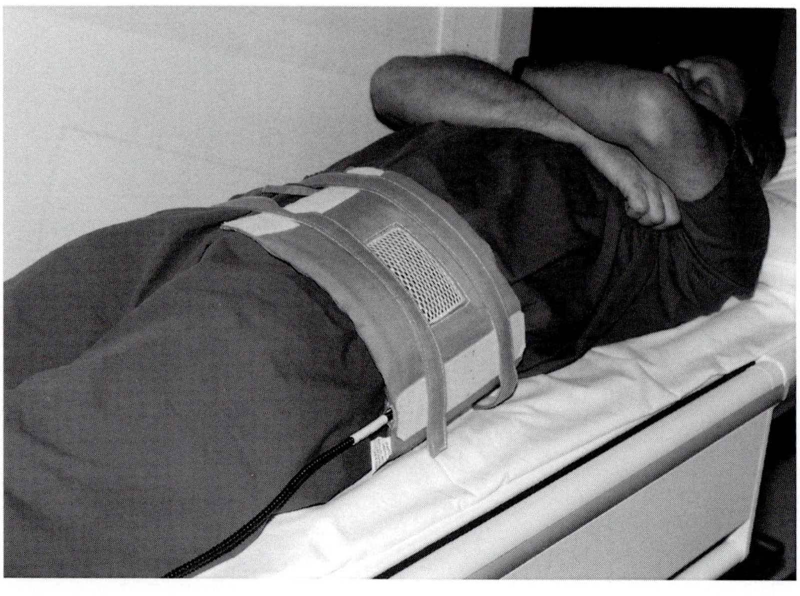

Figure 3–1
5 × 11-in. flexible coil is used for imaging of the hip.

MRI ANATOMY

MRI anatomy of the hip is well displayed in the axial and coronal planes (Figs. 3–2, 3–3, and 3–4).

The hip is composed of the acetabulum, femoral head, proximal femur, synovial hip joint, and supporting musculature of the pelvis and proximal thigh. The acetabulum is

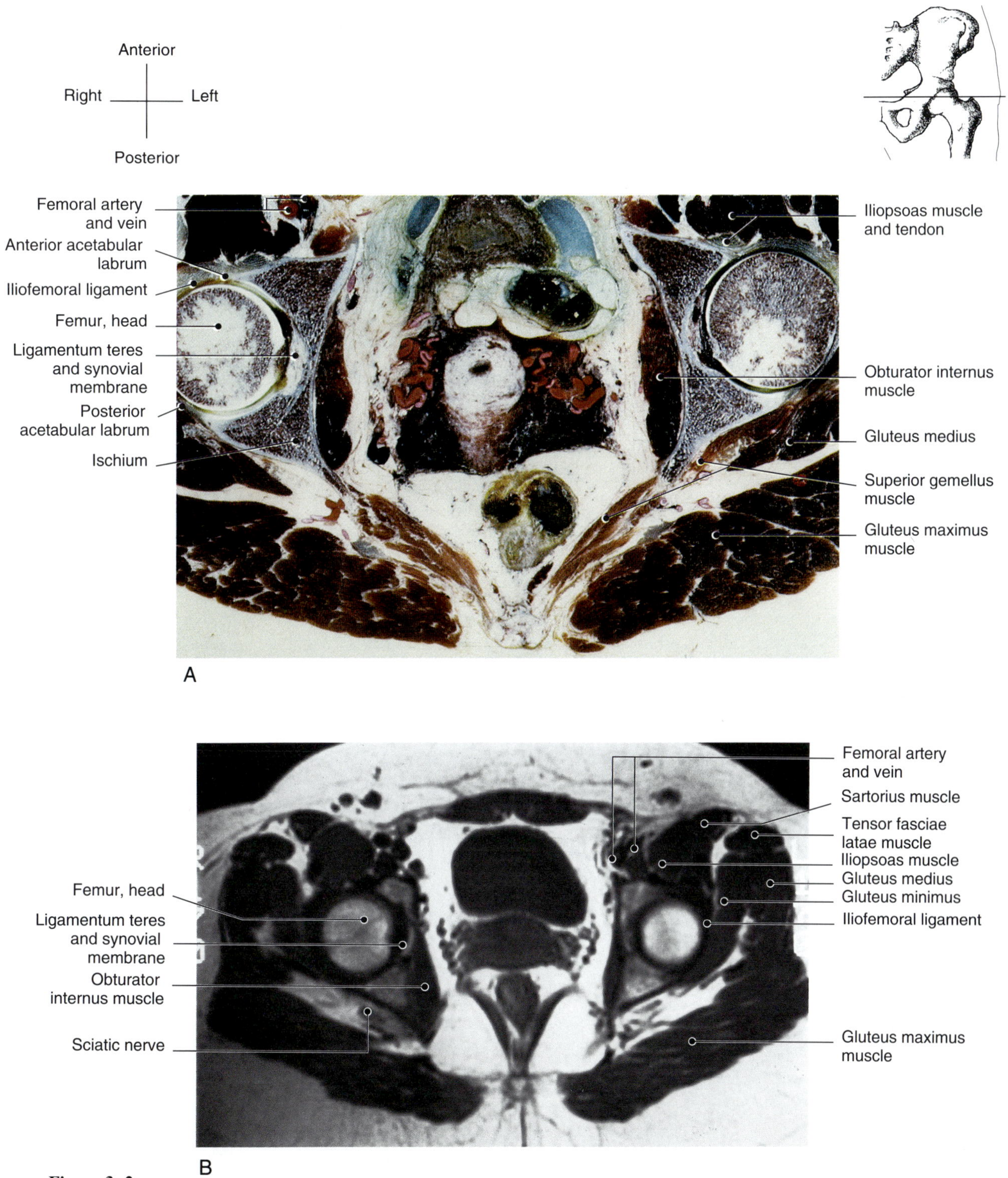

Figure 3–2
Axial cryoplaned section (A) *and magnetic-resonance image (TR, 600 ms; TE, 20 ns)* (B) *of the hip at the level of the femoral head. (From Chan WP, Rauschning W, Wu CY, et al. Magnetic resonance imaging anatomy and cryomicrotome atlas.* In *Chan WP, Lang P, Genant HK, eds. MRI of the Musculoskeletal System. Philadelphia: WB Saunders, 1994.)*

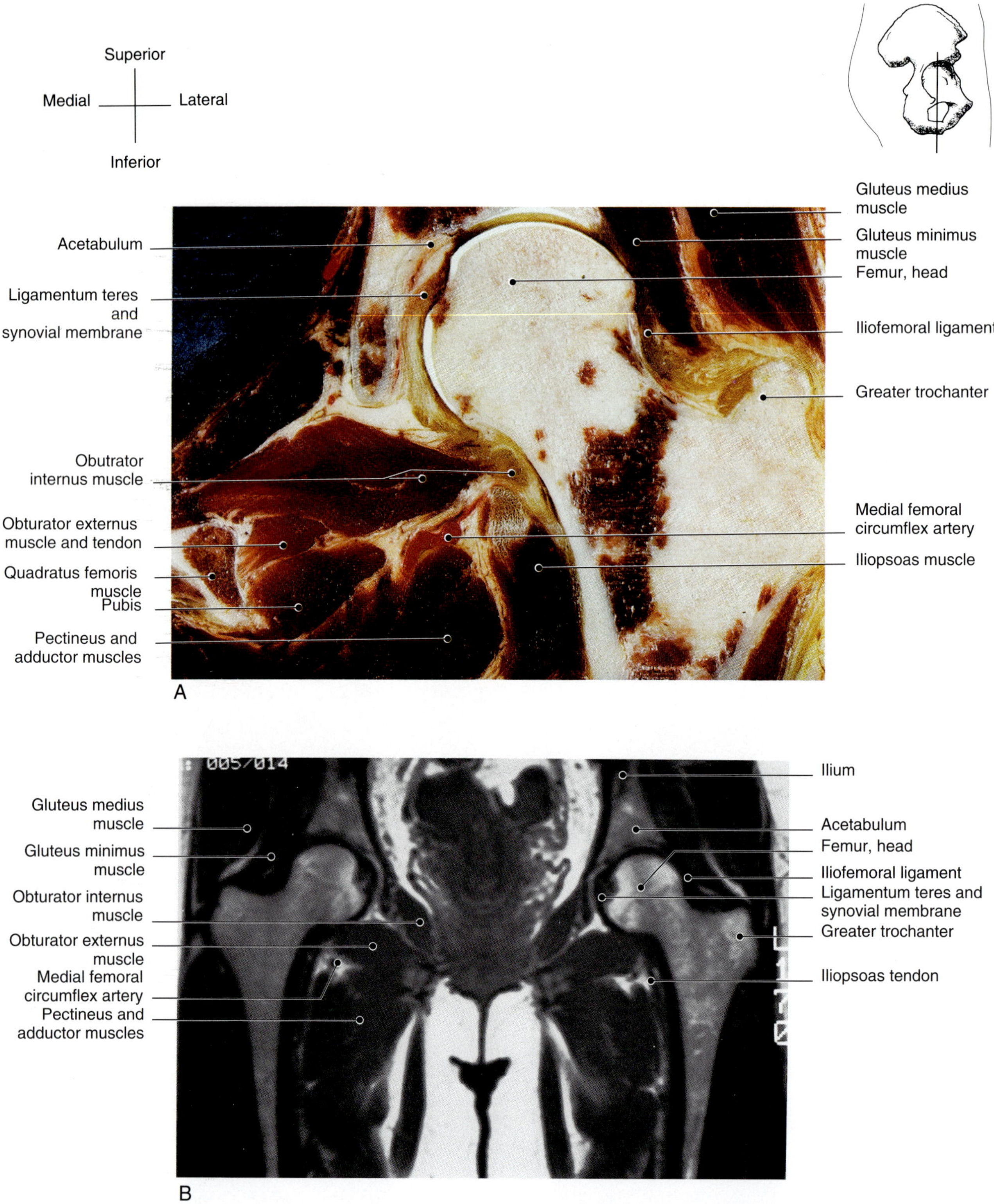

Figure 3–3

Anterior coronal cryoplaned section (A) *and magnetic resonance image (TR, 600 ms; TE, 20 ns)* (B) *of the hip. (From Chan WP, Rauschning W, Wu CY, et al. Magnetic resonance imaging anatomy and cryomicrotome atlas.* In *Chan WP, Lang P, Genant HK, eds. MRI of the Musculoskeletal System. Philadelphia: WB Saunders, 1994.)*

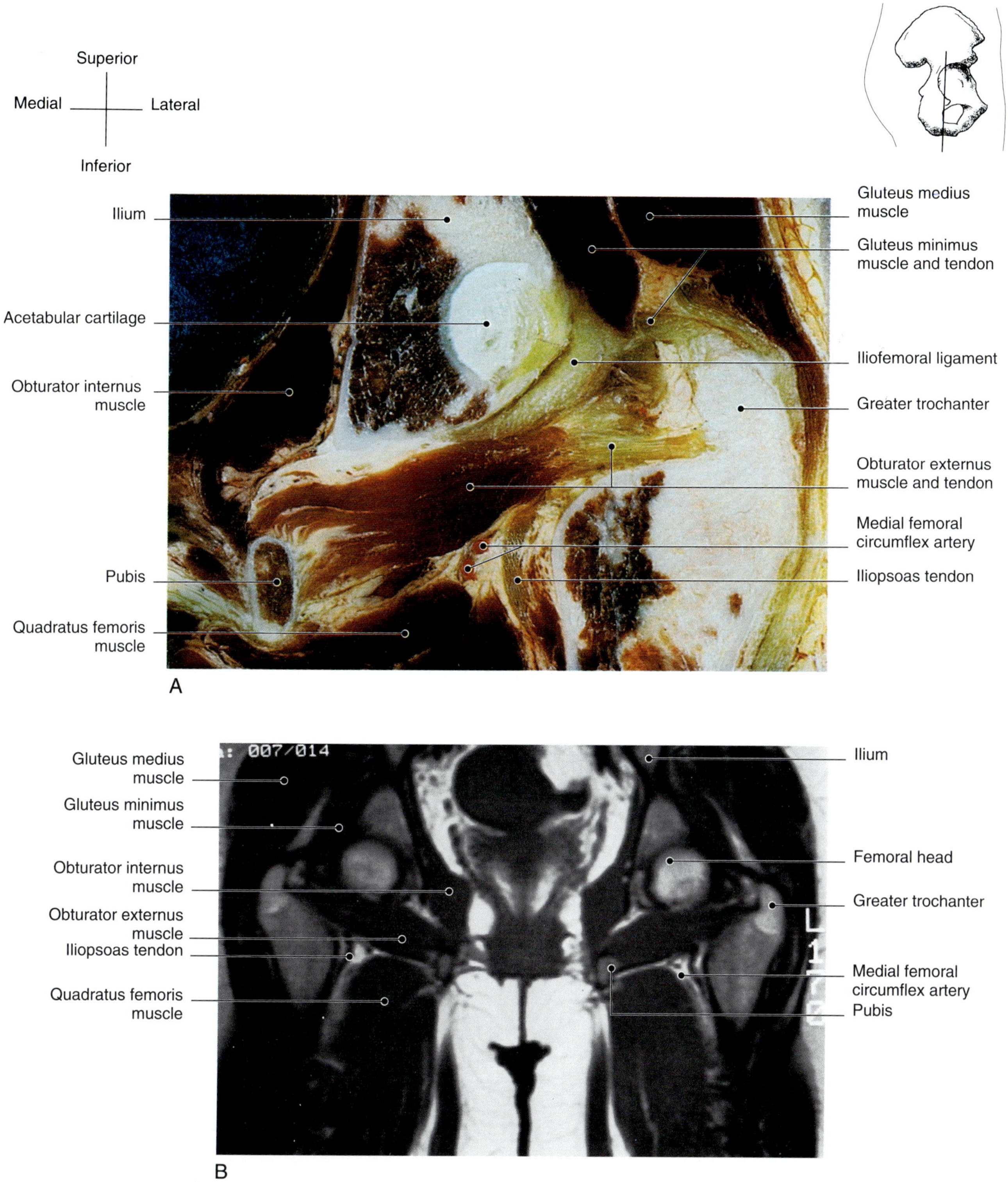

Figure 3–4

Posterior coronal cryoplaned section (A) *and magnetic resonance image (TR, 600 ms; TE, 20 ns)* (B) *of the hip. (From Chan WP, Rauschning W, Wu CY, et al. Magnetic resonance imaging anatomy and cryomicrotome atlas.* In *Chan WP, Lang P, Genant HK, eds. MRI of the Musculoskeletal System. Philadelphia: WB Saunders, 1994.)*

formed by the pubis, ilium, and ischium. Its articular surface is lined by hyaline cartilage that is 1 to 3 mm thick. The central area is devoid of cartilage and serves as the attachment site of the ligamentum teres. The bony acetabular rim serves as the site of attachment for the synovial membrane and the labrum. The fibrocartilaginous labrum extends the acetabular cup and prevents hip displacement. This labrum is low and intermediate in signal on the SE and gradient recalled-echo sequences, respectively. The femoral head is entirely covered by articular cartilage except for the fovea centralis, the insertion site of the ligamentum teres. The synovial joint capsule extends from the acetabular rim to the femoral neck; therefore, the head and neck are largely devoid of periosteum. A small amount of fluid is visible in most normal hip joints. Generally, fluid does not extend to surround the femoral neck or distend the joint. The supporting ligaments about the hip include the capsular ligament and the ligamentum teres. The anterior joint is reinforced by the iliofemoral ligament, a thick band of fibers that arise from the anterior iliac spine and extend anteriorly and inferiorly to insert on the intertrochanteric line of the femur. The proximal femur and neck are oriented to provide maximal freedom of movement and still support the body in the upright position. Prominent buttressing trabeculae within the neck are evident in fan-like array. This is appreciated as a vertically oriented, low-signal band extending from the superomedial aspect of the femoral head to the inferolateral aspect of the femoral neck. It appears dark because it contains relatively more calcium than the adjacent fatty marrow.[4, 10]

The MRI appearance of the proximal femur depends on the bone-marrow composition. Yellow marrow, which is hematopoietically inactive, is composed predominantly of fat cells. Hematopoietically active red marrow contains only 40% fat and has a richer vascular network. Both age and systemic disease affect its appearance. The cartilaginous capital epiphysis does not contain any marrow until it ossifies early in life and is replaced by yellow marrow. Thus, in the very young child the femoral capital epiphysis demonstrates moderate-high signal, a reflection of the high water content of non-ossified epiphyseal cartilage. As the capital epiphysis matures, fatty marrow forms in the center of the cartilage anlage and gradually enlarges to occupy the entire epiphysis. This results in progressively higher signal on the T1 sequence with time. In children and teenagers, fatty yellow marrow and hematopoietic red marrow are distributed heterogeneously within the femoral neck and intertrochanteric region. The femoral epiphysis and trochanters are filled with yellow marrow. The yellow marrow has high signal on the T1 sequence and intermediate signal on the T2 sequence (Fig. 3–5). The red marrow has intermediate signal on T1 and T2 se-

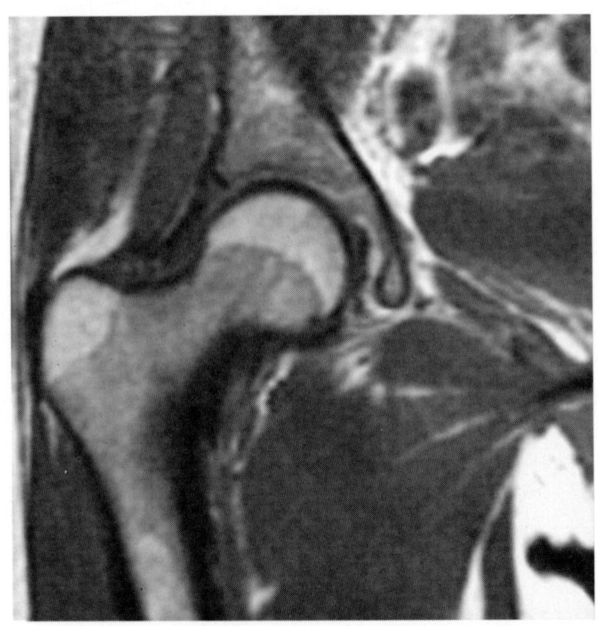

Figure 3–5
Coronal T1 image in a 16-year-old male. *Note the brighter signal of yellow marrow in the femoral epiphysis and apophysis of the greater trochanter.*

quences. By the third decade of life, the red marrow converts to yellow marrow within the femoral neck, and the amount of red marrow within the proximal femoral diaphysis and intertrochanteric region varies. Conversion to yellow marrow is complete by the sixth decade.[4, 10]

The muscular anatomy is complex. The muscles can be divided into anterior, medial, posterior, and lateral groups. Several bursae are important. The most important is the iliopsoas bursa, which is located between the iliopsoas, pectineus, and femoral neurovascular bundle. The trochanteric bursa is located about the greater trochanter.[4, 10]

PATHOLOGY

Avascular Necrosis

MRI has been shown to be the most sensitive and specific technique for the diagnosis of AVN of the hip.[2, 7, 9] MRI plays several important roles in the diagnosis and outcome of AVN of the femoral head. First, the clinical diagnosis may not be obvious, even in persons with known risk factors. Second, MRI can determine the extent of the AVN process. When involvement of the femoral head weight-bearing surface exceeds 25%, collapse is highly likely. Finally, MRI permits accurate surveillance of those at risk for AVN and for monitoring therapeutic intervention in patients with AVN.

Four classes of abnormal signal in the femoral head have been correlated with histopathologic features. Class-A lesions have fatty bone-marrow signal, except at the periphery of the lesion (Fig. 3–6). The signal of Class-B lesions is similar to that of blood—that is, high signal on the T1 and T2 sequences. The signal of Class-C lesions is similar to that of simple fluid—that is, low signal on the T1 sequence and high signal on the T2 sequence. The signal of Class-D lesions is similar to that of fibrous tissue—that is, low signal on the T1 and T2 sequences. Because both MRI and bone scintigraphy may yield false-negative results, both may be complementary in cases of strong clinical suspicion because their errors only partially overlap.[9] The lesions of most symptomatic hips and even more asymptomatic hips are considered Class A at initial MRI examination. The majority also manifest the "double-line" sign, which could represent reparative granulation tissue (Fig. 3–7).

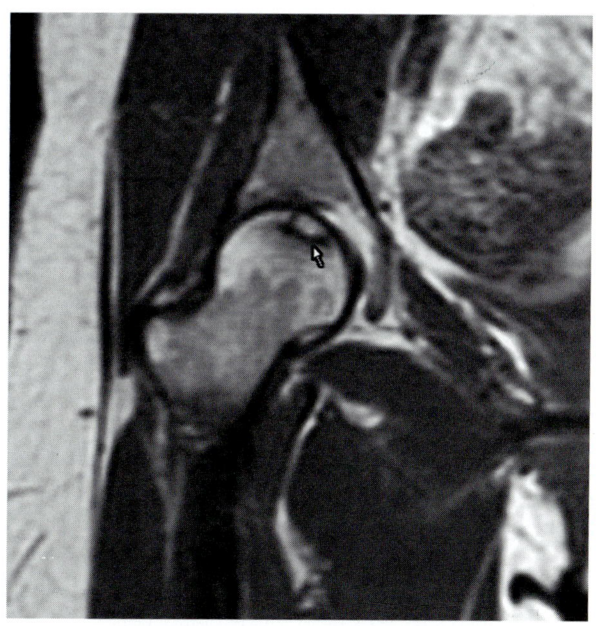

Figure 3–6
Coronal T1 image. *Class-A lesion is characterized by fatty bone marrow in the AVN lesion except at the periphery* (arrow).

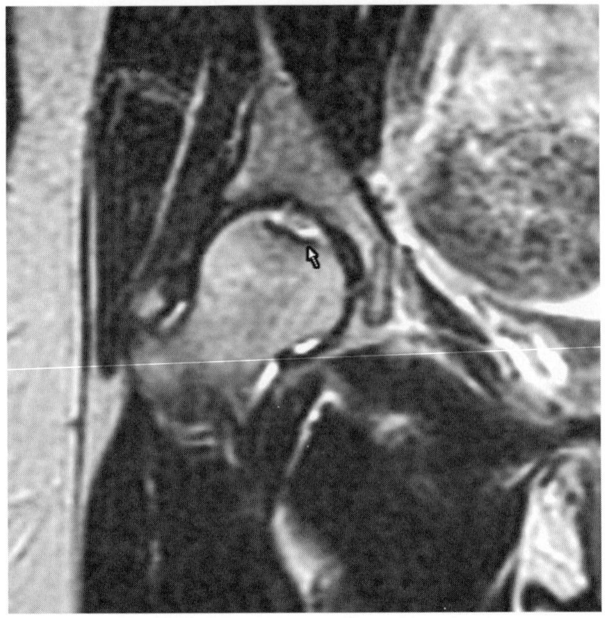

Figure 3–7
Coronal FSE T2 image. *"Double-line" sign denoted by adjacent bright and dark signal at the periphery of the AVN lesion* (arrow).

A therapeutic staging system (Stage 0 to Stage 6) is used to classify lesions at presentation.[6] Stage 0 describes a mild abnormality on MRI and normal results on plain radiography and scintigraphy. Stage 1 describes positive findings on both MRI and bone scintigraphy and normal results on plain radiography. Stage 2 is the earliest presentation on plain radiography, usually showing increased density in the involved area of the femoral head. Stage 3 is the earliest evidence of mechanical failure manifested by a crescent sign or subtle collapse. Stage 4 describes femoral-head flattening and a normal acetabulum. Stage 5 involves the acetabulum manifested by degenerative findings. Stage 6 describes advanced degenerative findings of the hip joint. Stages 0, 1, and 2 are generally treated conservatively with core decompression. Hemiarthroplasty and total joint replacement may be required for Stages 3, 4, 5, and 6.

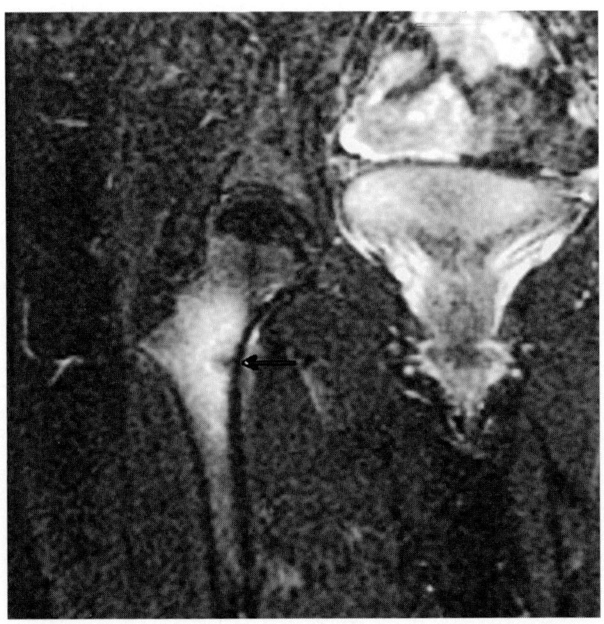

Figure 3–8
Coronal STIR image. *A small linear area of dark signal* (arrow) *denotes a stress fracture with surrounding bright signal in the bone marrow from edema.*

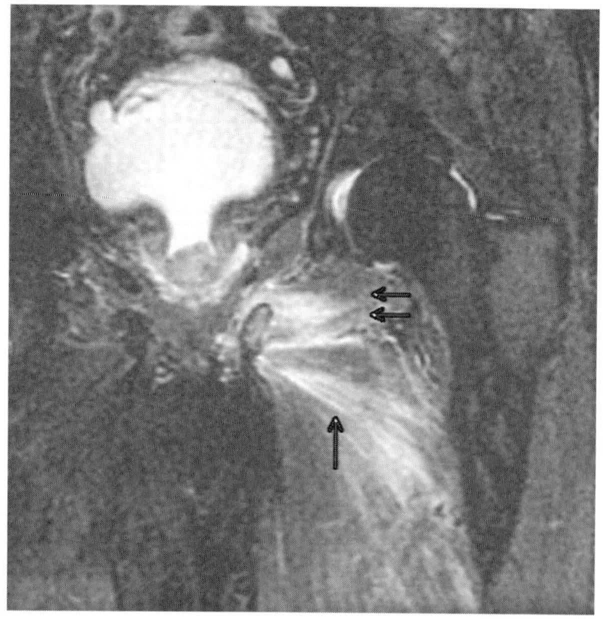

Figure 3–9
Coronal STIR image. *There is diffuse increased signal in the pectineus and adductor muscles* (arrow) *and obturator externus muscle* (arrows) *from edema resulting from muscular injury.*

Trauma

MRI is useful in detection of trauma to the hip region. Fracture lines appear as low-signal bands on the T1 and T2 sequence with varying degrees of edema. Similarly, MRI demonstrates insufficiency fractures along the medial aspect of the femoral neck in osteoporotic persons, as well as stress fractures of the femoral neck and proximal femur (Fig. 3–8). Bursitis and muscle strains are nicely demonstrated by high signal on the T2 or STIR sequences (Fig. 3–9). The signal of a hematoma varies more widely, depending on its age (Fig. 3–10).[5, 8]

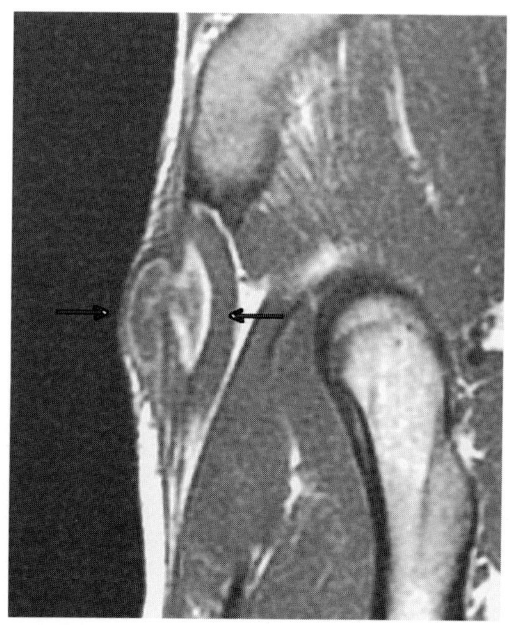

Figure 3–10
Sagittal FSE T2 image. *A heterogeneous signal mass is associated with the rectus femoris muscle* (arrows) *from a hematoma after a direct injury to the muscle.*

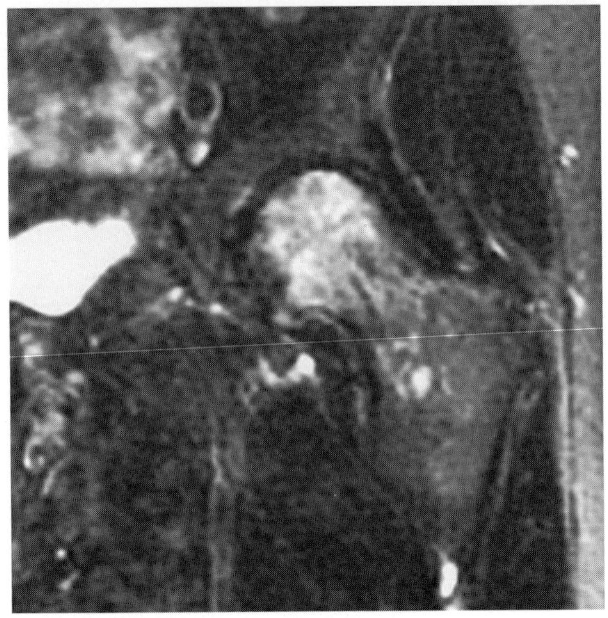

Figure 3–11
Coronal FSE T2 image. *There is increased signal in the bone marrow of the femoral head, neck, and shaft in this patient with transient osteoporosis.*

Miscellaneous Bone-Marrow Disorders

Early arthritis, early osteomyelitis, sickle cell crisis, transient osteoporosis (Fig. 3–11), and osteoid osteoma can all present with nonspecific pain, normal results on plain radiography, but an abnormal bone-marrow pattern on MRI.[1, 3, 11] Widespread bone-marrow edema yields low signal on the T1 sequence, high signal on the T2 sequence, and pronounced bright signal on the STIR sequence. These characteristics are not too different from those of AVN; therefore, additional clinical factors must be considered for management. Bone scintigraphy can help in that findings usually are positive in osteomyelitis, arthritis, and osteoid osteoma. Transient osteoporosis, early AVN, and sickle cell crisis usually yield normal results on bone scintigraphy.

References

1. Beltran J, Caudill JL, Herman LA, et al. Rheumatoid arthritis: MR imaging manifestations. Radiology 1987; 165:153-157.
2. Beltran J, Herman LJ, Burk JM, et al. Femoral head avascular necrosis: MR imaging with clinicopathologic and radionuclide correlation. Radiology 1988; 166:215-220.
3. Bloem JL. Transient osteoporosis of the hip: MR imaging. Radiology 1988; 167:753-755.
4. Chan WP, Rauschning W, Wu CY, et al. Magnetic resonance imaging anatomy and cryomicrotome atlas. *In* Chan WP, Lang P, Genant HK, eds. MRI of the Musculoskeletal System. Philadelphia: WB Saunders, 1994.
5. Deutsch AL, Mink JH, Waxman AD. Occult fractures of the proximal femur: MR imaging. Radiology 1989; 170:113-116.
6. Ficat RP. Idiopathic necrosis of the femoral head: Early diagnosis and treatment. J Bone Joint Surg (Br) 1985; 67:3-10.
7. Glickstein MF, Burk DL, Scheibler ML, et al. Avascular necrosis versus other diseases of the hip: Sensitivity of MR imaging. Radiology 1988; 169:213-215.
8. Lee JK, Yao L. Stress fractures: MR imaging. Radiology 1988; 169:217-220.
9. Mitchell DG, Rao VM, Dalinka MK, et al. Femoral head avascular necrosis: Correlation of MR imaging, radiographic staging, radionuclide imaging, and clinical findings. Radiology 1987; 162:709-715.
10. Stoller DW, Maloney WJ. The hip. *In* Stoller DW, ed. Magnetic Resonance Imaging in Orthopaedics and Sports Medicine. Philadelphia: JB Lippincott, 1993.
11. Unger E. Diagnosis of osteomyelitis by MR imaging. AJR 1988; 150:605-610.

Hip Arthroscopy

Although Burman is credited with the first hip arthroscopy, performed in cadavers in 1931,[1] hip arthroscopy is far less popular than knee and shoulder arthroscopy. Gross suggested a practical use for hip arthroscopy in the pediatric population as early as 1977,[8] but its use in adults, pioneered by Glick and coworkers,[6] is only now becoming common. Erikson and associates,[5] Johnson,[9] Dvorak and colleagues,[4] Byrd,[2] and others have made recent advances in hip arthroscopy.

INDICATIONS

The indications for hip arthroscopy are more limited than for other joints. Because of its anatomy, the hip joint is difficult to access via arthroscopy, and maneuverability is difficult. Arthroscopy may be indicated for cases of loose bodies, torn labral tissue, articular cartilage lesions, synovial or ligamentum teres impingement, and refractory pain of undetermined etiology. Arthroscopy can be used in the young arthritic population to delay the need for total joint replacement.[7]

POSITIONING AND PORTAL PLACEMENT

Two positions are popular for hip arthroscopy, the supine and the lateral decubitus positions. The lateral decubitus position, developed by Glick[6] after his initial dissatisfaction with the supine position, is performed with the patient on his or her side with the involved hip on top. The patient is placed in the lateral decubitus position on a fracture table with a peroneal post, and traction is applied via the foot plate, skeletal traction, or a commercially available external traction device. The leg is abducted 45 degrees and forward-flexed 10 degrees.[6] Approximately 50 lbs of traction is necessary to distract the hip 8 to 10 mm for arthroscopic visualization.[7] The supine position has been reintroduced by Byrd,[2] who also utilizes a fracture table. A padded peroneal post is lateralized to the operative side, the hip is positioned in extension and 25 degrees of abduction, and traction is applied. Fluoroscopy is recommended for either position to confirm entry into the joint (Fig. 3–12).

Portals are similar for both positions and include the anterior, anterolateral (anterior trochanteric), and posterolateral (posterior trochanteric) portals (Fig. 3–13). The anterior portal is established at the intersection of a sagittal line drawn distally from the anterior superior iliac spine and a transverse line across the superior margin of the greater trochanter. The arthroscope can be inserted in this portal in a direction 45 degrees cephalad and 30 degrees toward the midline. Although this portal places the lateral femoral cutaneous nerve at risk, studies demonstrate that the nerve, which arborizes before this point, lies lateral to this portal.[3] The other two portals are established at the anterior and posterior margins of the superior edge of the greater trochanter. These portals lie approximately 4 cm below the superior gluteal nerve, and the posterolateral portal is approximately 3 cm superior to the sciatic nerve.[3]

Special extra-long cannulas and sheaths ($5\frac{1}{4}$ in.) have been developed for hip arthroscopy. Surgical instruments and the arthroscope can be easily exchanged with these cannulas. Cannulated trocars are also commercially available to allow insertion over a guidewire that can be introduced through a large-diameter spinal needle, which facilitates portal placement (Fig. 3–14).

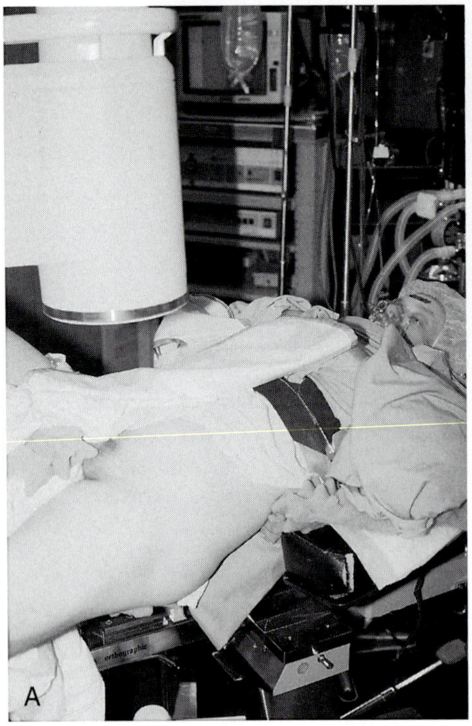

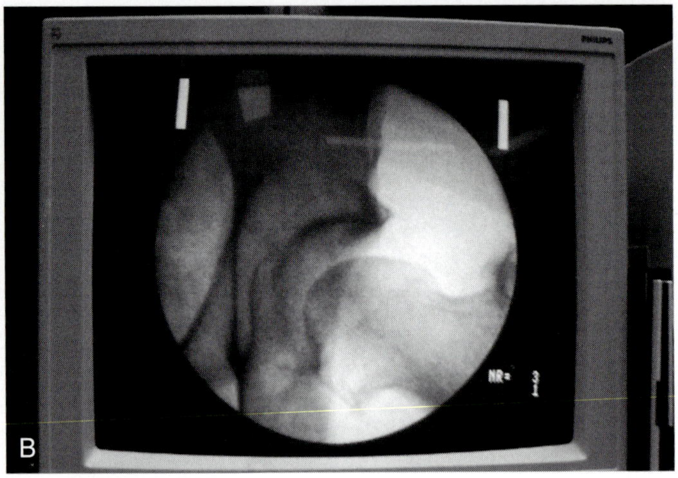

Figure 3–12
Fluoroscopy used for hip arthroscopy. A, *Operating room set-up.* B, *Fluoroscopic image with 1-cm distraction of the affected hip.*

ARTHROSCOPIC ANATOMY

Most of the hip joint can be visualized with the arthroscope (Fig. 3–15).[10] Eighty percent or more of the femoral head can be seen, and the insertion of the ligamentum teres into the anteromedial portion of the femoral head is a readily identifiable landmark. The acetabulum is also well visualized with the horseshoe-shaped, lunate surface of the acetabulum that extends to the peripheral labrum and central acetabular fossa. The acetabular fossa extends inferiorly and is filled with vascular adipose tissue extending to the transverse ligament. Viewing the joint through different portals helps evaluate all forms of hip pathology.

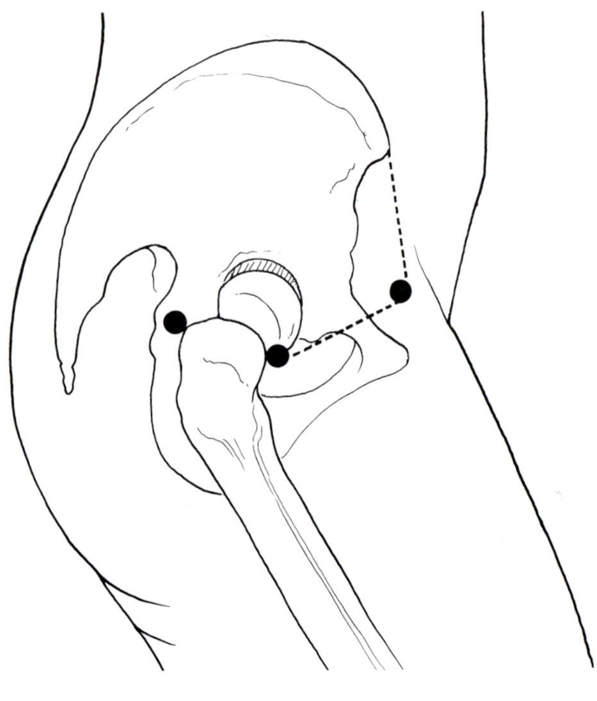

Figure 3–13
Portals for hip arthroscopy *include the anterior portal and two portals adjacent to the superior edge of the greater trochanter. (From Miller MD, Cooper DE, Warner JJP. Review of Sports Medicine and Arthroscopy. Philadelphia: WB Saunders, 1995.)*

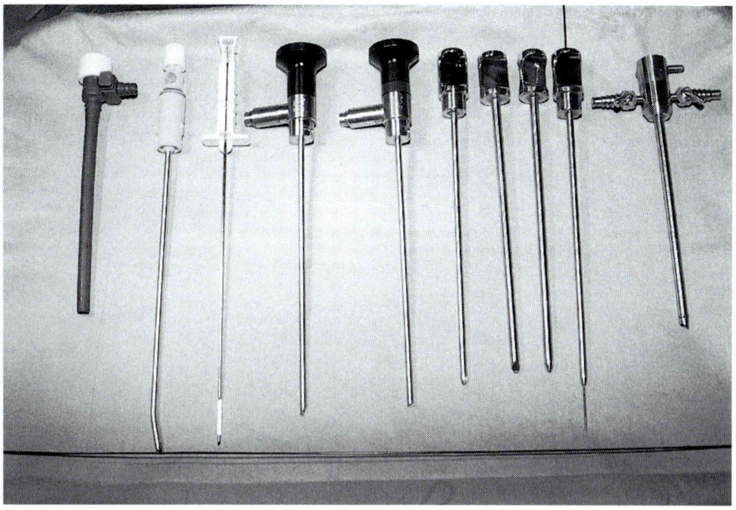

Figure 3–14
Instruments used for hip arthroscopy. Left to right, *long disposable cannula, long curved shaver blade, 14-gauge spinal needle, 70-degree arthroscope, 30-degree arthroscope, cannulated cannulas without and with guidewire, and arthroscopic sheath. Guidewire is shown at the bottom of the figure.*

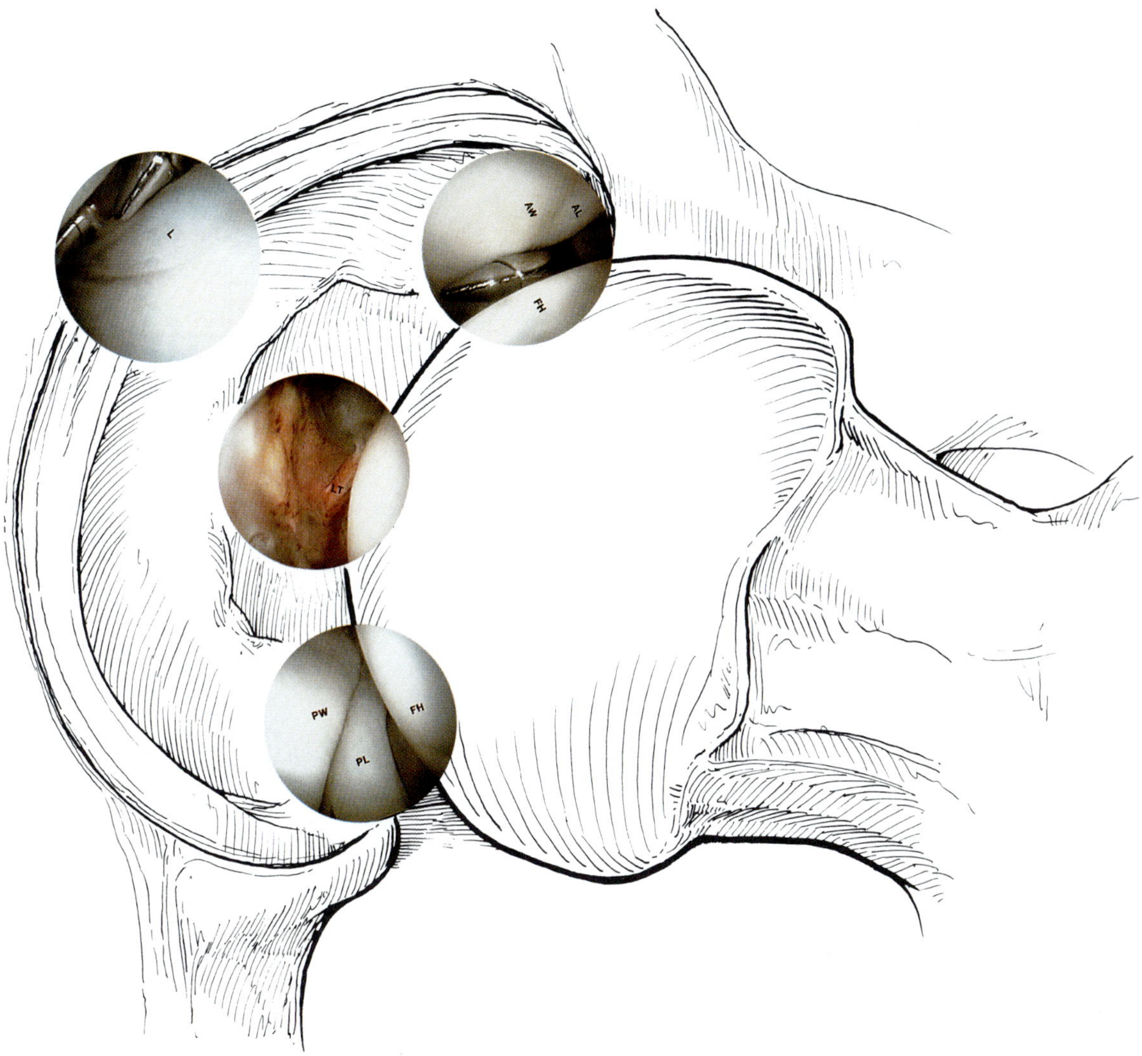

Figure 3–15
Arthroscopic anatomy of the hip (L = labrum; AL = anterior labrum; AW = wall of acetabulum; FH = femoral head; PL = posterior labrum; PW = posterior wall; LT = ligamentum teres).

COMPLICATIONS

Most of the complications reported for hip arthroscopy include nerve traction palsies and articular cartilage injury. Neuropraxias are usually transient and can be reduced by carefully padding the peroneal post, limiting the traction time, and using specialized distracters. Adequate care should be taken in and around the joint to avoid articular cartilage injury. Neurovascular injury can be avoided by careful portal placement and introduction of cannulas and sleeves over cannulated introducers.

References

1. Burman MS. Arthroscopy or the direct visualization of joints. J Bone Joint Surg 1931; 4:669-695.
2. Byrd JWT. Hip arthroscopy utilizing the supine position. Arthroscopy 1994; 10:275-280.
3. Byrd JWT, Pappas JN, Pedley MJ. Hip arthroscopy: An anatomic study of portal placement and relationship to the extra-articular structures. Arthroscopy 1995; 11:418-423.
4. Dvorak M, Duncan C, Day B. Arthroscopic anatomy of the hip. Arthroscopy 1990; 6:264-273.
5. Erikson E, Arvidsson I, Arvidsson H. Diagnostic and operative arthroscopy of the hip. Orthopedics 1986; 9:169-176.
6. Glick J, Sampson T, Gordon R, et al. Hip arthroscopy by the lateral approach. Arthroscopy 1987; 37:223-231.
7. Glick JM. Hip arthroscopy. *In* McGinty JB, ed. Operative Arthroscopy. New York: Raven Press, 1991, pp 663-676.
8. Gross R. Arthroscopy in hip disorders in children. Orthop Rev 1977; 6:43-49.
9. Johnson LL. Diagnostic and Surgical Arthroscopy, 3rd ed. St. Louis: CV Mosby, 1986, pp 1491-1519.
10. Keene GS, Villar RN. Arthroscopic anatomy of the hip: An in vivo study. Arthroscopy 1994; 10:392-399.

Illustrative Cases

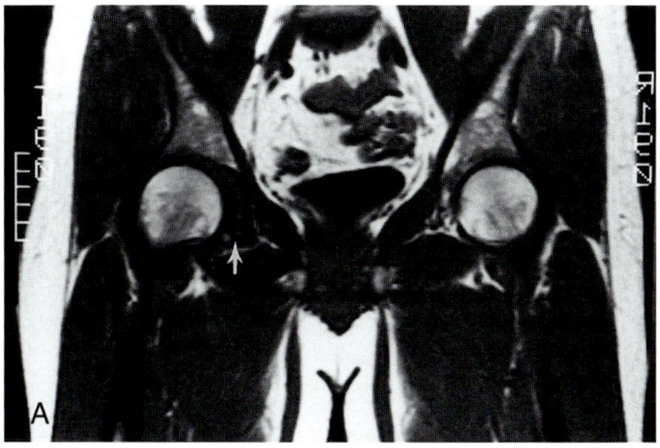

Figure 3–16. **Synovial Osteochondromatosis, Right Hip**
A, *Coronal T1-weighted SE image demonstrates a distended right hip joint medially with multiple small, high-signal osteochondral loose bodies* (arrow), *consistent with osteochondromatosis.* B, *Arthroscopic figure demonstrates multiple loose bodies in the right hip.*
Case courtesy of J.W. Thomas Byrd, M.D., F.A.C.S.

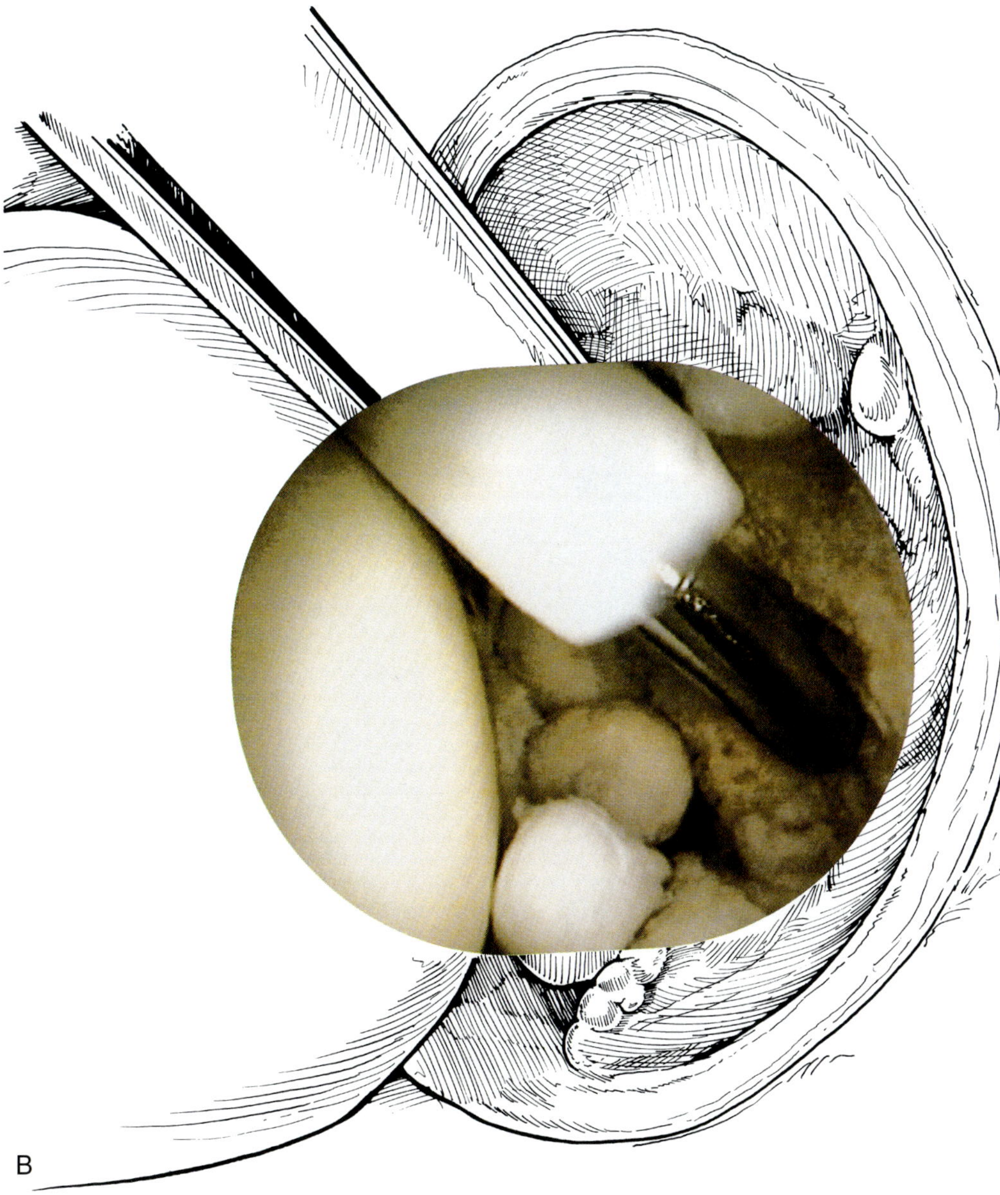

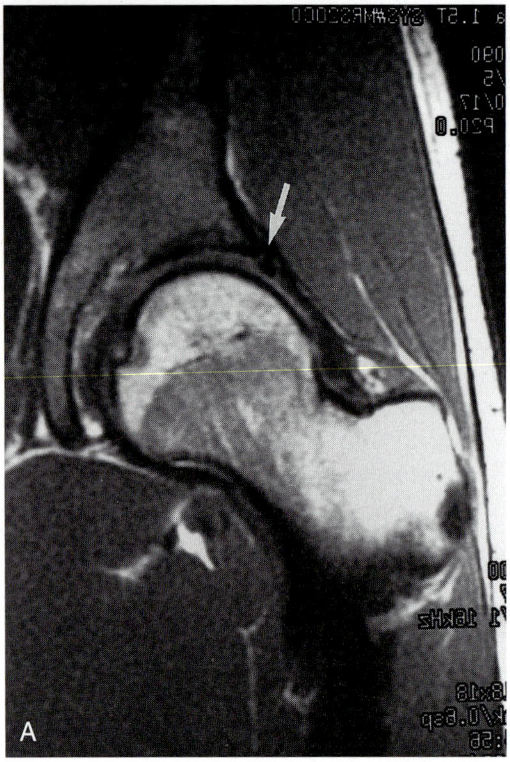

Figure 3–17. **Superior Labral Tear, Left Hip**
A, *Coronal T1-weighted SE image shows linear bright signal* (arrow) *traversing the superior labrum, corresponding to a labral tear.*
B, *Arthroscopic figure shows a tear* (arrow) *in the superior labrum.*
Case courtesy of J.W. Thomas Byrd, M.D., F.A.C.S.

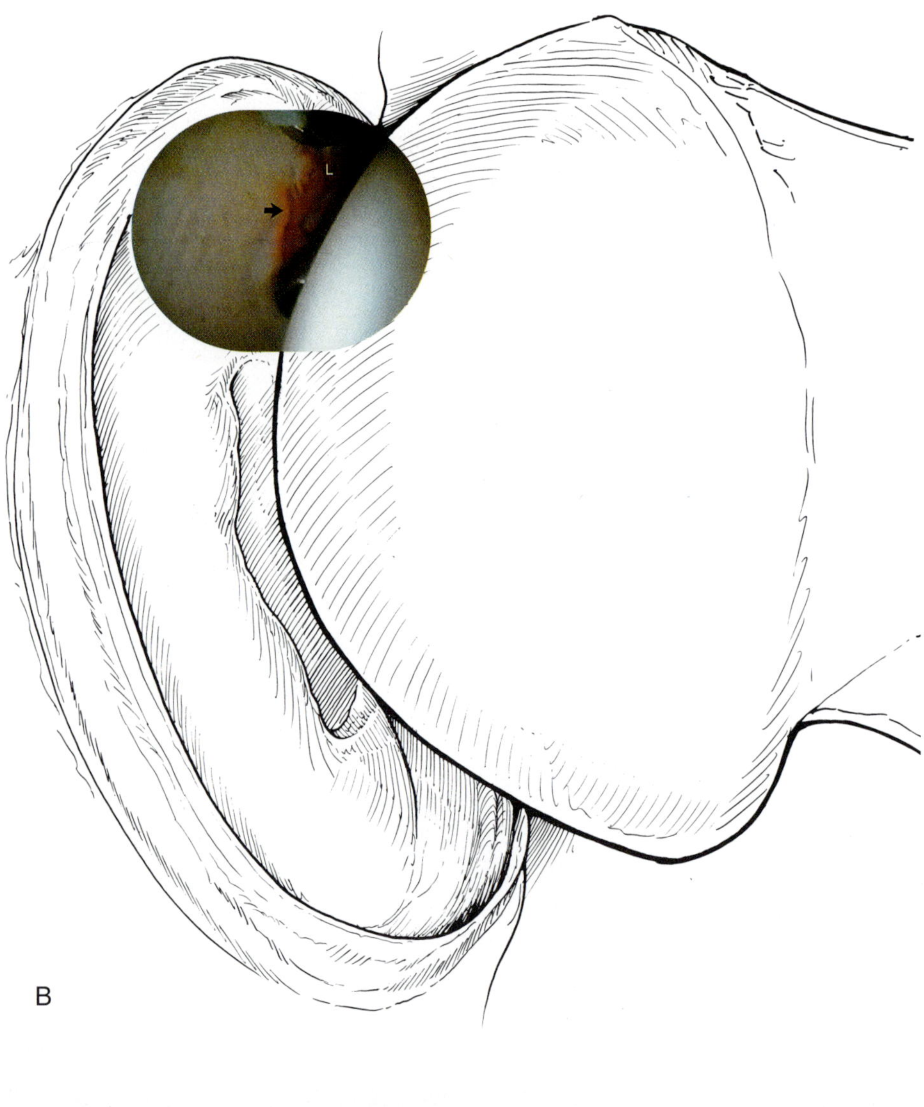

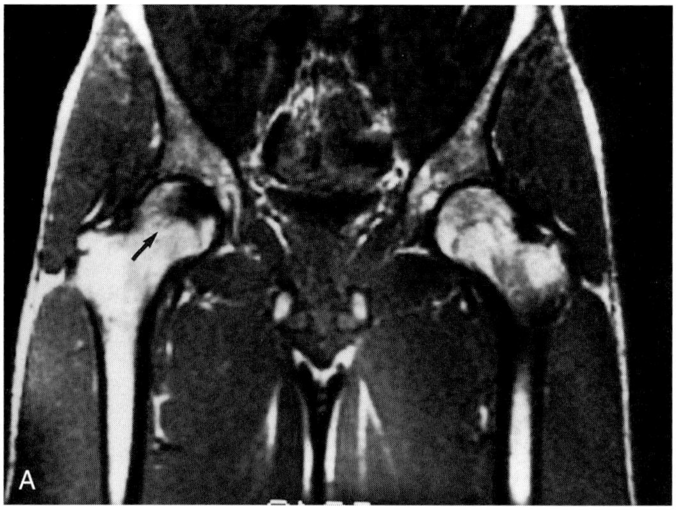

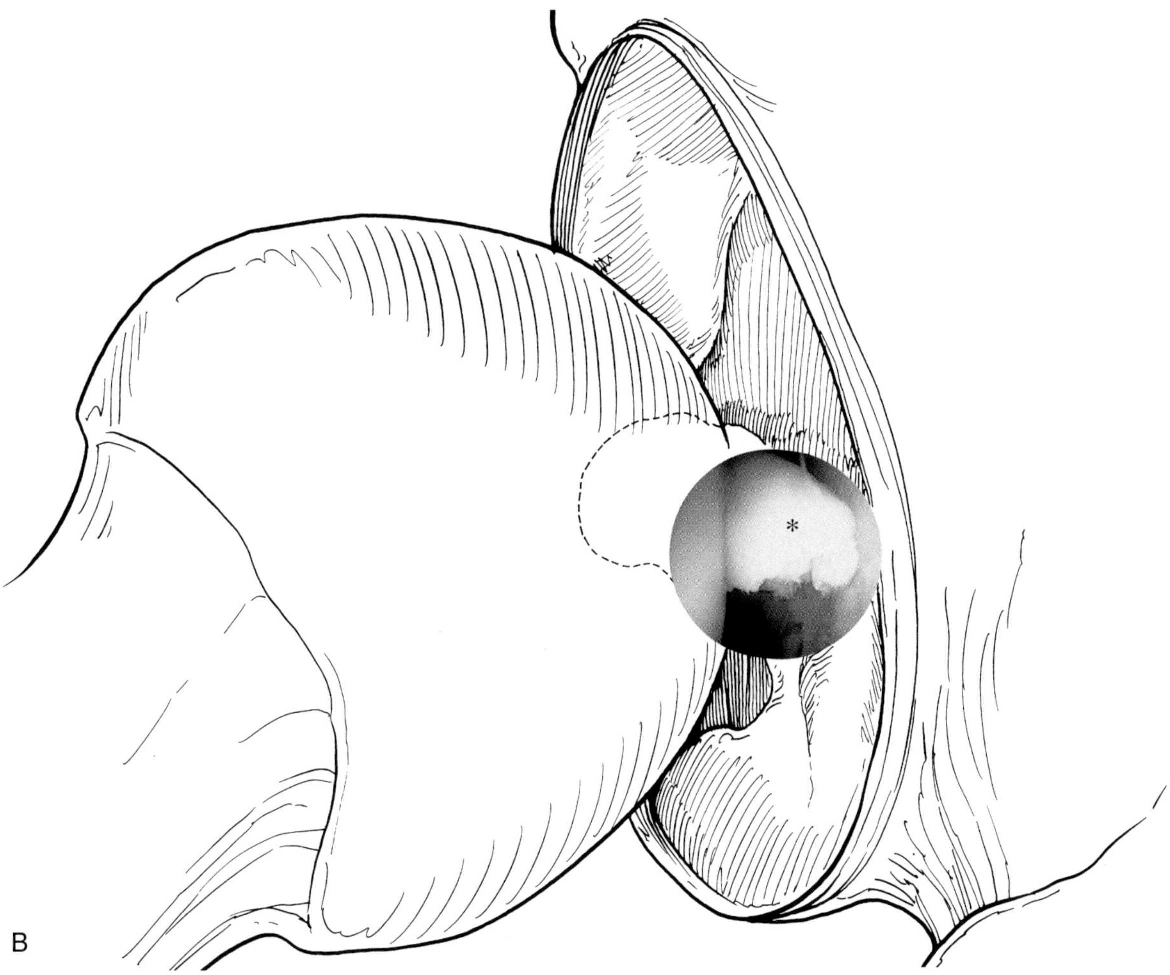

Figure 3–18. **Osteochondral Injury, Right Hip**
A, *Coronal T1-weighted SE image reveals large low-signal area beneath the articular surface of the femoral head* (arrow), *consistent with an osteochondral injury.* B, *Arthroscopic photo shows a large flap tear of the articular cartilage of the femoral head* (*).
Case courtesy of J.W. Thomas Byrd, M.D., F.A.C.S.

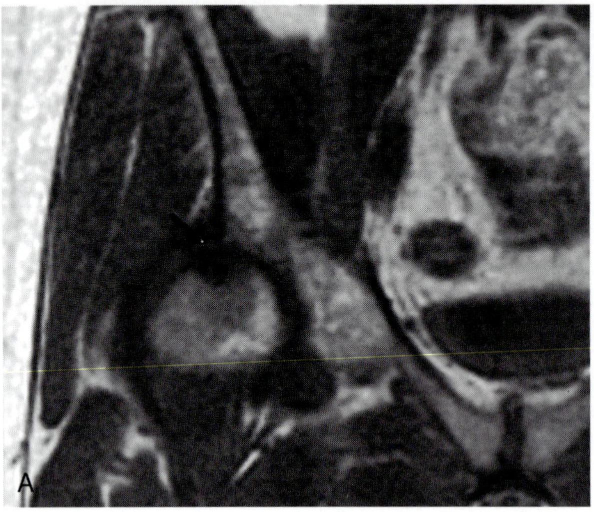

A

Figure 3–19. **Advanced Chondrosis/AVN, Right Femoral Head**

A, *Coronal T1-weighted image reveals a focus of decreased signal* (arrow) *adjacent to the articular surface of the femoral head.* B, *Arthroscopic view demonstrates a large area of exposed bone adjacent to normal articular cartilage.*

Case courtesy of G. Bradford Wright, M.D.

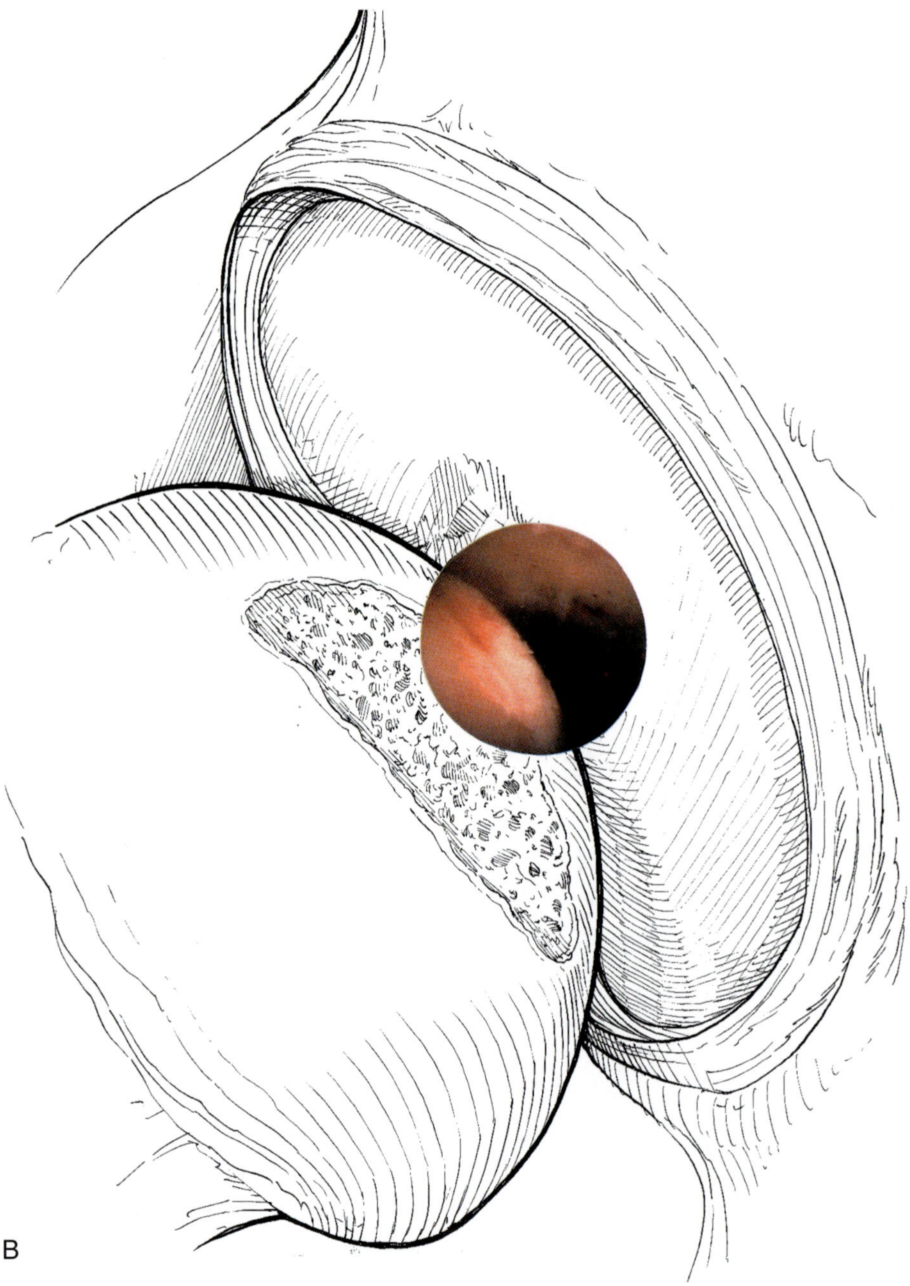

B

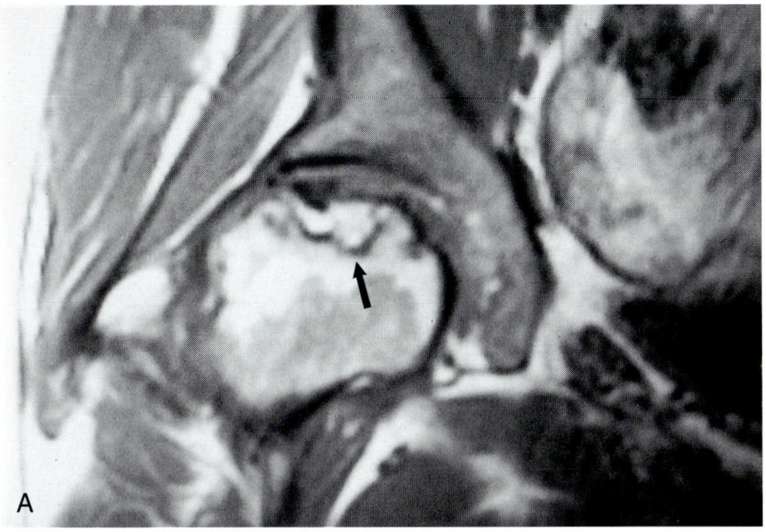
A

Figure 3–20. **Osteocartilaginous Defect/"Burned out" Right Hip**
A, *Coronal T1-weighted image shows osteonecrosis. Note the subchondral collapse with irregularity of the articular surface of the femoral head with a central focus of bright signal outlined by serpiginous dark signal* (arrow). B, *Arthroscopic figure demonstrates an area of articular cartilage defect with exposed bone.*
Case courtesy of James M. Glick, M.D.

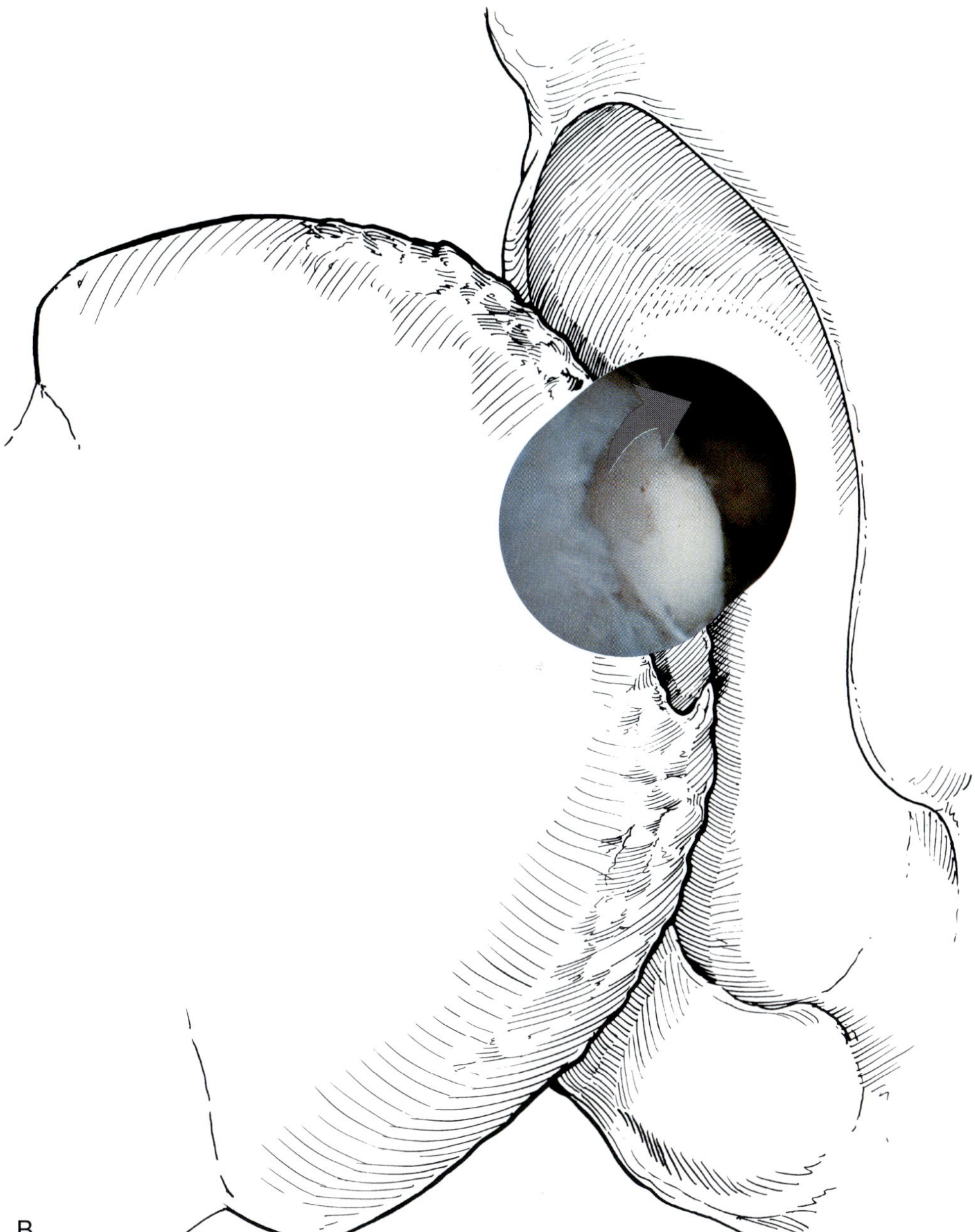
B

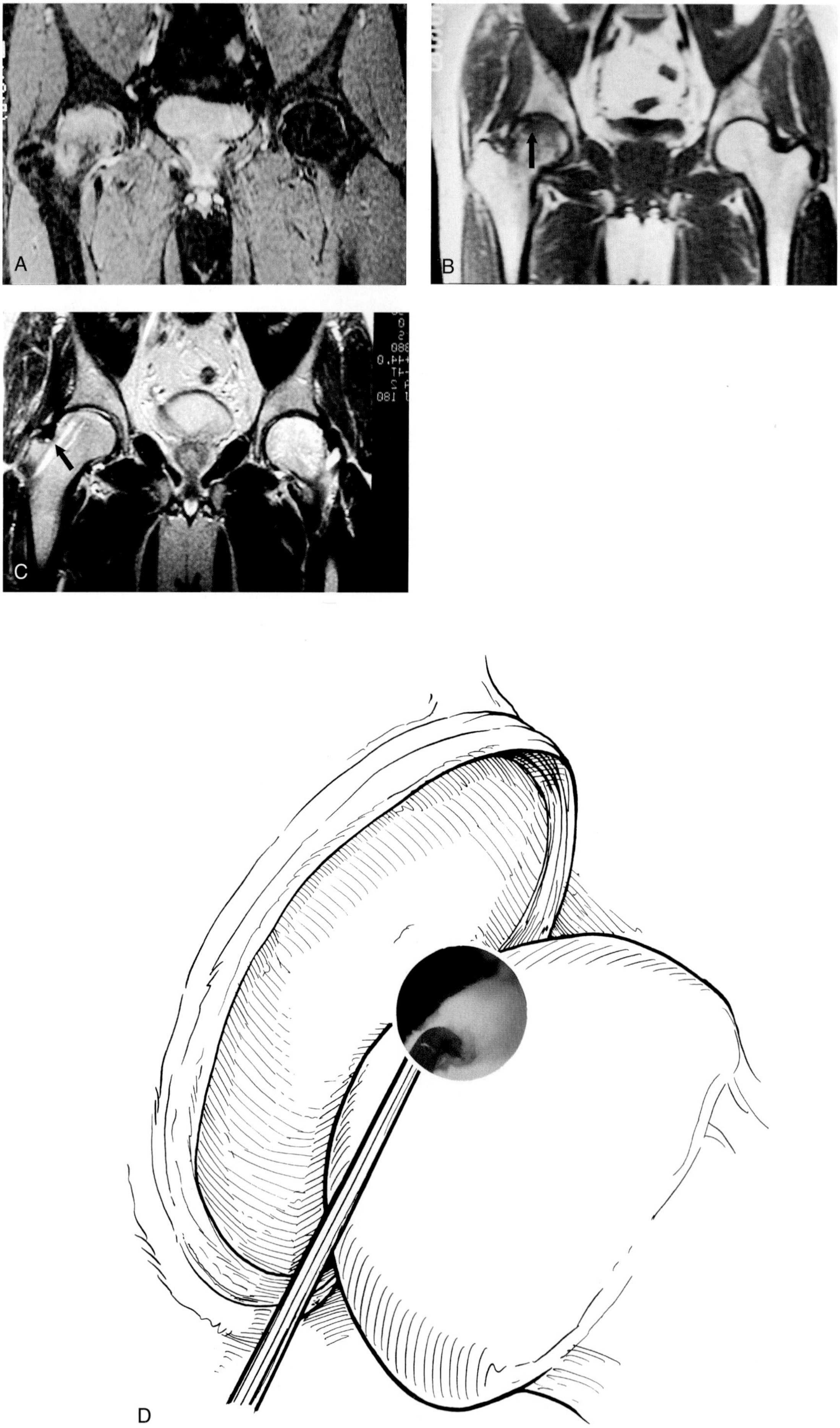

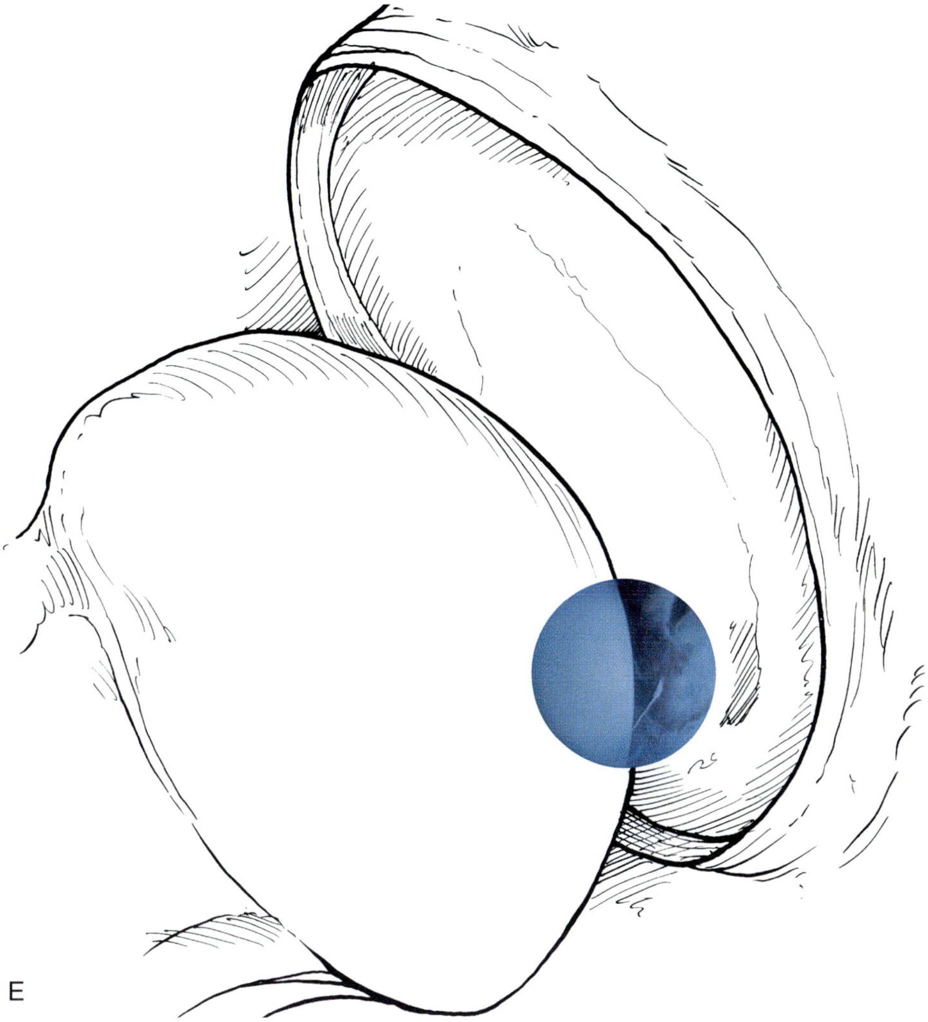

E

Figure 3–21. **Moderate Avascular Necrosis (AVN), Right Hip, Early AVN, Left Hip**

A, *Coronal STIR image reveals diffuse bright signal throughout the right femoral head and neck of the right hip. The left hip is normal.* B, *Coronal T1-weighted image demonstrates diffuse low signal within the bone marrow. A small focus of bright signal is outlined by dark signal* (arrow) *at the articular surface.* C, *Coronal T2-weighted image obtained 6 months following the initial study reveals diffuse bright signal within the left femoral head without focal findings to suggest a more advanced stage of osteonecrosis. Note the linear track of bright signal within the right femoral head and neck* (arrow) *from prior core decompression.* D, *Arthroscopic view of the left hip demonstrates focal defect in the articular cartilage of the femoral head.* E, *Right-arthroscopy was normal.*

Case courtesy of James M. Glick, M.D.

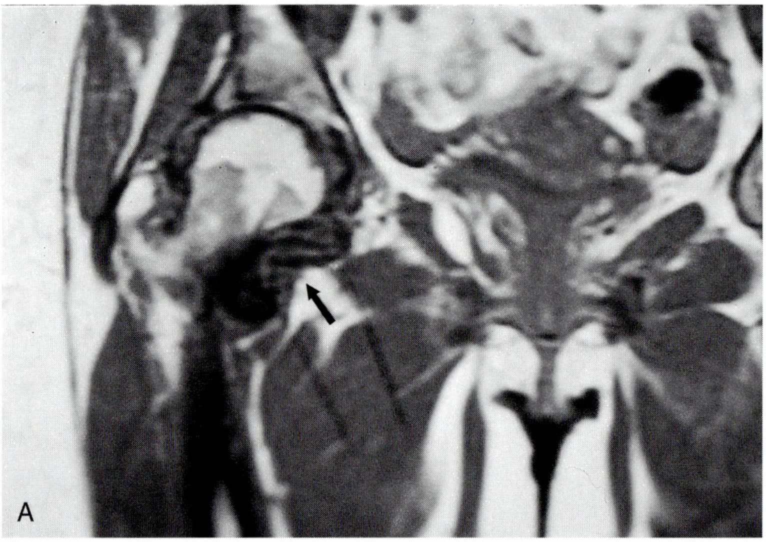

A

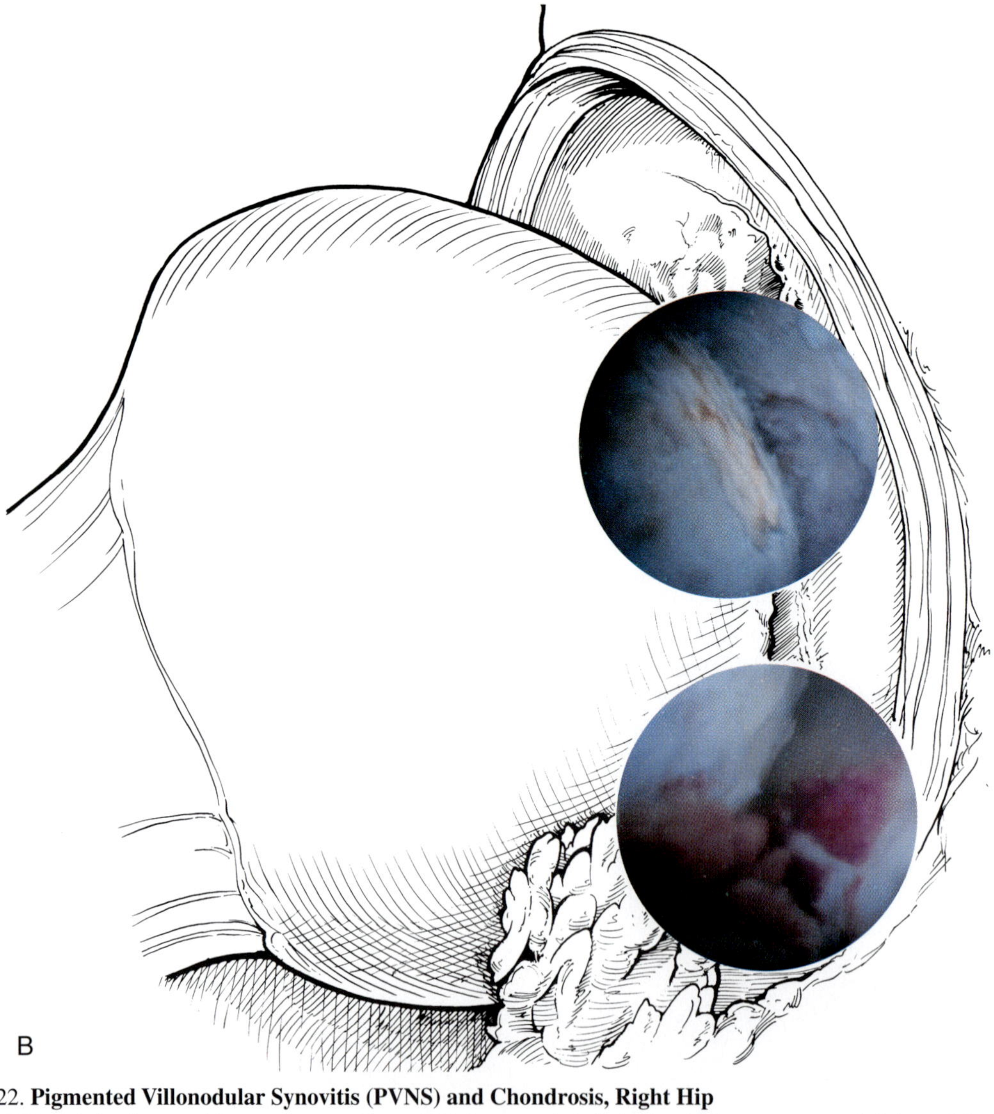

B

Figure 3–22. **Pigmented Villonodular Synovitis (PVNS) and Chondrosis, Right Hip**
A, *Coronal T1-weighted coronal image shows a distended joint capsule inferiorly with heterogeneous bright and dark signal intensity* (arrow) *indicative of synovial inflammation, hemosiderin deposits, and capsular effusion. Note also the superior joint space narrowing, the attenuated intermediate signal intensity of the articular cartilage, and the small, low-signal-intensity subchondral cysts* (arrows). B, *Arthroscopic view of PVNS in the inferior portion and advanced chondrosis in the superior portion of the femoral head.*
Case courtesy of James M. Glick, M.D.

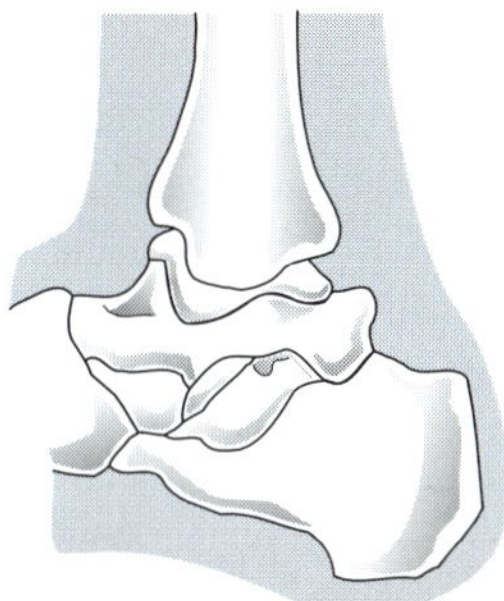

CHAPTER

4

Ankle

MRI of the Ankle and Foot

MRI of the ankle and foot can contribute significantly to several osseous, articular, and soft tissue abnormalities of the ankle. MRI is particularly indicated in tendon and ligamentous injuries, osteochondral injuries, sinus tarsi syndrome, tarsal tunnel syndrome, plantar fasciitis, and diabetic foot disorders. This section reviews the MRI anatomy, imaging technique, and pathology applicable to this anatomic region.

TECHNIQUE

Ankle imaging is performed with the patient lying supine; the foot is in a neutral position, securely placed in an extremity coil (Fig. 4–1). Routine imaging is performed in three planes to include the coronal, axial, and sagittal orientations. The oblique axial plane is an additional orientation that optimizes visualization of some tendinous and ligamentous anatomy. High resolution is obtained with a field of view of 10 to 14 cm and a slice thickness of 3 to 4 mm. A combination of T1 and T2 spin-echo sequences is the mainstay, although gradient recalled-echo, fast spin-echo (FSE), and short tau inversion recovery (STIR) sequences are valuable adjuncts to the protocol, which is tailored to the clinical concern. A T1 sequence and fat suppression with gadolinium contrast also highlights osseous, articular, and soft tissue abnormalities for appropriate indications such as infection, soft tissue neoplasm, or a synovial process.

MRI ANATOMY

MRI anatomy of the ankle and foot are well displayed in the axial, coronal, and sagittal planes (Figs. 4–2 through 4–6).

Text continued on page 118

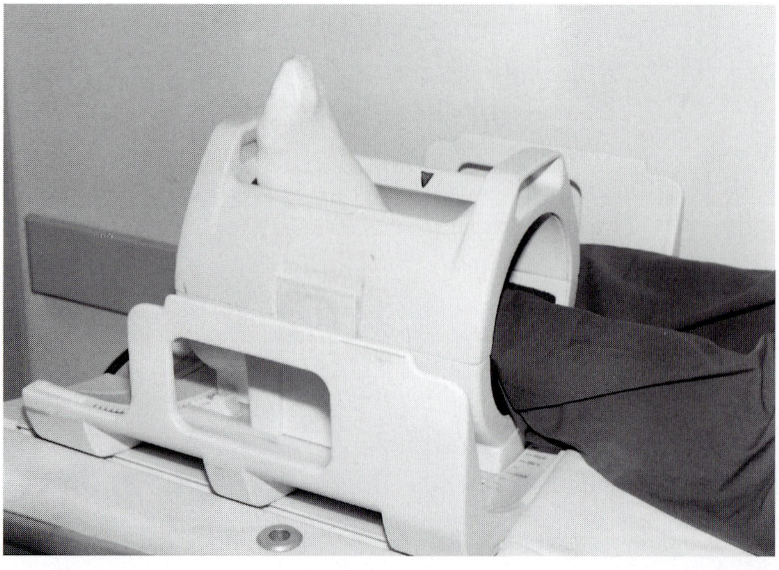

Figure 4–1
Extremity coil (transmit/receive) for imaging the ankle.

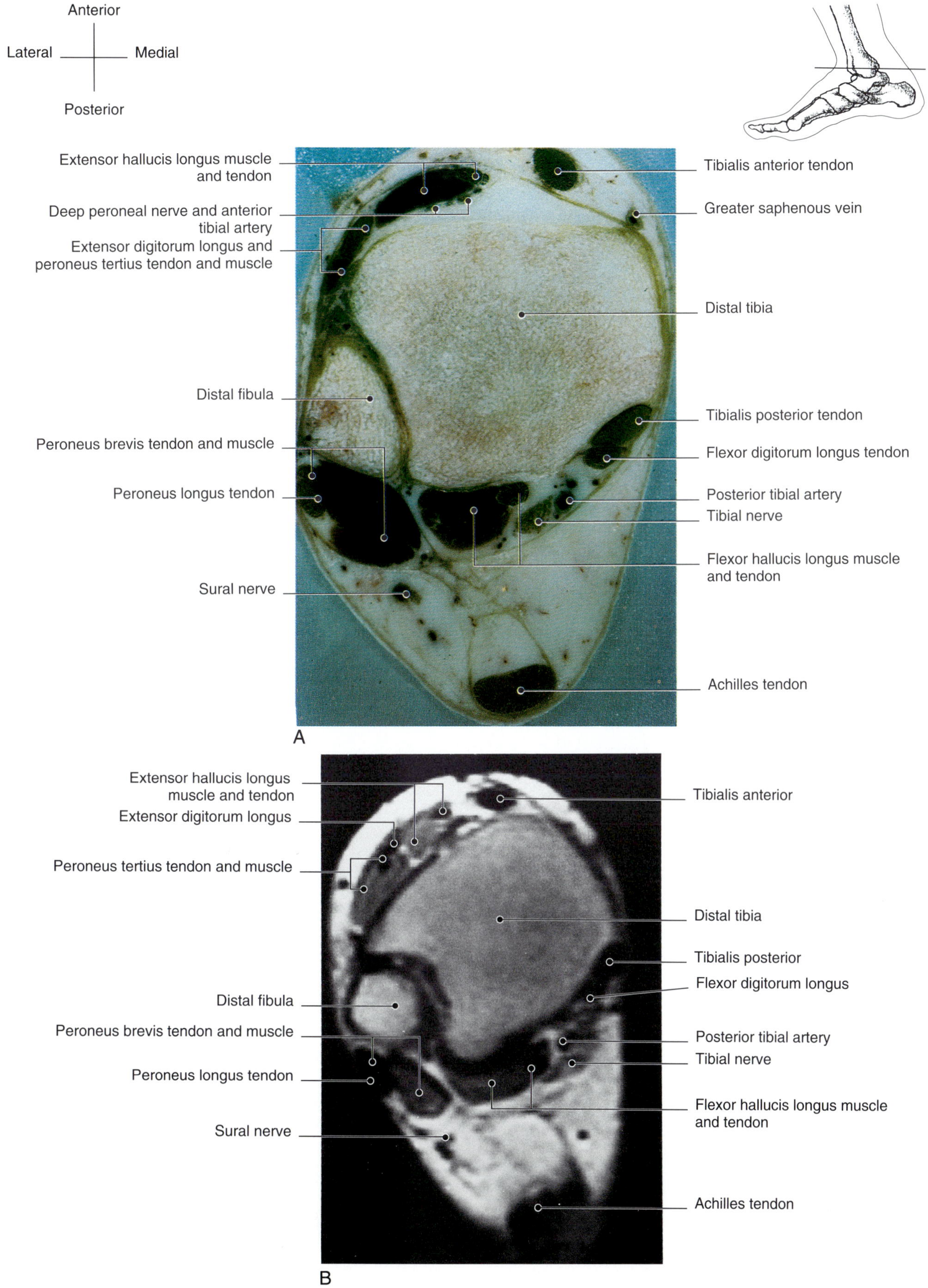

Figure 4–2

Axial cryoplaned section (A) *and magnetic-resonance image (TR, 2000 ms; TE, 20 ns)* (B) *of the ankle at the level of the distal tibia and fibula. (From Chan WP, Raushning W, Wu Cy, et al. Magnetic resonance imaging anatomy and cryomicrotome atlas.* In *Chan WP, Lang P, Genant HK, eds. MRI of the Musculoskeletal System. Philadelphia: WB Saunders, 1994.) [Case A courtesy of Scott J. Erickson, M.D., and G.F. Carrera, M.D.]*

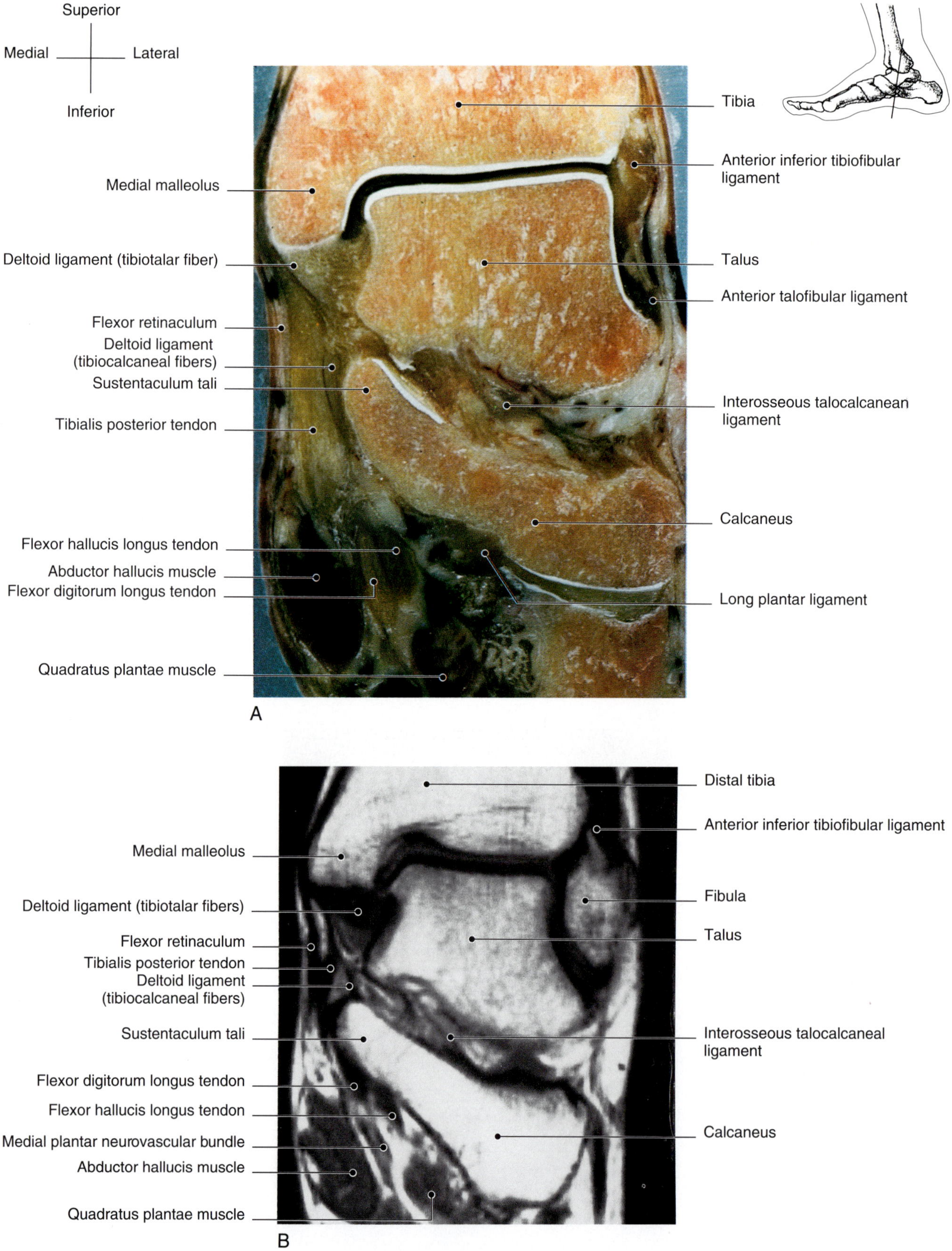

Figure 4–3

Midcoronal cryoplaned section (A) *and magnetic-resonance image (TR, 500 ms; TE, 20 ns)* (B) *of the ankle. (From Chan WP, Raushning W, Wu Cy, et al. Magnetic resonance imaging anatomy and cryomicrotome atlas.* In *Chan WP, Lang P, Genant HK, eds. MRI of the Musculoskeletal System. Philadelphia: WB Saunders, 1994.) [Case A courtesy of Scott J. Erickson, M.D., and G.F. Carrera, M.D.]*

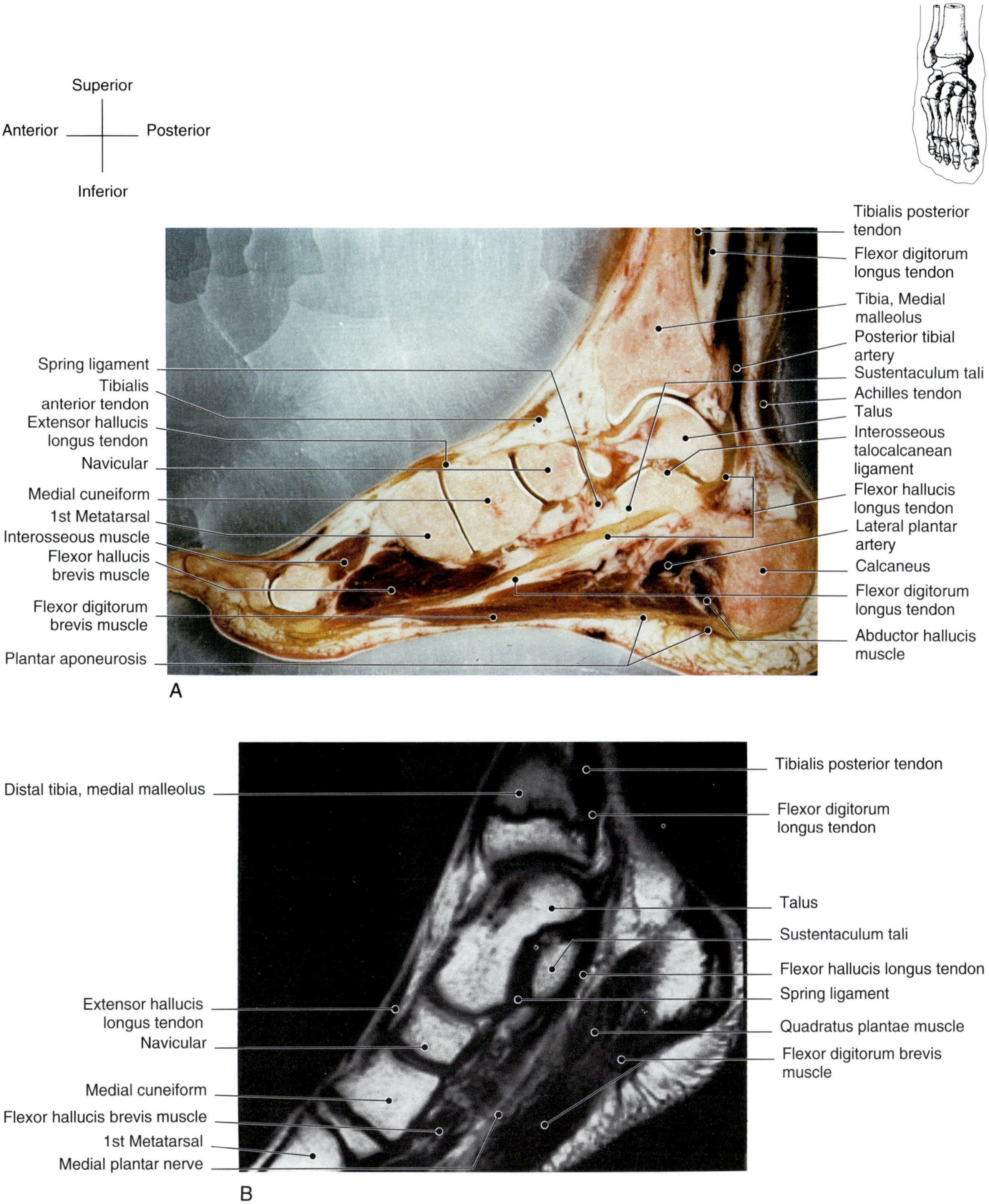

Figure 4–4

Paramedian sagittal cryoplaned section (A) *and magnetic resonance image (TR, 500 ms; TE, 20 ns)* (B) *of the ankle and foot through the medial compartment tendons. (From Chan WP, Raushning W, Wu Cy, et al. Magnetic resonance imaging anatomy and cryomicrotome atlas.* In *Chan WP, Lang P, Genant HK, eds. MRI of the Musculoskeletal System. Philadelphia: WB Saunders, 1994.) [Case A courtesy of Scott J. Erickson, M.D., and G.F. Carrera, M.D.]*

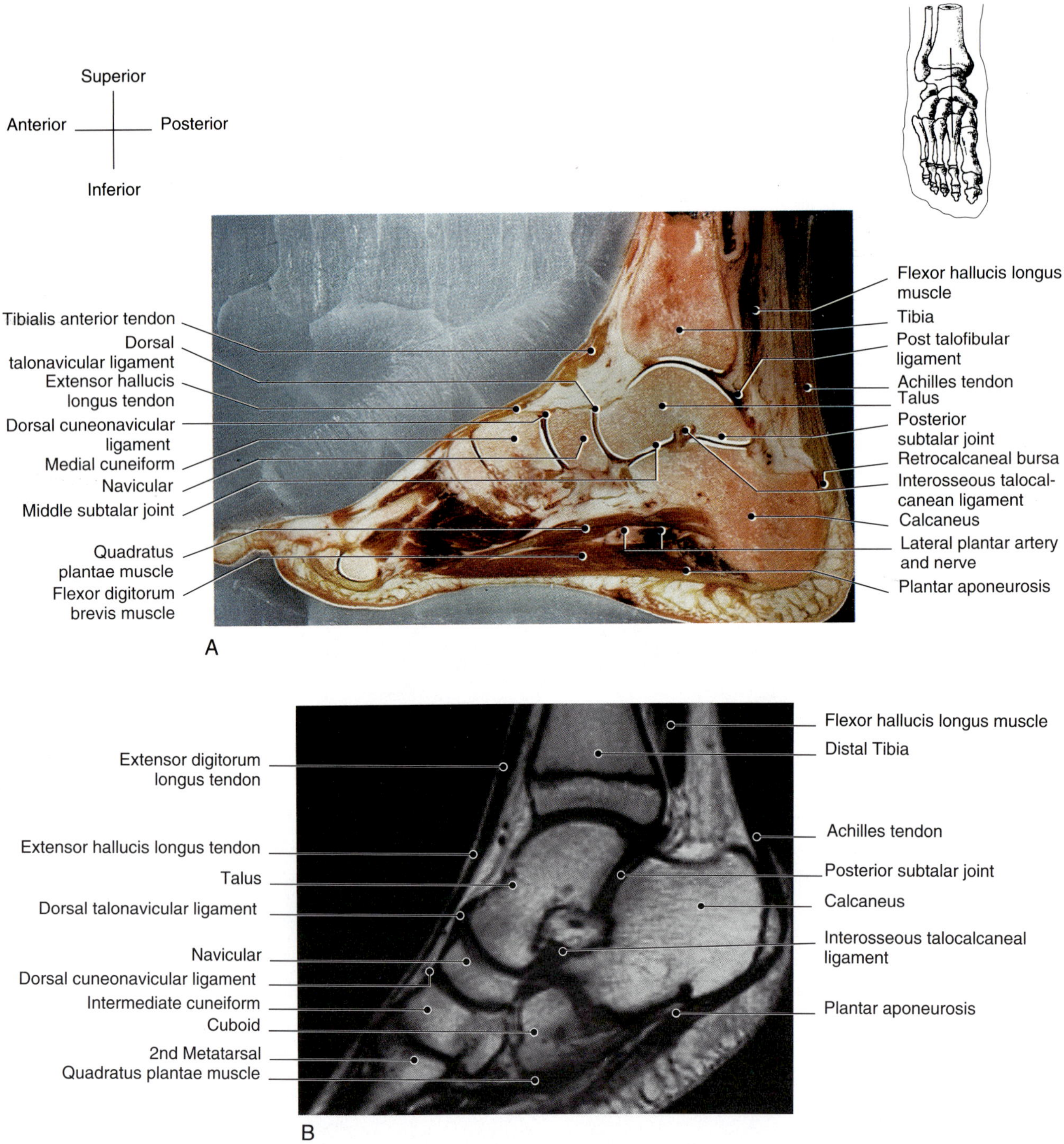

Figure 4–5
Midsagittal cryoplaned section (A) *and magnetic-resonance image (TR, 500 ms; TE, 20 ns)* (B) *of the ankle. (From Chan WP, Raushning W, Wu Cy, et al. Magnetic resonance imaging anatomy and cryomicrotome atlas.* In *Chan WP, Lang P, Genant HK, eds. MRI of the Musculoskeletal System. Philadelphia: WB Saunders, 1994.) [Case A courtesy of Scott J. Erickson, M.D., and G.F. Carrera, M.D.]*

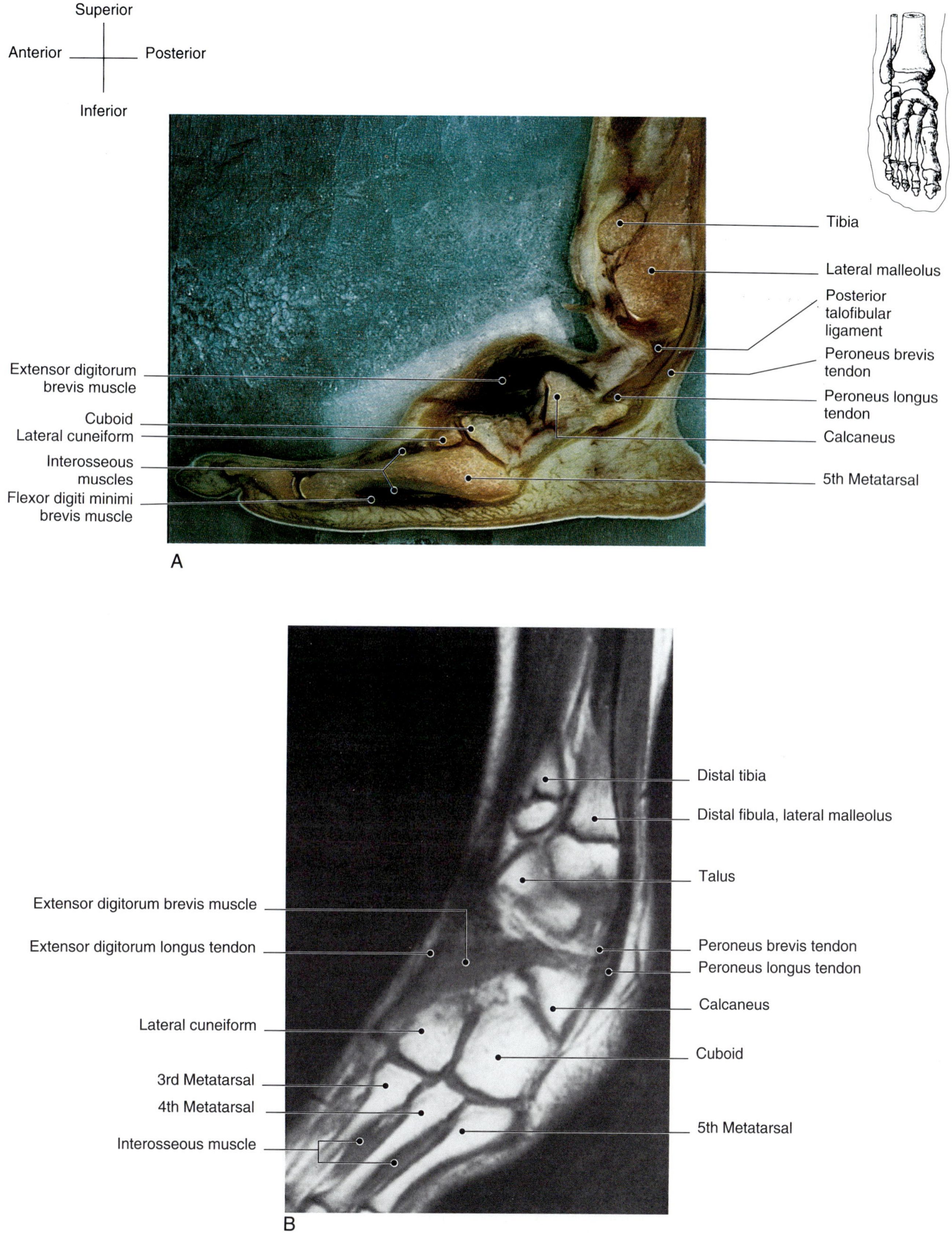

Figure 4–6

Paramedian sagittal cryoplaned section (A) *and magnetic resonance image (TR, 500 ms; TE, 20 ns)* (B) *of the ankle and foot through the lateral compartment tendons. (From Chan WP, Raushning W, Wu Cy, et al. Magnetic resonance imaging anatomy and cryomicrotome atlas.* In *Chan WP, Lang P, Genant HK, eds. MRI of the Musculoskeletal System. Philadelphia: WB Saunders, 1994.) [Case A courtesy of Scott J. Erickson, M.D., and G.F. Carrera, M.D.]*

Tendons

The ankle tendons can be divided into four groups: posterior (Achilles tendon), lateral (peroneal tendons), medial (flexor tendons), and anterior (extensor tendons). The one major posterior tendon, the Achilles tendon, inserts on the calcaneus. A second posterior tendon, the plantars tendon, present in 90% of persons, courses just medial to the Achilles tendon to insert onto the calcaneus or sometimes onto the Achilles tendon or flexor retinaculum. The Achilles tendon is normally flat or slightly concave anteriorly and should not exceed 8 mm in thickness. It is separated from the ankle by a fat pad.[4, 22]

Two lateral tendons course posteriorly to the lateral malleolus, which they utilize as a pulley. The peroneus brevis is the more anterior of the two tendons and it inserts on the base of the fifth metatarsal. The peroneus longus is posterior to the peroneus brevis tendon. It passes beneath the midfoot to insert on the base of the first metatarsal. These two tendons share a common sheath to the level of the fibular tip, where they diverge with separate tendon sheaths. The tendon positions are secured in place by the superior and inferior peroneal retinaculum.[4, 22]

There are three medial tendons from anterior to posterior: the tibialis posterior, just posterior to the medial malleolus; the flexor digitorum longus; and the flexor hallucis longus, which courses posteriorly to the talus and then inferiorly to the sustentaculum tali, which is a good landmark for its identification. These tendons pass through the tarsal tunnel along with the posterior tibial nerve in a closely spaced group covered by the flexor retinaculum. The neurovascular bundle, comprising the posterior tibial nerve, artery, and vein, courses between the flexor digitorum longus and the flexor hallucis longus tendons in the tarsal tunnel. The posterior tibialis, the largest of the three tendons with twice the cross-sectional area as the other two tendons, uses the medial malleolus as a pulley. It inserts on the navicular, medial, and intermediate cuneiforms and the second through fourth metatarsal bases. The flexor digitorum longus inserts on the fifth metatarsal. The flexor hallucis longus courses beneath the sustentaculum tali, which it uses as a pulley to insert on the base of the distal phalanx of the great toe after passing between two sesamoids under the first metatarsal.[4, 22]

There are four anterior tendons, which are, from medial to lateral: the tibialis anterior, the extensor hallucis longus, the extensor digitorum longus, and the peroneus tertius tendons. They are covered by an overlying extensor retinaculum. The anterior tibial inserts on the medial surface of the medial cuneiform and the base of the first metatarsal. The extensor hallucis longus inserts on the dorsal aspect of the base of the distal phalanx of the great toe. The extensor digitorum longus muscle divides into four tendons, which pass to the dorsal aspects of the toes. The peroneus tertius inserts on the proximal, dorsal aspect of the fifth metatarsal.[4, 22]

The axial plane is best for evaluation of the tendons to the level of the medial malleolus. More distally, all tendons but the Achilles tendon turn obliquely and are best seen in true cross-section in an oblique axial plane. The sagittal plane is optimal for evaluation of the Achilles tendon.

Normal tendons are hypointense on all sequences; however, portions of tendons that course at or near 55 degrees relative to the static magnetic field display increased signal on T1 sequences because of the "magic angle" phenomenon (discussed later).[7] Repositioning of the ankle and foot or noting an absence of the signal on T2 sequences helps to differentiate this artifact from a true abnormality. Small amounts of fluid are commonly seen in tendon sheaths as increased signal on T2 sequences.[4, 22]

Ligaments

The ankle joint is stabilized by three sets of ligaments: the medial collateral (deltoid) ligament, the lateral collateral ligament, and the distal tibiofibular syndesmotic complex. Ankle sprains injuring the lateral collateral ligaments are most common (Fig. 4–7). First-degree sprains display a focal area of high signal around the ligament on T2 sequences. Second-degree sprains display partial discontinuity of the ligament, and third-degree

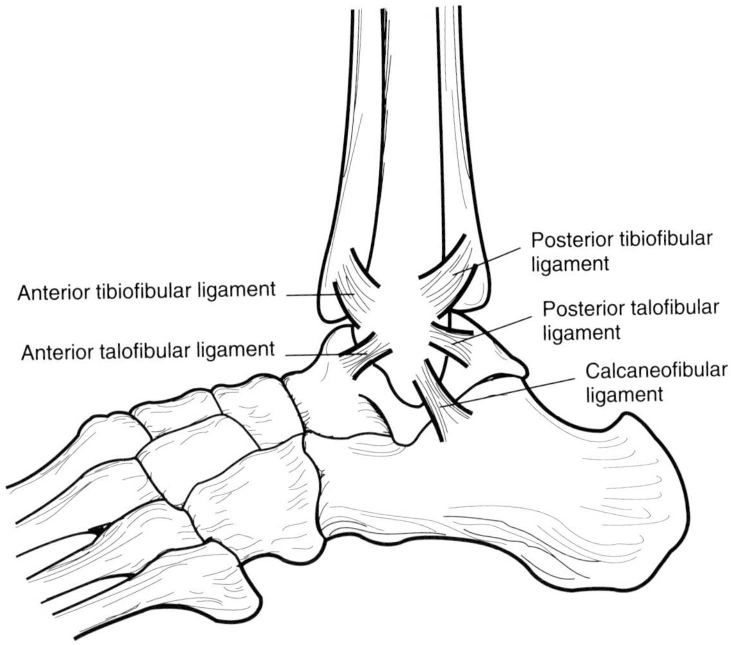

Figure 4–7
Lateral aspect of the ankle showing components of the lateral collateral ligament and the tibiofibular ligament. (From Chan WP, Peterfy C, Erickson SJ, et al. The ankle and foot. In *Chan WP, Lang P, Genant HK, eds. MRI of the Musculoskeletal System. Philadelphia: WB Saunders, 1994.)*

sprains display complete ligamentous disruption. Associated findings with any of these sprains may include thickening of the ligament or altered signal in any of the adjacent osseous or soft tissues. The anterior talofibular ligament, posterior talofibular ligament, and distal tibiofibular syndesmotic complex are best seen in the axial plane. Portions of the calcaneofibular ligament are seen in both axial and coronal planes.[4, 22]

The medial collateral (deltoid) ligament is located deep to the flexor tendons. It has components that extend from the medial malleolus to insert on the navicular, sustentaculum tali, and talus. There are superficial and deep components. The superficial component, the stronger of the two, courses more vertically. Its signal character tends to be homogeneously hypointense. The deep component (anterior and posterior tibiotalar subcomponents) courses horizontally. Its signal character tends to be heterogeneously intermediate to hypointense. Tears can present as nonvisualization, disruption, thinning, thickening, or beading.[21]

The lateral collateral ligament is composed of three structures: the anterior talofibular, posterior talofibular, and calcaneofibular ligaments. The malleolar fossa, an indentation on the medial aspect of the distal fibula, is a good marker for identifying these ligaments. The anterior talofibular extends from the anterior aspect of the fibula to the lateral talar neck. Its signal character tends to be homogeneously hypointense. The posterior talofibular extends from the distal aspect of the fibula to the posterior talar tubercle. Its signal character tends to be heterogeneously intermediate to hypointense, similar to the deltoid ligament. The calcaneofibular ligament extends obliquely just deep to the peroneal tendons.[4, 22]

The distal tibiofibular syndesmotic complex has three components: the anterior distal tibiofibular, posterior distal tibiofibular, and interosseous ligaments. Their signal character is also heterogeneous.

Bone

The ankle joint is composed of the distal tibia, distal fibula, and talar dome. The foot is subdivided into the hindfoot (talus and calcaneus), midfoot (tarsal navicular, three cuneiforms, and cuboid), and forefoot (metatarsals and phalanges). There are numerous accessory ossicles. The common ones include the os trigonum, os peroneum, accessory navicular, and os intermetatarseum. When an ossicle is small and completely within a tendon, its characteristic increased signal (due to fatty marrow on T1 sequences) might mimic a tendon injury.[4, 22]

Muscle

There are two muscles, the extensor digitorum brevis and extensor hallucis brevis, along the anterior aspect of the foot. The plantar aspect of the foot is more complex, with medial, lateral, and central compartments separated by fascial planes. The compartments normally communicate. An important communication between the central compartment and the leg allows proximal spread of infection.[4, 22]

PATHOLOGY

Tendon Disorders

Normal tendons usually have low signal on all pulse sequences, but this can vary with the magic-angle effect, which creates artificial increased signal in a tendon under certain circumstances (Fig. 4–8).[7] In the ankle, the posterior tibial and peroneal tendons are particularly susceptible to this effect. Absence of increased signal on T2 sequences and other associated pathologic findings help distinguish a normal from an abnormal tendon.

MRI is highly accurate in the evaluation of tendon injury. Tendon tears may be typed as follows: Type I is a partial tear with enlargement of the tendon; Type II is a partial tear with attenuation of the tendon; and Type III is a complete disruption with discontinuity of the tendon.[18] Generally, acute tears and tendinitis appear as a region of increased signal and focal swelling within a tendon. Subacute or chronic processes usually reveal focal or diffuse swelling with little alteration of signal in the tendon. In tenosynovitis, fluid completely surrounds a tendon or there is more fluid than is in the joint. A complete tear reveals a gap. A hematoma is seen in an acute tear, and fibrous tissue is seen in a chronic tear.[5]

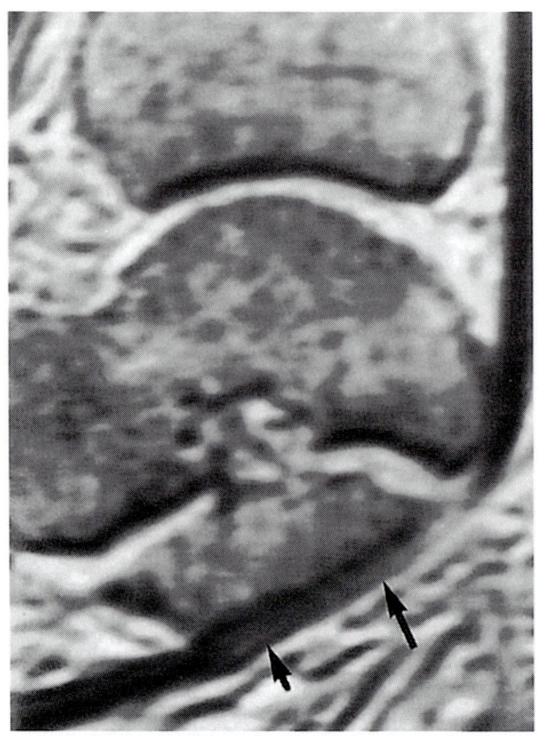

Figure 4–8
Reconstructed oblique sagittal image (TR/TE/flip = 37/min/15 degrees) in the long axis of the flexor hallucis tendon shows artifactual bright signal ("magic-angle" phenomenon) within a normal flexor hallucis longus as it passes beneath the sustentaculum talus (arrows). *(From Smith DK. Imaging of sports injuries of the ankle and foot. Oper Tech Sports Med 1995; 3:47-70.)*

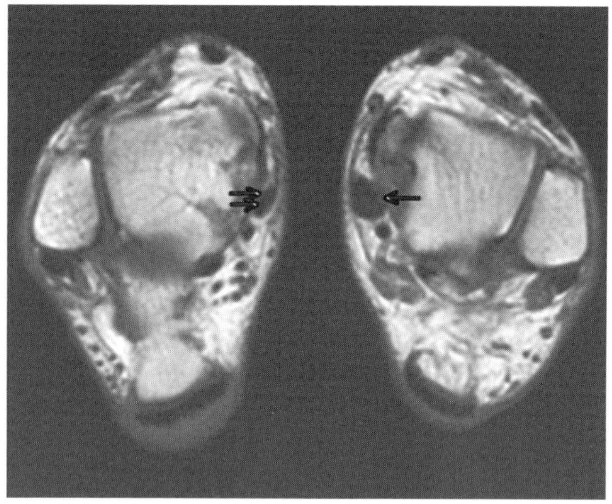

Figure 4–9
Axial T1 SE image, type-I posterior tibial tendon tear. *There is an enlarged left posterior tibial tendon with minimal intra-substance signal* (arrow). *Compare with normal right posterior tibial tendon* (arrows).

The posterior tibial tendon rupture classically occurs in women over the age of 50 who present with an acquired flatfoot deformity. Young athletes may also incur this injury in sports requiring rapid change in direction. Most tears occur between the medial malleolus and the navicular insertion. Early cases may be detected before complete disruption (Fig. 4–9). Several pitfalls exist. T1 sequences can show high signal because of fat between tendon slips inserting on the navicular. The tendon sheath itself ends 1 to 2 cm before the navicular insertion; therefore, fluid at that location is always abnormal. It is otherwise common for the sheath to have a small amount of fluid.[5, 18, 21]

The flexor hallucis longus tendon is particularly prone to inflammation (Fig. 4–10). Tenosynovitis and partial tears are especially common in ballet dancers. Similarly, tethering of the tendon between the posterior tibia and a prominent os trigonum may result in inflammation (os trigonum syndrome). Fluid is in the tendon sheath in 20% of normal persons with an ankle effusion; however, excessive fluid may indicate tenosynovitis. Clinical correlation is certainly important in this instance.[5, 22]

The anterior tibial tendon is frequently injured in downhill runners and hikers as an overuse phenomenon. Rupture is rare but may result in foot drop.[5]

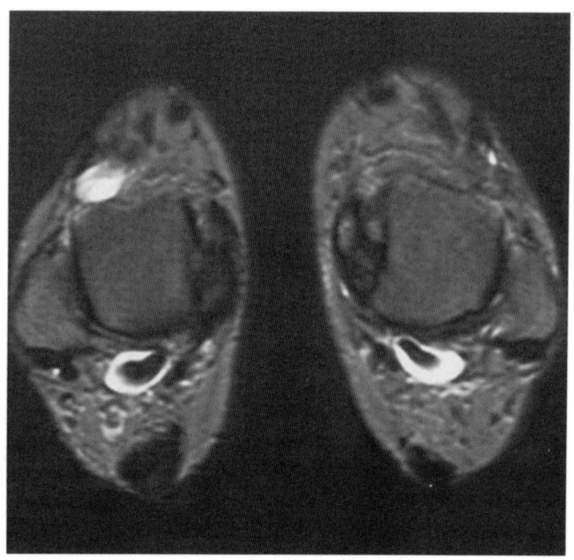

Figure 4–10
Axial T2 FSE image, bilateral flexor hallucis longus tenosynovitis. *Distention of both tendon sheaths of the flexor hallucis longus tendons is considerable and out of proportion to the amount of joint fluid seen at other levels.*

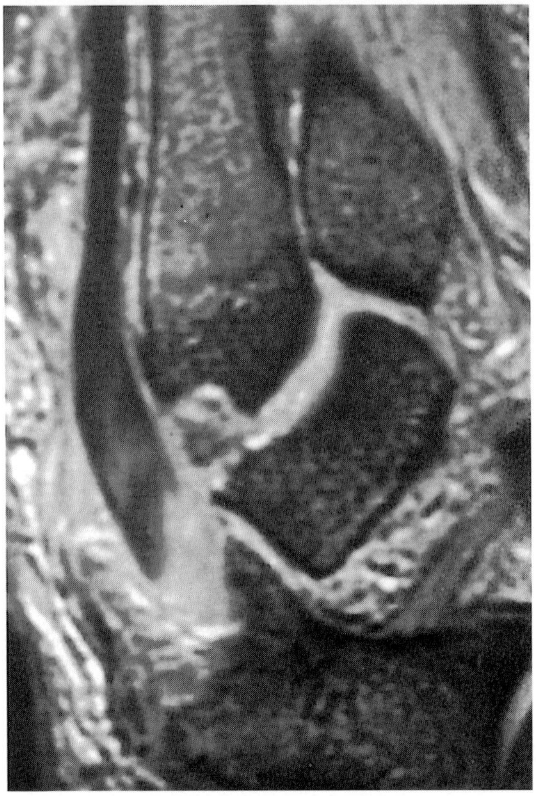

Figure 4–11
Reconstructed oblique sagittal image shows a full thickness tear of the peroneus brevis tendon with smooth enlargement and abrupt cut-off at the site of the tear. (From Smith DK. Imaging of sports injuries of the ankle and foot. Oper Tech Sports Med 1995; 3:47-70.)

The peroneal tendons are frequently afflicted with tenosynovitis. Fluid in the sheath may mimic a tear as it insinuates itself between the two tendons. These tendons are also prone to subluxation or dislocation with avulsion of the peroneal retinaculum, which can be sustained with either forced plantar flexion or dorsiflexion as might occur in skiing, soccer, or skating. A distal fibular fracture is common. A shallow or absent fibular groove also is possible. An injury to the peroneus brevis often occurs after an ankle sprain and is a frequent cause of chronic ankle pain following inversion injury (Fig. 4–11).[5, 22]

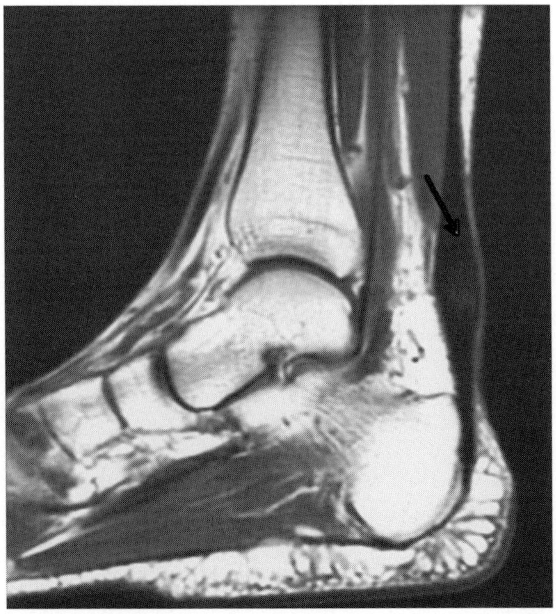

Figure 4–12
Sagittal T1 SE image, Achilles tendinitis. *There is fusiform swelling of the Achilles tendon* (arrow) *with minimal intra-substance signal.*

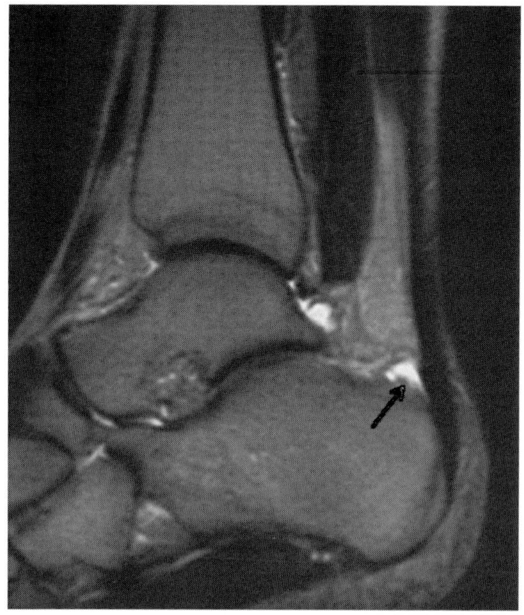

Figure 4–13
Sagittal T2 FSE image, retrocalcaneal bursitis. *There is a small focus of bright fluid* (arrow) *at the junction of the Achilles tendon and calcaneus.*

The Achilles tendon derives its fibers from the gastrocnemius and soleus muscles. It is the largest and strongest tendon. It has no tendon sheath. Tendinitis is common and occurs in running and jumping athletes (Fig. 4–12). Irritation near the insertion can result in retrocalcaneal bursitis, which mimics tendinitis (Fig. 4–13). A rupture of the tendon usually occurs in sedentary "weekend" athletes (Fig. 4–14). Both tendinitis and tears are most common in the least vascular portion of the tendon, several centimeters proximal to its calcaneal insertion. Sometimes it is difficult to clinically distinguish between complete and partial tendon ruptures and to determine the exact location of the rupture. MRI can offer the clinician the necessary information for appropriate management.[17, 21]

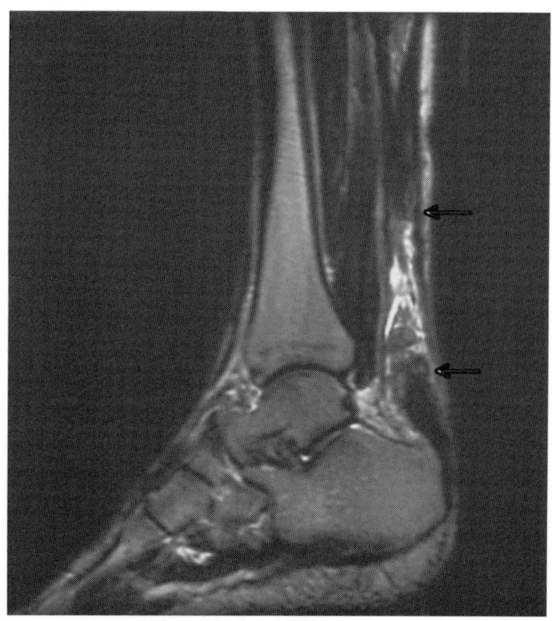

Figure 4–14
Sagittal T1 SE image, Achilles tendon rupture. *A large gap between the ends of the torn Achilles tendon* (arrows) *is filled with hematoma and fluid.*

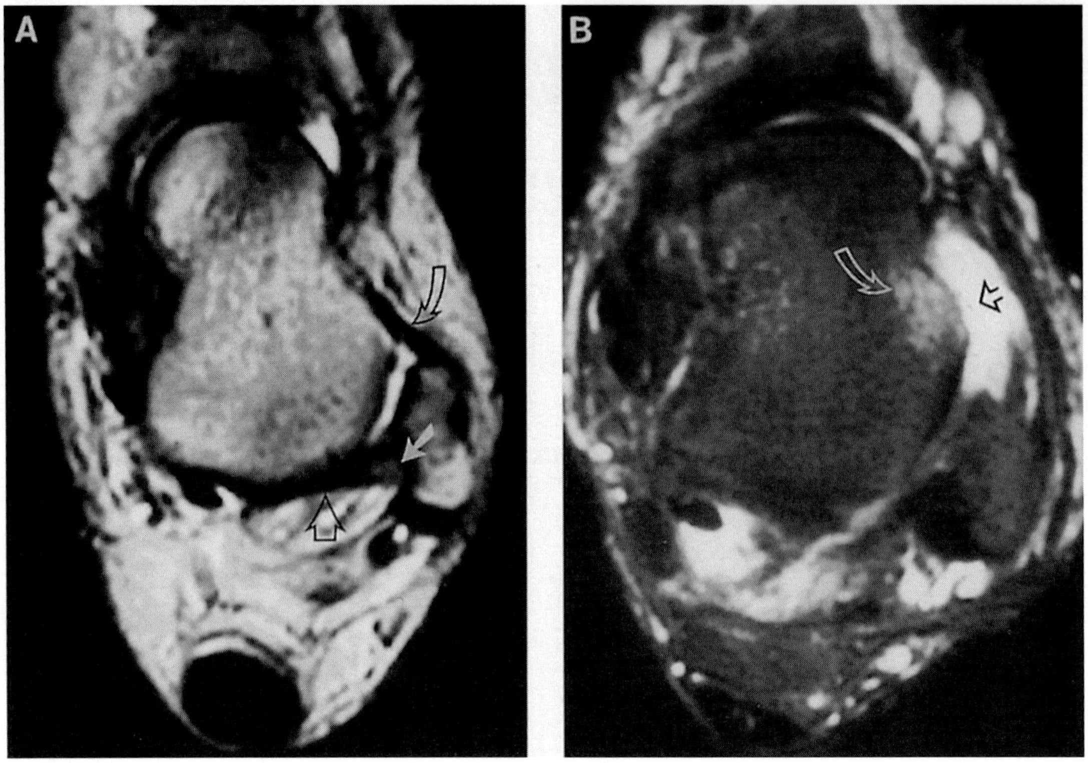

Figure 4–15
A, *Axial FSE T2-weighted magnetic-resonance image through the posterior concavity* (white arrow) *of the fibula at the level of the talar body shows intact anterior* (curved open arrow) *and posterior* (straight open arrow) *talofibular ligaments. Note that the fluid in the ankle joints abuts the posterior surface of the anterior talofibular ligament.* B, *Axial FSE T2-weighted magnetic-resonance image with fat suppression shows disrupted anterior talofibular ligament (ATFL,* open arrow*) with marrow edema* (curved open arrow: bright signal of the lateral talus). *(From Smith DK. Imaging of sports injuries of the ankle and foot. Oper Tech Sports Med 1995; 3:47-70.)*

Ligament Disorders

MRI findings of ligamentous injury include attenuation, thickening, irregularity, discontinuity, and complete absence of the ligament. Acutely, the soft tissues show high signal secondary to edema and hemorrhage on T2 sequences. Chronically, the soft tissues show low signal mass.[13, 19, 20]

The common ankle sprain results in injury to the lateral collateral ligament following inversion stress. The anterior talofibular, calcaneofibular, and posterior talofibular ligaments are injured progressively in accord with the severity of the sprain. Anterior talofibular ligament tears are equally frequent at the midsubstance of the tendon and at its insertion on the talus (Fig. 4–15).[9, 13, 19, 20]

The medial collateral (deltoid) ligament is injured less frequently. Tears, when they do occur, are often associated with ankle fractures. Sometimes the ligaments remain relatively intact, and a bony avulsion occurs. Such avulsion injuries may be easily overlooked using MRI alone (Fig. 4–16).[13, 14, 19, 20]

The anterior and posterior tibiofibular ligaments are usually associated with ankle fractures and other ligamentous injuries. They are rarely seen in isolation. A potential pitfall is that their appearance in cross-section on a sagittal image may mimic loose bodies.[13, 19, 20]

Tarsal Tunnel Syndrome

The tarsal tunnel is an osseofibrous tunnel bounded by the flexor retinaculum superficially and by the medial surfaces of the talus and calcaneus on its deep margin. The tunnel contents include the three flexor tendons on the medial aspect of the ankle and the posterior

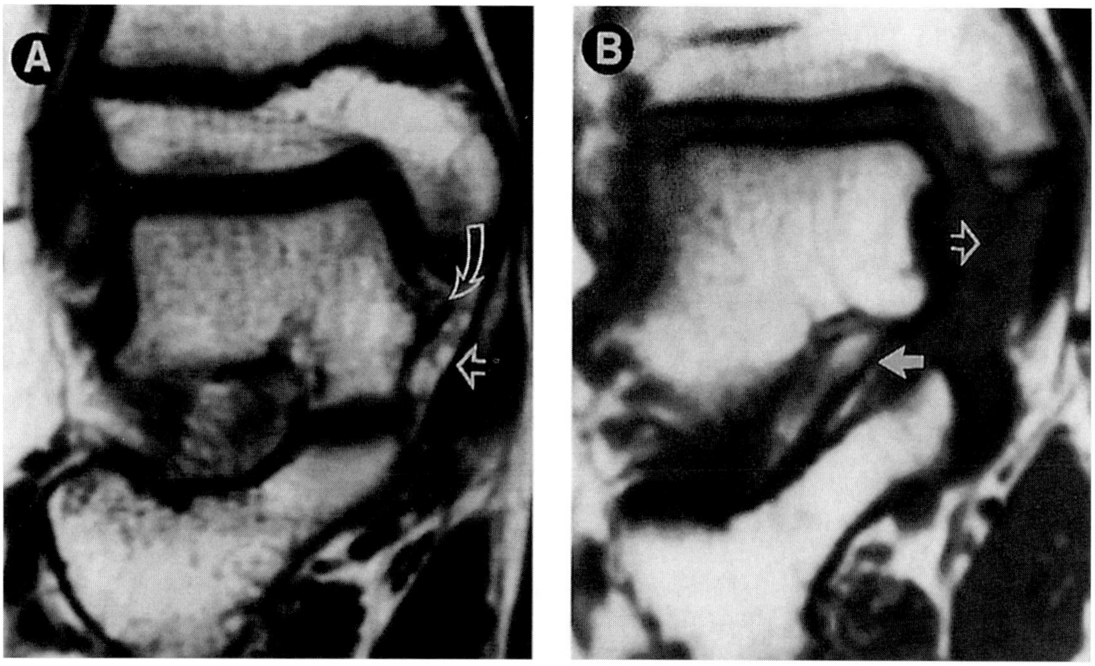

Figure 4–16
A, *Coronal T1-weighted image shows the normal attachment of the superficial deltoid ligament* (straight open arrow) *between the medial malleolus and sustentaculum talus, and the deep deltoid ligament* (curved open arrow) *between the medial malleolus and the medial aspect of the talus.* B, *Coronal T1-weighted image shows disruption of the superficial and deep deltoid fibers* (open arrow) *following ankle eversion injury. The talocalcaneal interosseous ligament* (closed arrow) *supports the subtalar joint along with the cervical ligament. (From Smith DK. Imaging of sports injuries of the ankle and foot. Oper Tech Sports Med 1995; 3:47-70.)*

tibial nerve, artery, and vein, as well as their branches. The axial and oblique axial planes are best for evaluation. Entrapment of the posterior tibial nerve or its branches beneath the flexor retinaculum is known as the tarsal tunnel syndrome. Symptoms include paresthesias in the heel and toes. MRI can accurately demonstrate the contents of the tunnel. Masses are responsible for the syndrome in approximately half of cases (Fig. 4–17). These masses include neural tumors, ganglia, and accessory muscles. Other causes include flexor tenosynovitis, post-traumatic fibrosis, thickening of the retinaculum, muscular hypertrophy, subtalar coalition, and varicose veins.[8, 12]

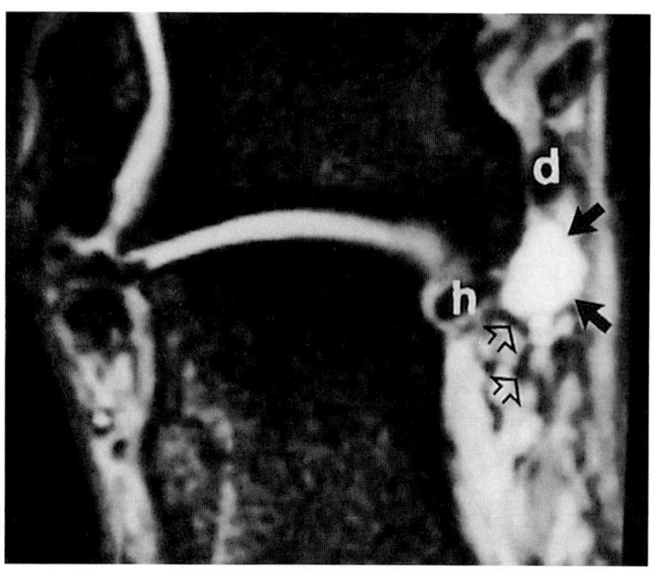

Figure 4–17
Coronal GRE image, ganglion. *A round cystic mass* (closed arrows) *is in the tarsal tunnel between the flexor digitorum* (d) *and the flexor hallucis* (h) *tendons. Plantar nerves* (open arrows) *are displaced inferiorly. (From Smith DK. Imaging of sports injuries of the ankle and foot. Oper Tech Sports Med 1995; 3:47-70.)*

Sinus Tarsi Syndrome

The tarsal sinus and canal is a cone-shaped area between the posterior subtalar joint and the talocalcaneonavicular joint. Internal structures are surrounded by fat and include five ligaments, most prominently the cervical and interosseous ligaments, as well as arteries, nerves, and joint capsule. The sinus tarsi syndrome usually is secondary to inflammation and hemorrhage from prior inversion injuries. Inflammatory arthritis is responsible for a smaller percentage of cases. The syndrome causes lateral foot pain that is increased with pressure over the lateral opening of the sinus tarsi. There is also a sense of instability of the hindfoot. MRI shows diffuse infiltration from fibrosis, chronic synovitis, synovial cysts, tears of the interosseous or cervical ligaments, or subchondral cysts at the insertion of the ligaments (Fig. 4–18).[15, 21]

Bone Trauma

MRI can detect not only the presence of an osteochondral lesion but also the stability of the fragment. Osteochondral injuries of the talus often are secondary to inversion injury with impaction of either the medial or the lateral talar dome against the tibia or fibula, respectively. These injuries, which are not typically diagnosed until after the initial injury, are distributed fairly evenly. Radiographic staging follows the criteria of Berndt and Harty.[3] Stage I is a compression fracture. Stage II is a partially avulsed bone fragment. Stage III is a totally avulsed but nondisplaced bone fragment. Stage IV is a completely avulsed and displaced bone fragment. On MRI, T1 and T2 sequences are useful in the evaluation. Fracture fragments are unstable if there is high signal between the fragment and the talar dome on T2 sequences (Fig. 4–19), or if there are subchondral cysts. One should look for high signal fluid, then, when assessing for Stage-II through Stage-IV injuries. On MRI, Stages II, III, and IV are suggested when fluid partially surrounds the fragment, completely surrounds the fragment, and fills the empty donor site, respectively. An intra-articular loose body should be sought in Stage-III cases.[3, 6]

Stress fractures occur in the foot and ankle. Common sites include the medial and lateral malleoli, calcaneus, navicular, and metatarsals. On MRI, stress fractures have a characteristic band of low signal surrounded by high-signal edema and hemorrhage on T2 sequences.

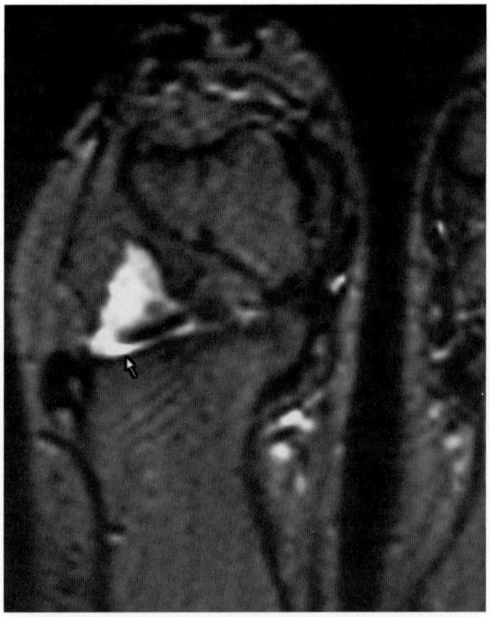

Figure 4–18
Coronal T2 FSE image, sinus tarsi syndrome. *The sinus tarsi is filled with bright signal fluid* (arrow), *presumably from chronic inflammation.*

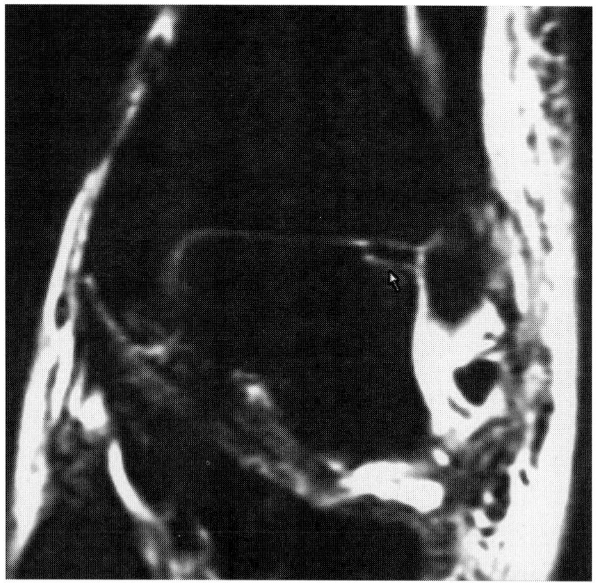

Figure 4–19
Coronal short tau inversion recovery (STIR) image, unstable OCD. *There is bright fluid* (arrow) *undermining the osteochondral defect fragment.*

Avascular Necrosis

Post-traumatic avascular necrosis of the talus and head of the second metatarsal can be well detected with MRI. Avascular necrosis can affect the talus as a complication of a fracture that interrupts the blood supply to the proximal talus. Spontaneous avascular necrosis can occur bilaterally in the tarsal navicular in patients with prior pes planus deformity. The MRI appearance is similar to that of lesions elsewhere, such as the femoral head. Such injuries typically reveal hypointense margins on T1 sequences and a double-line sign consisting of adjacent increased and decreased signal regions on T2 sequences.[10]

Tarsal Coalition

Calcaneonavicular and talocalcaneal coalition are the two most common types of coalition. Tarsal coalition is better studied with computed tomography, but MRI shows continuity of the cortex and bone marrow with their respective low and high signals on T1 sequences. A fibrous or cartilaginous coalition reveals relatively low-signal tissue on all sequences (Fig. 4–20).

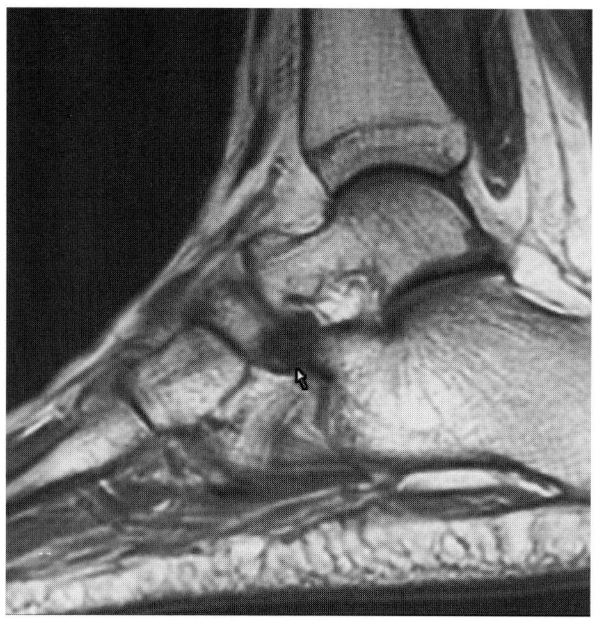

Figure 4–20
Sagittal T1 SE image, tarsal coalition. *An intermediate signal soft tissue fullness* (arrow) *spans the articulation of the calcaneus with the navicular tarsal bone.*

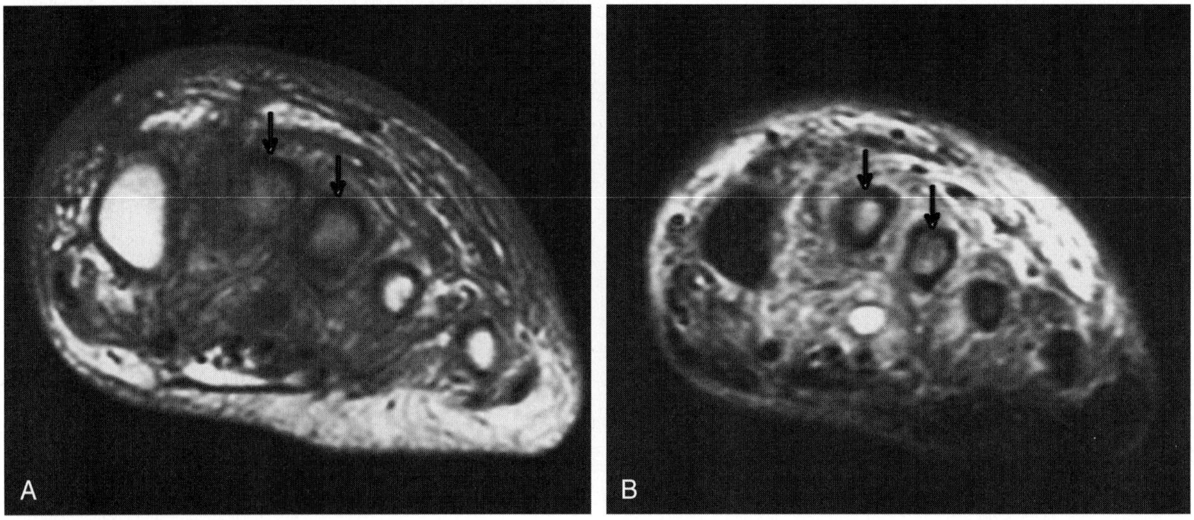

Figure 4–21
A, ***Coronal T1 SE image, osteomyelitis.*** *Signal from the bone marrow of the second and third metatarsals is depressed* (arrows). B, ***Coronal short tau inversion recovery (STIR) image.*** *The second and third metatarsals now reveal increased signal within the bone marrow* (arrows). *Also note the cellulitis.*

Osteomyelitis

Osteomyelitis typically occurs in diabetics with coexisting cellulitis and soft tissue edema. MRI is sensitive to this process (Fig. 4–21). Infected bone shows decreased signal in the bone marrow on the T1 sequence and increased signal on the T2 sequence. Signal visibility is improved with fat-saturation techniques on the proton-density or T2 sequence, the STIR technique, or fat saturation of the T1 sequence with utilization of gadolinium. Extensive bone-marrow involvement suggests osteomyelitis until proven otherwise. Minimal bone-marrow involvement may indicate only sympathetic edema from adjacent soft tissue infection.[1, 23]

Neoplasms

MRI is excellent in detecting neoplasms and delineating their extent—for example, whether they are confined to one compartment or extend to multiple compartments. Hemangiomas, aggressive fibromatosis, and sarcomas are typical foot neoplasms. The hemangioma characteristically appears as a striated or serpentine mass that is high in signal on the T1 sequence with respect to muscle and high in signal on the T2 sequence with respect to muscle and fat (Fig. 4–22). Small foci of low signal may represent phleboliths.[24] Aggressive fibromatosis is a benign lesion that presents as an ill-defined mass with regions of low signal on both T1 and T2 sequences attributed to dense collagen deposits.[16] Synovial sarcomas are relevant in the differential diagnosis of masses in this region because of their predilection for anatomic regions that have many tendons. Synovial sarcomas have been described as well circumscribed and uniformly high in signal on the T2 sequence.[11]

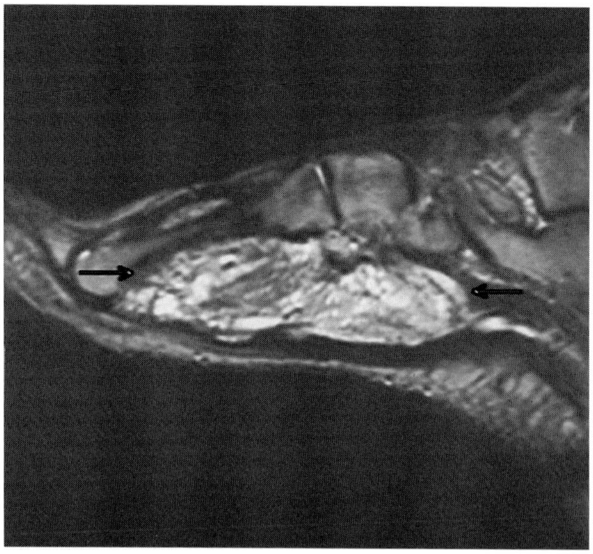

Figure 4–22
Sagittal T2 FSE image, hemangioma. *A large, high-signal soft tissue mass is in the plantar aspect of the foot* (arrows). *Plain radiography revealed soft tissue phleboliths.*

Plantar Fasciitis and Fibromatosis

Patients with plantar fasciitis complain about focal tenderness and heel pain over the medial calcaneal tuberosity. The plantar aponeurosis originates from the calcaneal tuberosity and is low in signal on MRI. The sagittal and coronal planes are best for MRI evaluation of this anatomy. Plantar fasciitis thickens the fascia, commonly at its insertion site to the medial calcaneal tuberosity. With respect to muscle, the fasciitis typically is similar in terms of signal on the T1 sequence and relatively low in signal on the T2 sequence. Any focal high signal on the T2 sequence likely indicates focal inflammation and edema (Fig. 4–23).[2]

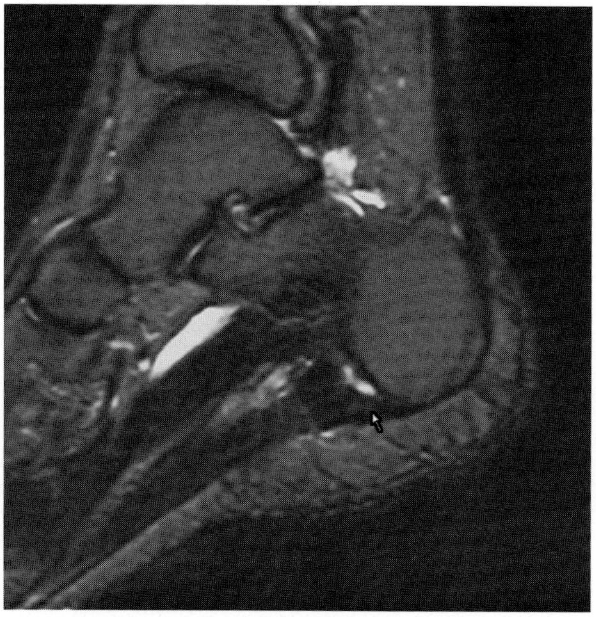

Figure 4–23
Sagittal T2 FSE image, plantar fasciitis. *A bright focus of signal is at the medial aspect of the plantar aponeurosis* (arrow), *suggesting inflammation.*

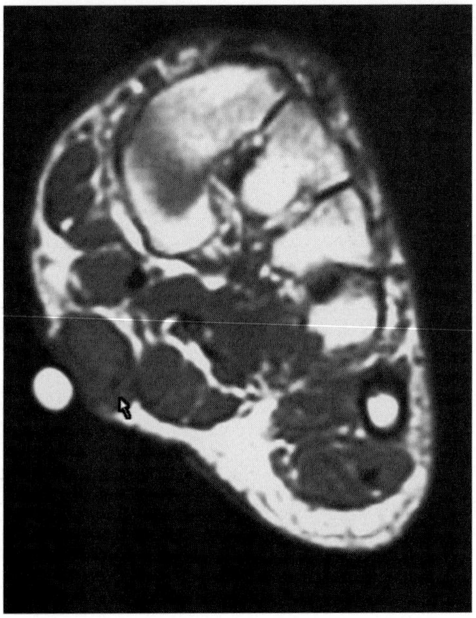

Figure 4–24
Coronal T1 SE image, plantar fibroma. *There is an intermediate-signal soft tissue mass* (arrow) *with small foci of dark signal, likely representing collagen deposits.*

Plantar fibromatosis is a benign condition. The course of the plantar fascia undergoes nodular thickening that is often evident clinically. MRI reveals a mass with low-signal regions on both T1 and T2 sequences secondary to dense collagen deposits (Fig. 4–24).

Morton's Neuroma

Morton's neuromas are common entities that are well evaluated by either ultrasonography or MRI. The neuroma is a focal mass of fibrosis due to swelling and neuritis of the plantar digital nerves secondary to compression between the metatarsal heads. MRI reveals a small mass low in signal on both the T1 and the T2 sequences at this level. They are relatively easier to see on the T1 sequence, although edema and intermetatarsal bursal distention are best seen on the T2 sequence. The appearance of these neuromas is enhanced following intravenous administration of gadolinium, and they are well delineated on the T1 sequence with fat suppression (Fig. 4–25).

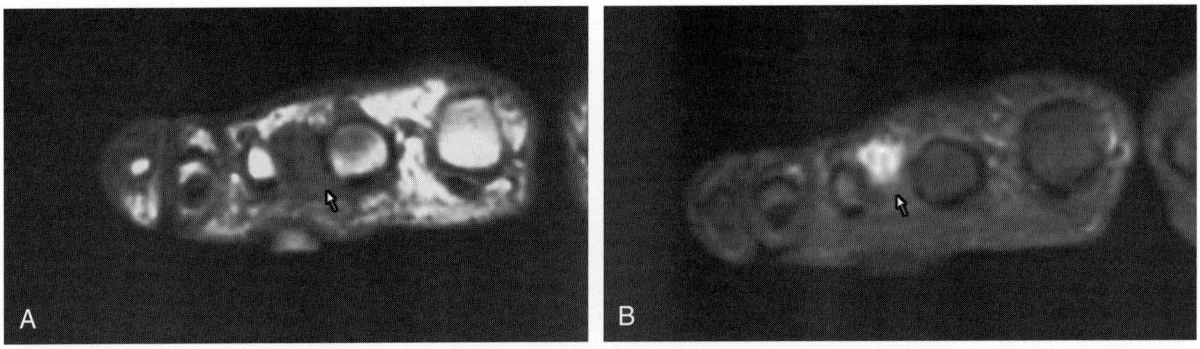

Figure 4–25
A, ***Coronal T1 SE image, Morton's neuroma.*** *A region of intermediate-signal mass* (arrow) *is between the second and third intermetatarsal spaces.* B, ***Coronal T1 SE image with fat suppression after the intravenous administration of gadolinium.*** *This intermetatarsal mass is now enhanced* (arrow).

References

1. Beltran J, Campanini DS, Knight C, et al. The diabetic foot: Magnetic resonance imaging evaluation. Skel Radiol 1990; 19:37-41.
2. Berkowitz JF, Kier R, Rudicel S. Plantar fasciitis: MR imaging. Radiology 1991; 179:665-667.
3. Berndt AL, Harty M. Transchondral fractures (osteochondritis dissecans) of the talus. J Bone Joint Surg [Am] 1959; 41:988-1020.
4. Chan WP, Rauschning W, Wu CY. Magnetic resonance imaging anatomy and cryomicrotome atlas. *In* Chan WP, Lang P, Genant HK, eds. MRI of the Musculoskeletal System. Philadelphia: WB Saunders, 1994.
5. Cheung Y, Rosenberg ZS, Magee T, et al. Normal anatomy and pathologic conditions of ankle tendons: Current imaging techniques. Radiographics 1992; 12:429-444.
6. DeSmet AA, Fisher DR, Burnstein MI, et al. Value of MR imaging in staging osteochondral lesions of the talus (osteochondritis dissecans): Results in 14 patients. AJR 1990; 154:555-558.
7. Erickson SJ, Cox IH, Hyde JS, et al. Effect of tendon orientation on MRI signal intensity: A manifestation of the "magic angle" phenomenon. Radiology 1991; 181:389-392.
8. Erickson SJ, Quinn SF, Kneeland JB, et al. MR imaging of the tarsal tunnel and related spaces: Normal and abnormal findings with anatomic correlation. AJR 1990; 155:323-328.
9. Erickson SJ, Smith JW, Ruiz ME, et al. MR imaging of the lateral collateral ligament of the ankle. AJR 1991; 156:131-136.
10. Haller J, Sartoris DJ, Resnick D, et al. Spontaneous osteonecrosis of the tarsal navicular in adults: Imaging findings. AJR 1988; 151:355.
11. Keigley BA, Haggar AM, Gaba A, et al. Primary tumors of the foot: MR imaging. Radiology 1989; 171:755-759.
12. Kerr R, Frey C. MR imaging in the tarsal tunnel syndrome. J Comput Assist Tomogr 1991; 15:280-286.
13. Kier R, Dietz MJ, McCarthy SM, et al. MR imaging of the normal ligaments and tendons of the ankle. J Comput Assist Tomogr 1991; 15:477-482.
14. Klein MA. MR imaging of the ankle: Normal and abnormal findings in the medial collateral ligament. AJR 1994; 162:377-383.
15. Klein MA, Spreitzer AM. MR imaging of the tarsal sinus and canal: Normal anatomy, pathologic findings, and features of the sinus tarsi syndrome. Radiology 1993; 186:233-240.
16. Quinn SF, Erickson SJ, Dee PM, et al. MR imaging in fibromatosis: Results in 26 patients with pathologic correlation. AJR 1991; 156:539-542.
17. Quinn SF, Murray WT, Clark RA, et al. Achilles tendon: MR imaging at 1.5T. Radiology 1987; 164:767-770.
18. Rosenberg ZS, Cheung Y, Jahss M, et al. Rupture of the posterior tibial tendon: CT and MR imaging with surgical correlation. Radiology 1988; 169:229-235.
19. Schneck CD, Mesgarzadeh M, Bonakdarpour A, et al. MR imaging of the most commonly injured ankle ligaments. Part I. Normal anatomy. Radiology 1992; 184:499-506.
20. Schneck CD, Mesgarzadeh M, Bonakdarpour A, et al. MR imaging of the most commonly injured ankle ligaments. Part II. Ligament injuries. Radiology 1992; 184:507-512.
21. Steinbach LS, Tirman PF. MRI of the ankle. Radiologist 1995; 2:111-125.
22. Stoller DW. The ankle and foot. *In* Stoller DW, ed. Magnetic Resonance Imaging in Orthopaedics and Sports Medicine. Philadelphia: JB Lippincott, 1993.
23. Yuh WT, Corson JD, Baraniewski HM, et al. Osteomyelitis of the foot in diabetic patients: Evaluation with plain film, ^{99m}TC-MDP bone scintigraphy, and MR imaging. AJR 1989; 152:795-800.
24. Yuh WT, Kathol MH, Sein MA, et al. Hemangiomas of skeletal muscle: MR findings in five patients. AJR 1987; 149:765-768.

Ankle Arthroscopy

Ankle arthroscopy is now a well-established diagnostic and therapeutic tool. The popularity of this technique may have been delayed because placing and maneuvering the arthroscope is difficult in this joint. Advances in distraction devices and arthroscopic equipment and techniques have extended the indications for arthroscopy of the ankle. Drez and associates,[1] Ferkel,[4] Guhl,[6] Morgan,[8] and others have done much to advance ankle arthroscopy.

INDICATIONS

The most accepted indication for ankle arthroscopy is removal of loose bodies. This is uncommon but may be a result of osteochondritis dissecans or traumatic osteochondral injuries. These lesions, recently reclassified,[7] can be debrided or repaired with arthroscopic techniques (Fig. 4–26). Synovial or osteophytic impingement is perhaps the most common indication for ankle arthroscopy.[2, 5, 10] Another procedure that is gaining acceptance is

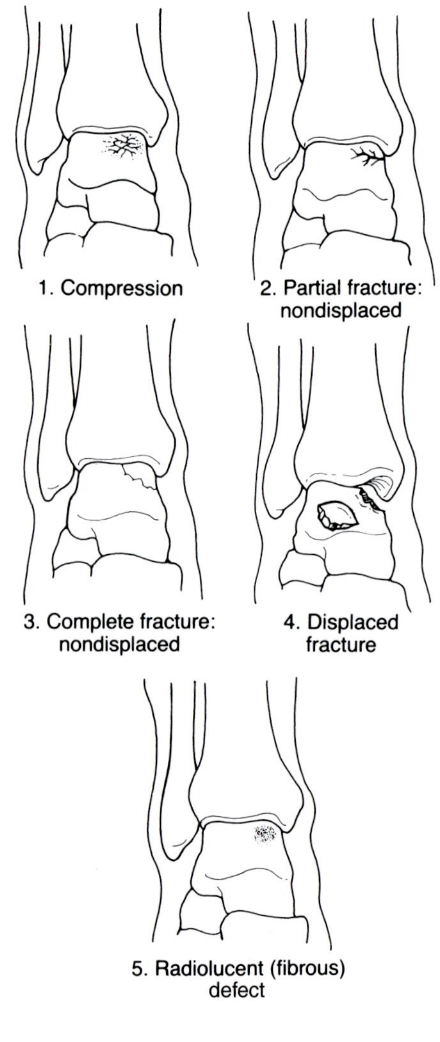

Figure 4–26
Loomer and associates' modification to the Berndt-Harty classification of osteochondral lesions of the talus. (From Miller MD, Cooper DE, Warner JJP. Review of Sports Medicine and Arthroscopy. Philadelphia: WB Saunders, 1995.)

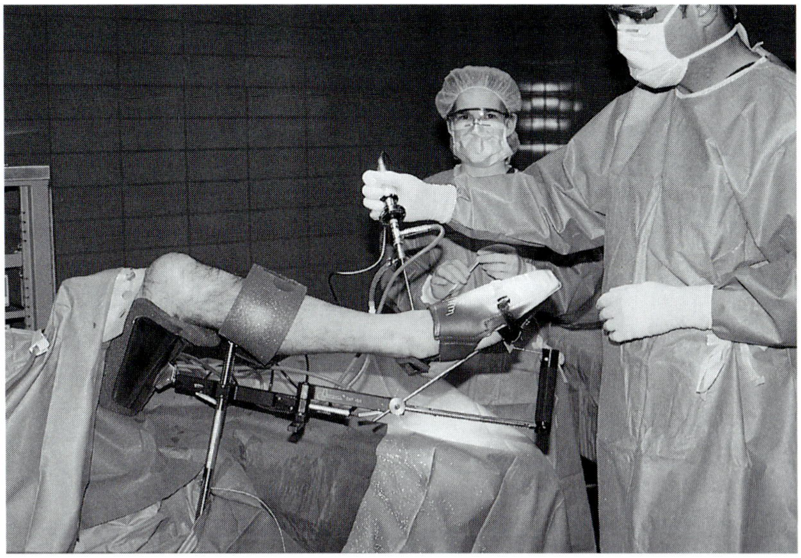

Figure 4–27
Commercially available ankle distractor in place.

arthroscopically assisted tibiotalar arthrodesis.[9] Other relative indications for ankle arthroscopy include adjunctive treatment of fractures, stabilization procedures, and synovectomy for rheumatologic conditions.

POSITIONING AND PORTAL PLACEMENT

Most surgeons perform ankle arthroscopy with the patient supine. Several commercially available ankle distracters are available and provide enough distraction for adequate visualization (Fig. 4–27). Alternatively, the patient's knee and leg can be positioned over the end of the operating table, and a gauze-bandage loop can be fashioned as the surgeon's foot provides a distraction force.[11] The standard 4.0-mm arthroscope can be used for most procedures, although smaller arthroscopes (2.7-mm) may be helpful for areas that are more difficult to visualize (e.g., the posterior ankle). A 3.5-mm diameter shaver is often helpful for ankle arthroscopy.

The most commonly used portals are the anteromedial and anterolateral portals.[3] The anteromedial portal is placed just medial to the tibialis anterior tendon at the level of the ankle joint. A spinal needle helps to localize this site and instill saline into the joint. The anterolateral portal is established just lateral to the peroneus tertius tendon at the joint line level (Fig. 4–28). The "nick and spread" technique helps to establish these portals in order to ensure that superficial nerves and veins are avoided. A posterolateral portal, placed just lateral to the Achilles tendon, can be used for outflow or occasionally to visualize the posterior ankle. A 70 degree arthroscope placed through an anterior portal usually provides adequate visualization of the posterior ankle, however. Because of significant neurovascular risk, the anterocentral (dorsalis pedis and deep peroneal nerve) and posteromedial (posterior tibial artery, tibial nerve) portals are usually not recommended.

ARTHROSCOPIC ANATOMY

The anterolateral portal is most commonly used for visualization. The joint should be systematically evaluated (Fig. 4–29). The lateral sulcus and tip of the fibula can usually be visualized. The medial sulcus and tip of the medial malleolus is best seen with the arthroscope placed in the anteromedial portal. Pathology is addressed as necessary.

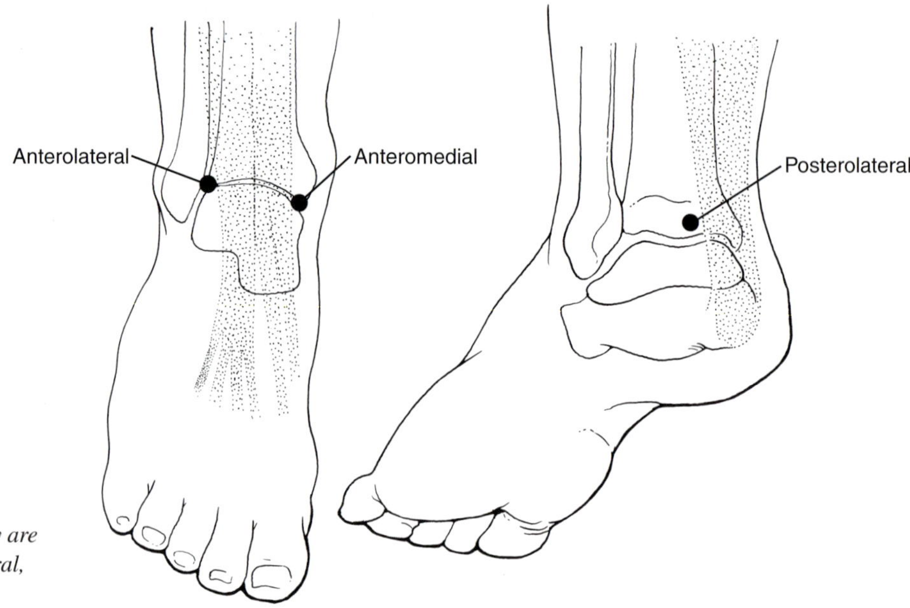

Figure 4–28
Portals for ankle arthroscopy are the anteromedial, anterolateral, and posterolateral.

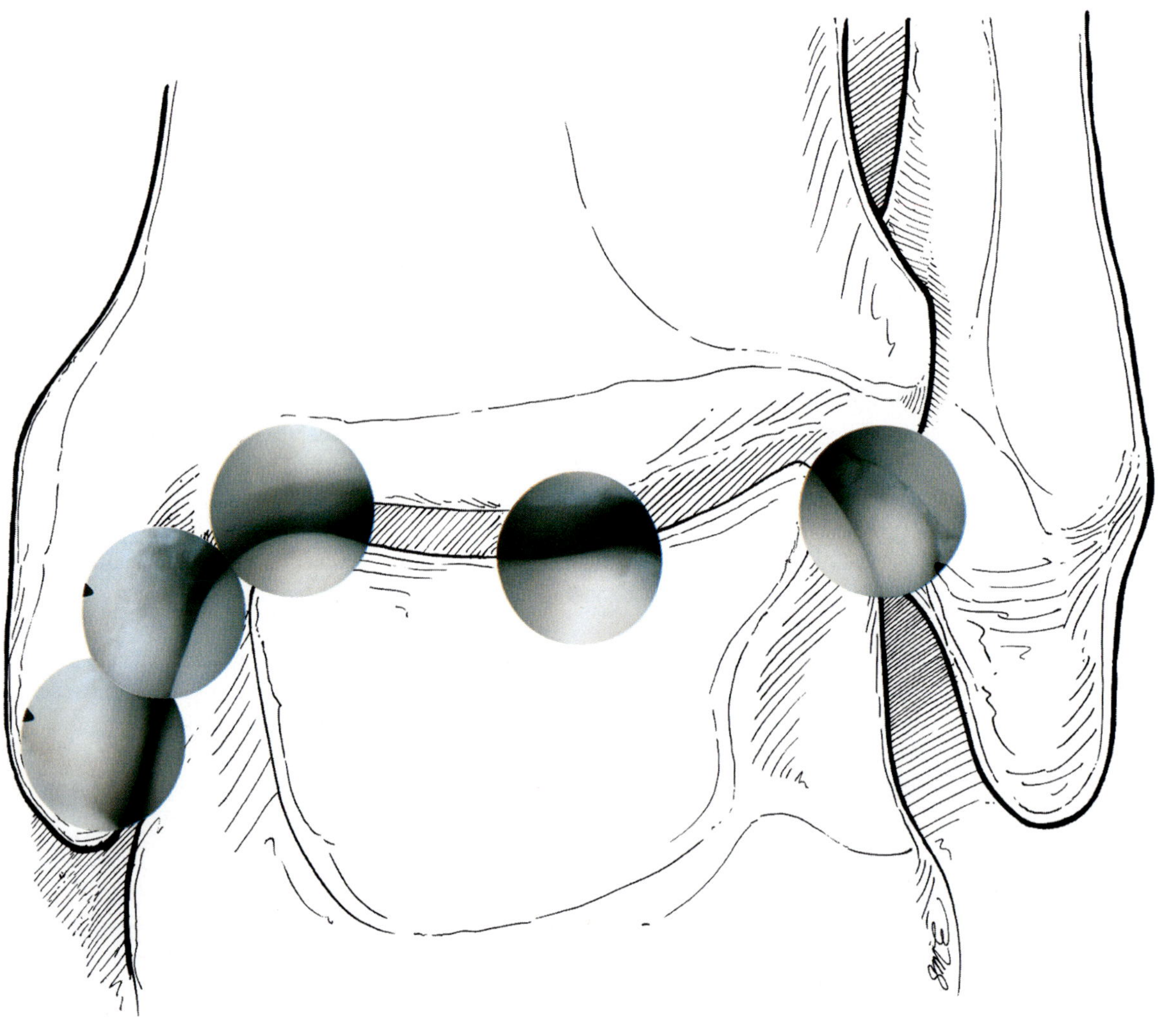

Figure 4–29
Arthroscopic anatomy of the ankle.

COMPLICATIONS

Complications may be related to portal placement. Injury to sensory nerves, especially the intermediate branch of the superficial peroneal nerve, can be a problem. Synovial fistulas are more common than in the knee because of a smaller soft tissue envelope. The use of a bulky soft tissue dressing for a week reduces the risk of synovial fistulas.[3] Articular cartilage injury can easily occur in this joint, also because of the lack of maneuverability. Additional care is required.

References

1. Drez D, Guhl JF, Gollehon DL. Ankle arthroscopy: Technique and indications. Foot Ankle 1981; 2:138-142.
2. Ewing JW. Arthroscopic management of transchondral talar dome fractures (osteochondritis dissecans) and anterior impingement lesions of the ankle joint. Clin Sports Med 1991; 10:677-687.
3. Ewing JW, Tasto JA, Tippett JW. Arthroscopic surgery of the ankle. Inst Course Lect 1995; 44:325-340.
4. Ferkel RD, Fischer SP. Progress in ankle arthroscopy. Clin Orthop 1989; 240:210-220.
5. Ferkel RD, Karzel RP, Del Pizzo W, et al. Arthroscopic treatment of anterolateral impingement of the ankle. Am J Sports Med 1991; 19:440 446.
6. Guhl JF. Arthroscopic advances: New techniques for arthroscopic surgery of the ankle. Orthopedics 1986; 9:261-269.
7. Loomer R, Fisher C, Lloyd-Smith R, et al. Osteochondral injuries of the talus. Am J Sports Med 1993; 21:13-19.
8. Morgan CD. Gross and arthroscopic anatomy of the ankle. *In* McGinty JB, ed. Operative Arthroscopy. New York: Raven Press, 1991, pp 677-694.
9. Ogilvie-Harris DJ, Lieverman I, Fitsalos D. Arthroscopically assisted arthrodesis for osteoarthritic ankles. J Bone Joint Surg [Am] 1993; 75:1167-1174.
10. Thein R, Eichenblat M. Arthroscopic treatment of sports-related synovitis of the ankle. Am J Sports Med 1992; 20:496-499.
11. Yates C, Grana W. A simple distraction technique for ankle arthroscopy. Arthroscopy 1988; 4:103-105.

Illustrative Cases—Ankle

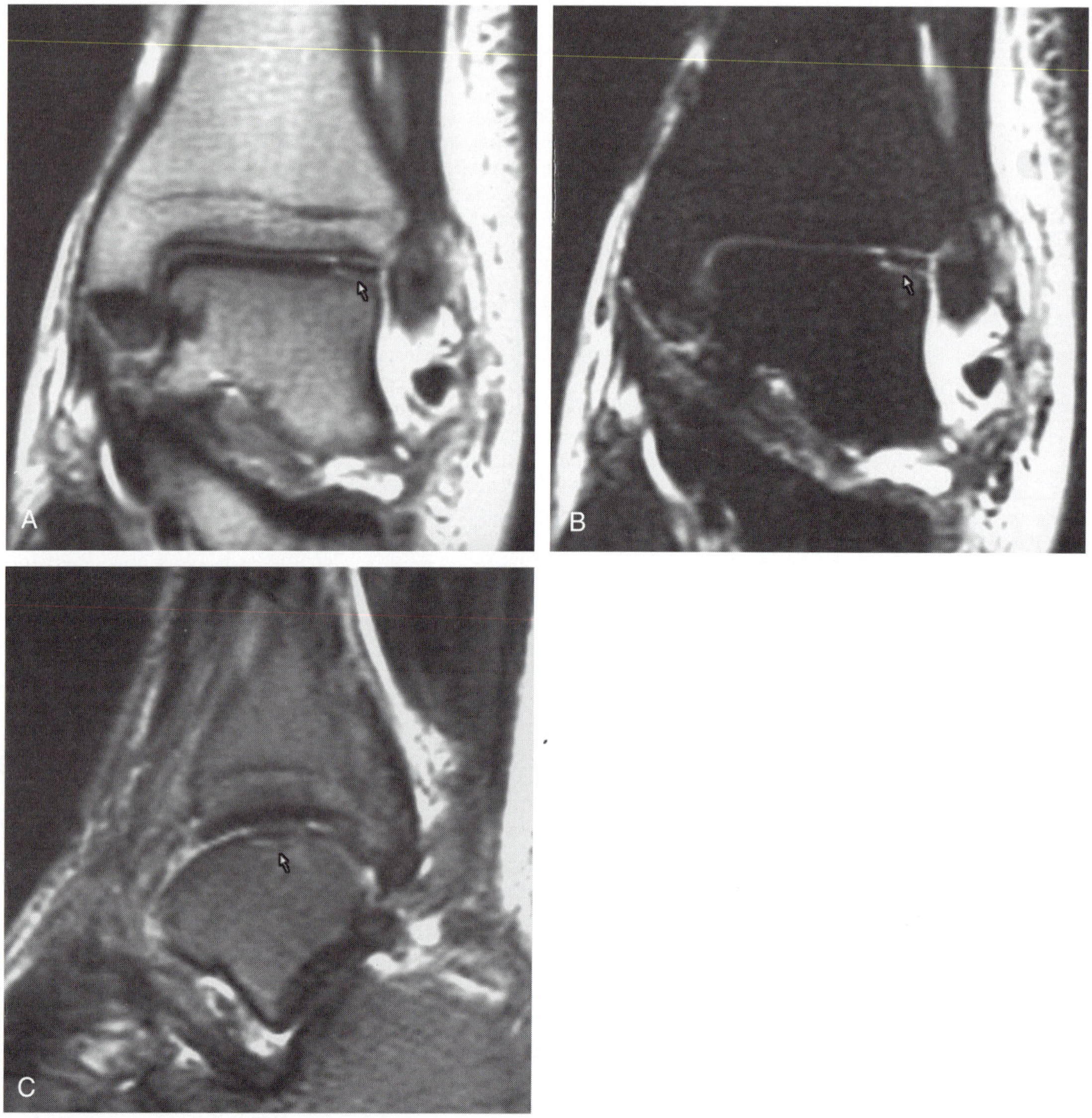

Figure 4–30. **Osteochondral Injury, Left Ankle**
A, *Coronal FSE T2-weighted image shows bright signal* (arrow) *surrounding dark signal in the osteochondral fragment, lateral talar dome.* B, *Coronal STIR image shows similar findings* (arrow). C, *Sagittal FSE T2 weighted image shows this injury* (arrow).

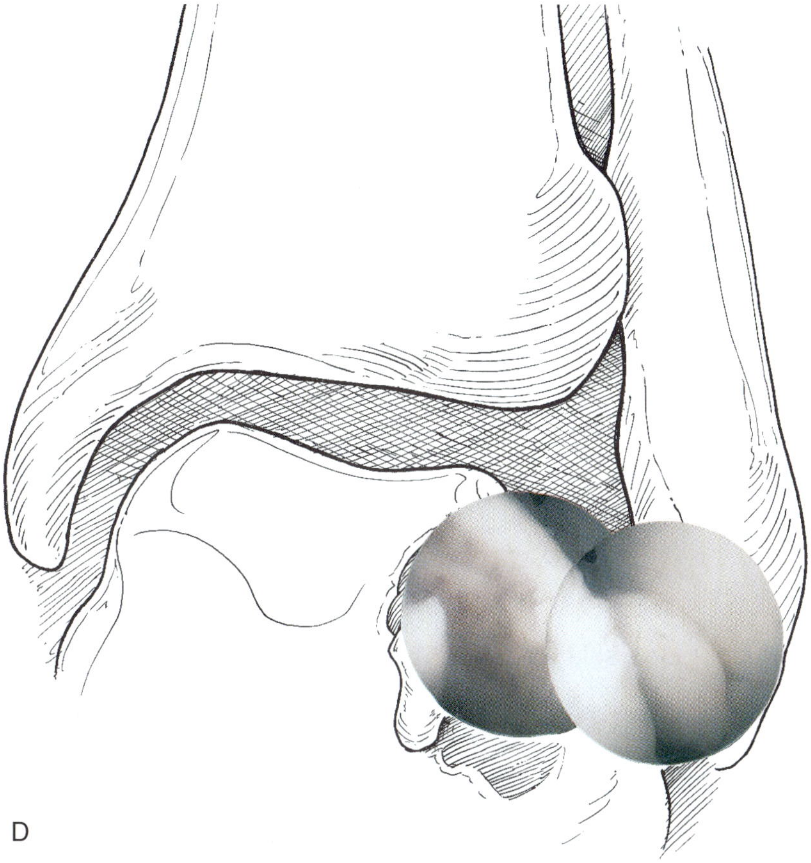

D

Figure 4–30. **Osteochondral Injury, Left Ankle, continued**
D, *Arthroscopic image demonstrates an osteochondral defect in the lateral talar dome.*

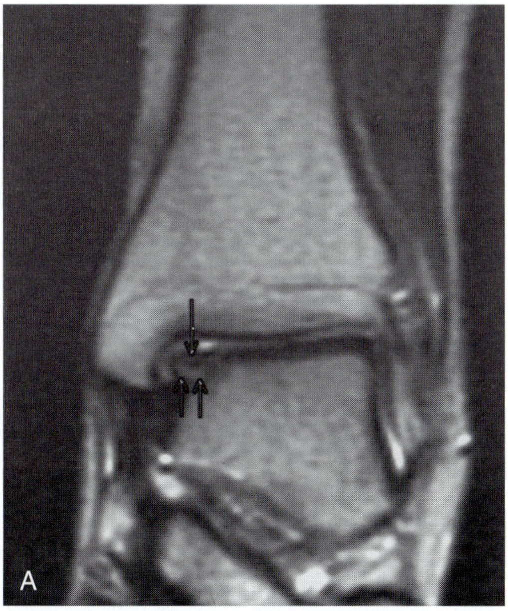

A

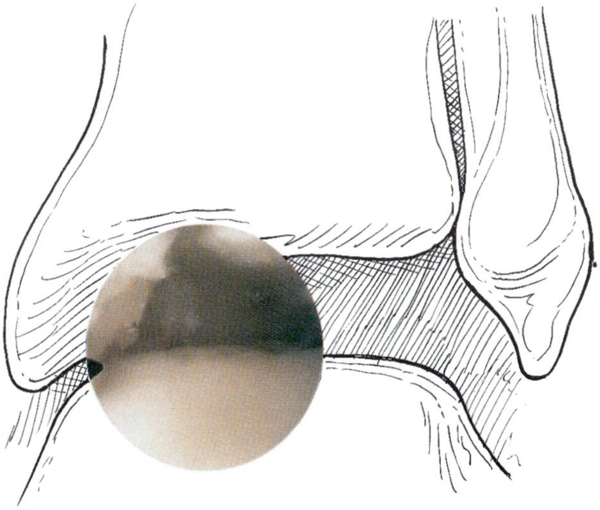

B

Figure 4–31. **Osteochondral Defect, Left Ankle**
A, *Coronal FSE T2-weighted image demonstrates an osteochondral flap* (arrow) *with dark signal intensity. Curvilinear bright signal (representing fluid) underlines the inferior aspect of the fragment* (double-arrow). B, *Arthroscopic image shows the osteochondral injury to the medial talar dome.*

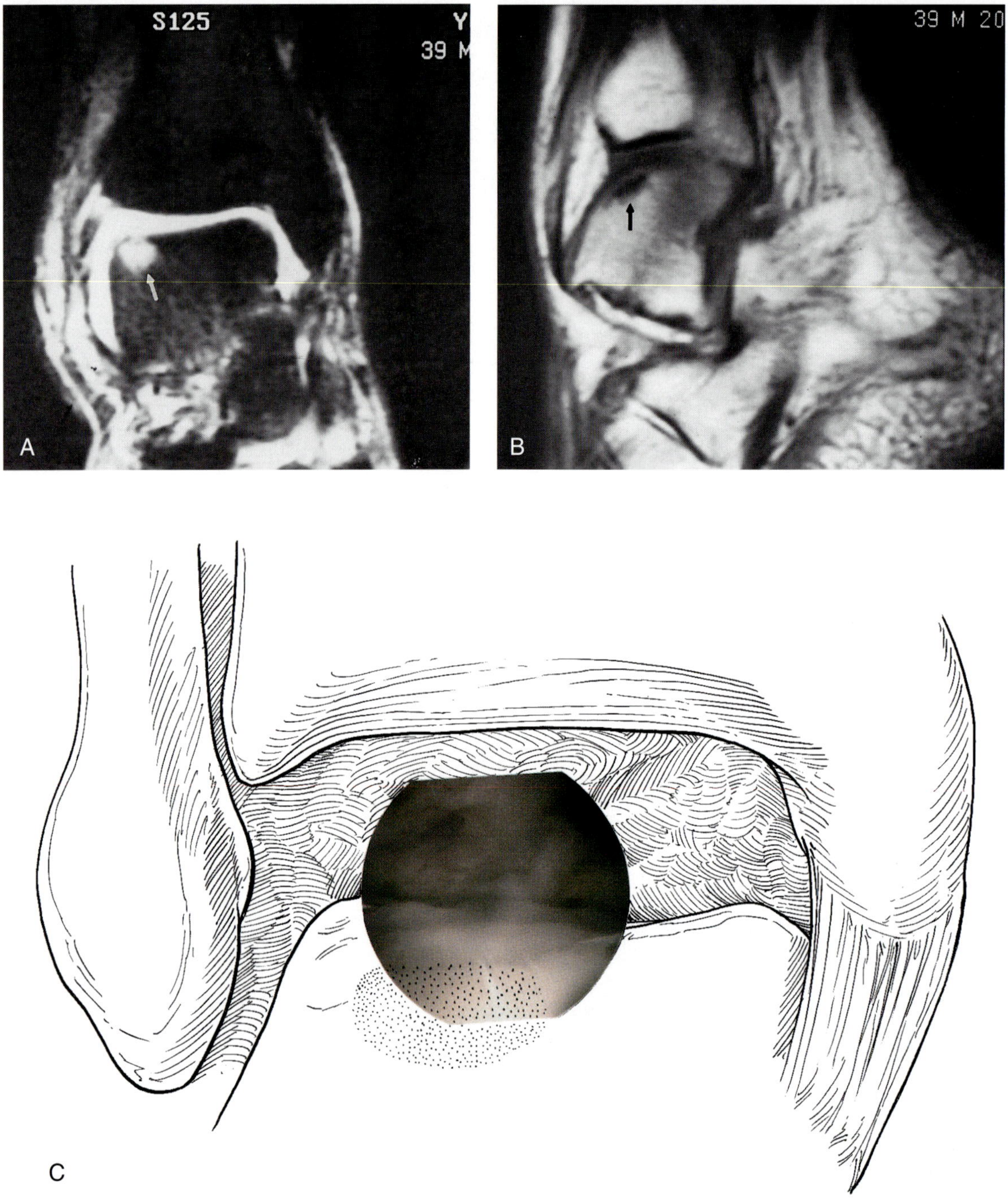

Figure 4–32. **Fibrous Osteochondral Defect, Right Ankle**
A, *Coronal STIR image shows round focus of bright signal* (arrow) *in the lateral talar dome. Note the subtle adjacent articular irregularity.* B, *Sagittal T1-weighted SE image shows a focal region of dark signal intensity* (arrow) *in this area.* C, *Arthroscopic view demonstrates the irregularity of the talar surface as viewed from the anteromedial portal.*
Case courtesy of Steven F. Conti, M.D.

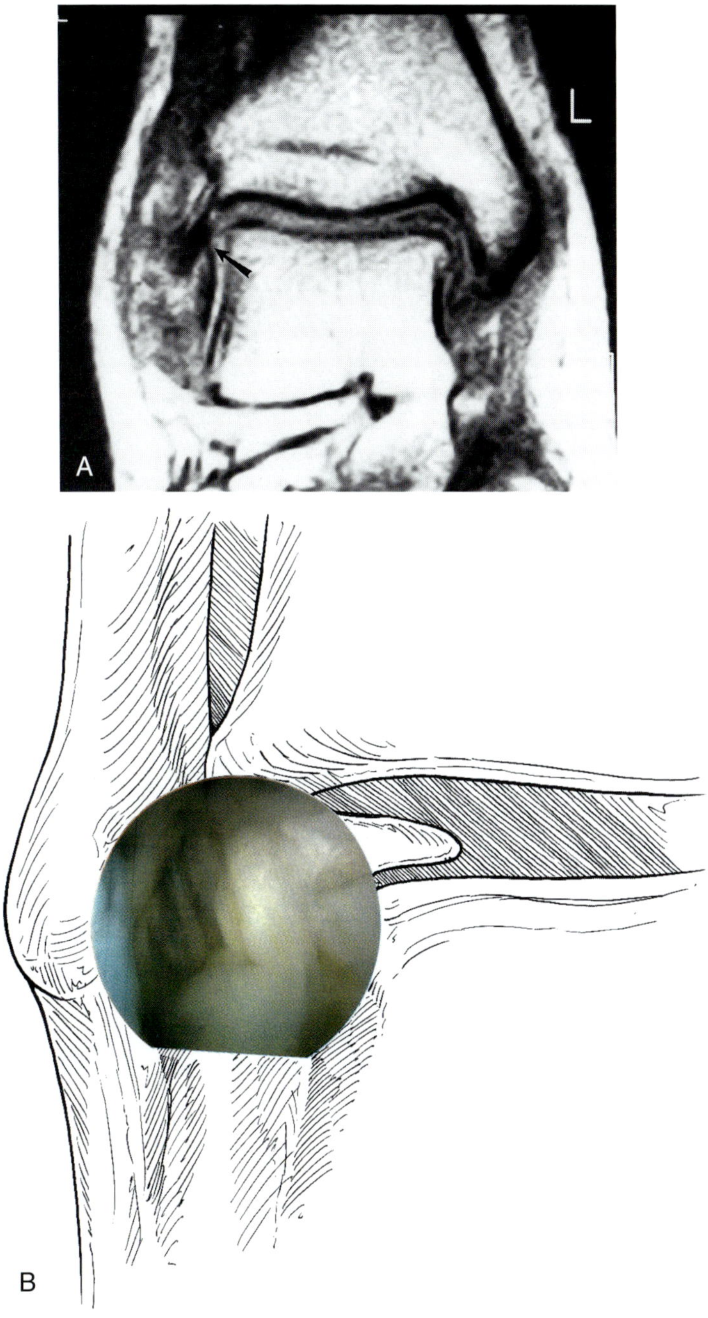

Figure 4–33. **Synovial Impingement "Meniscoid" Lesion, Right Ankle**
A, *Coronal T1-weighted SE image reveals a thickened area of intermediate signal intensity* (arrow) *between the lateral talar dome and the articular surface of the tibia.* B, *Arthroscopic image demonstrates the proliferative synovium and meniscoid or "Duke" lesion in the lateral talar dome.*
Case courtesy of Michael G. Maday, M.D.

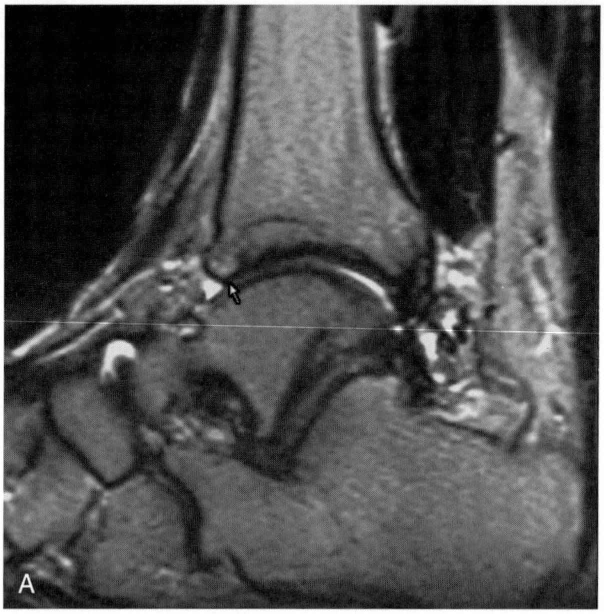

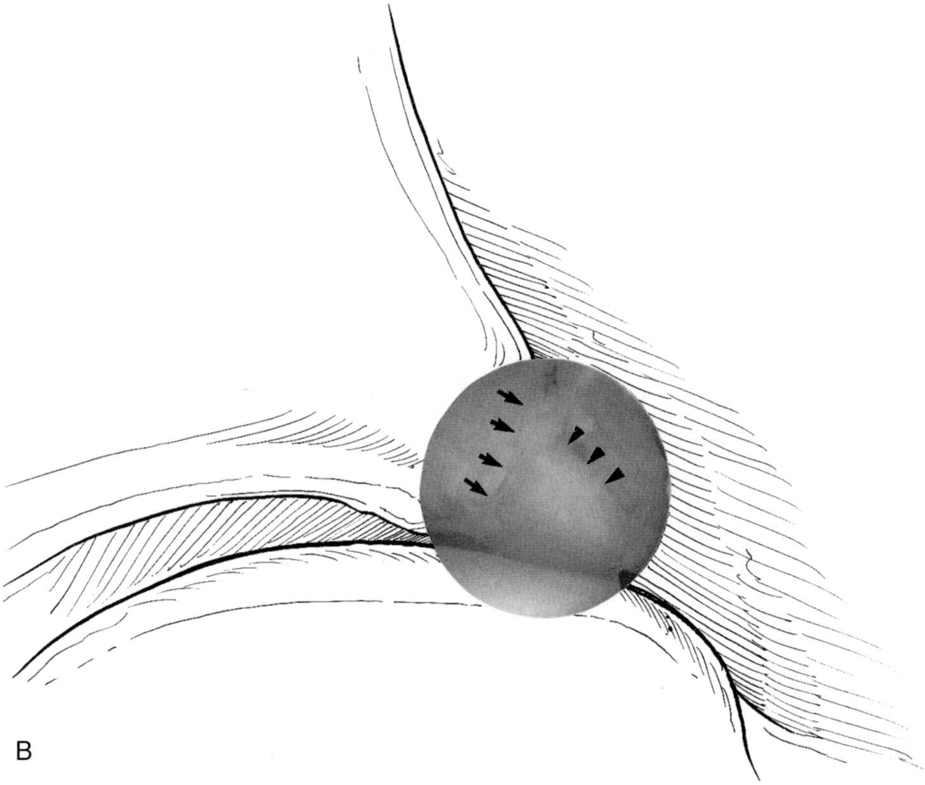

Figure 4–34. **Tibiotalar Impingement, Anterior Tibia (Spur), Right Ankle**
A, *Sagittal FSE T2-weighted image shows a bony prominence of the tibia* (arrow) *at the anterior margin of the tibiotalar joint.* B, *Arthroscopic view of large "shelf" off the anterior tibia. Arrows represent normal anterior aspect of the tibia. Arrowheads outline the anterior tibial spur.*

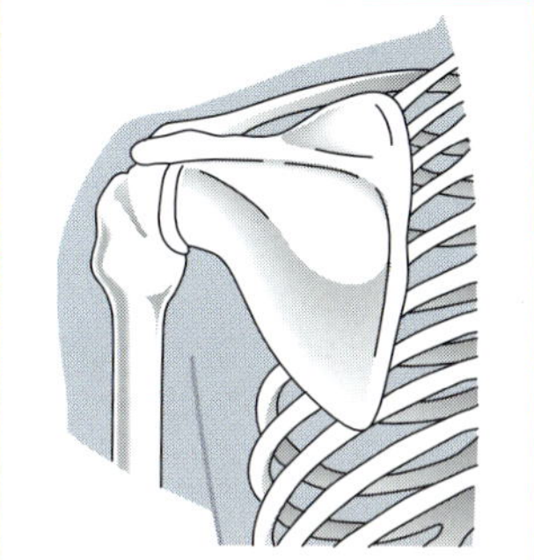

CHAPTER

5

Shoulder

MRI of the Shoulder

MRI is a reliable tool in the diagnosis of rotator cuff disease[7, 20] and labral tears.[12] It also helps in the diagnosis and evaluation of osteonecrosis, bone and soft tissue tumors, and other musculoskeletal disease in the shoulder region.

At times, it is difficult to know precisely which imaging method is best to evaluate the numerous problems arising in the shoulder region, but in all instances of shoulder pain, the initial examination should be routine radiography. MRI, as mentioned, is excellent for impingement, rotator cuff tear, and tendinitis. MRI, computed tomography, and arthrography probably have similar advantages for the evaluation of instability; therefore, the choice of modality might be a matter of preference or equipment availability. Arthrography is best for adhesive capsulitis.

Finally, although MRI is an excellent way to evaluate patients with refractory shoulder symptoms, it must be remembered that the information yielded by MRI can be detected in both symptomatic and asymptomatic persons; therefore, the clinical significance of this information can only be determined by the clinician.

TECHNIQUE

A standard MRI protocol utilizing three orthogonal planes is best for most examinations. Spin-echo coronal oblique, sagittal oblique, and axial sequences are adequate. The axial sequence is reviewed for the image that best depicts the supraspinatus muscle and tendon for orientation of the coronal oblique sequence. The sagittal oblique sequence is obtained in a plane perpendicular to that of the oblique coronal set.

A surface coil (Fig. 5–1), thin sections (3 to 4 mm), a small field of view (between 12 and 16 cm), and off-axis imaging are needed for good contrast and spatial resolution. The arm should be comfortably immobilized in neutral or slight external rotation. The precise sequence parameters—for example, fast spin-echo (FSE), gradient recalled-echo (GRE), and the use of fat saturation—depend on the protocol and equipment. The T1 and proton-density sequences provide excellent anatomic detail, and the T2 sequence indicates fluid

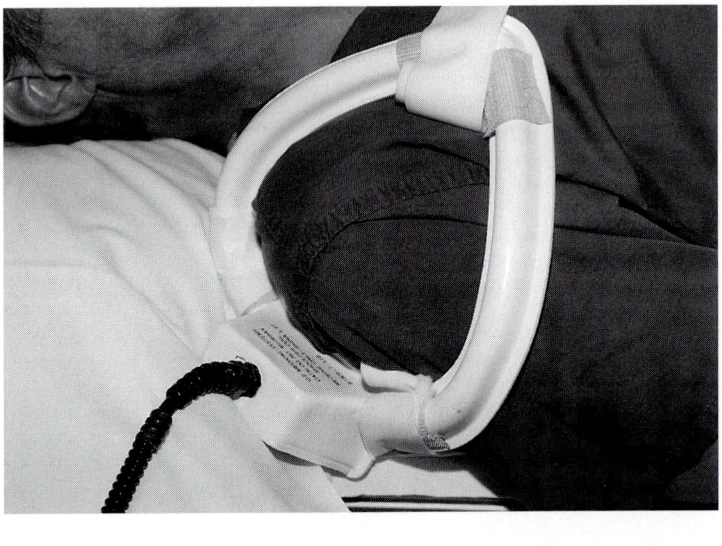

Figure 5–1
Shoulder surface coil (receive only).

location. Although most pathology is evident on the T2 sequence, at least one sequence should be T1 because of the possibility of unsuspected bone-marrow disease such as an infarct, a tumor, or infection. These entities are often most conspicuous on the T1 sequence.

Protocols may vary among institutions; therefore, a comment about alternative sequences, such as FSE, GRE, and fat suppression technique, is relevant.

FSE significantly reduces the image acquisition time, but these images are prone to edge-blurring artifacts that are worsened with shorter echo times, decreased phase encodings, and increased echo train lengths; therefore, FSE is not as good for anatomic detail on proton-density imaging. A 192 or 256 matrix and an echo train length of no more than 8 should be used to reduce image blurring. Also, fat can be confused with fluid if the repetition and echo times are similar to those used in conventional spin-echo imaging (2000/70). Longer repetition and echo times (3500/100) should be used to reduce fat-fluid isointensity.[2]

Fat-suppression or fat-nulling techniques have been applied to shoulder imaging to include fat-saturation and short tau inversion recovery techniques. Both techniques reduce the signal-to-noise ratio of the received signal. The fat-saturation technique works well with magnetic resonance arthrograms of the shoulder.[11]

The GRE sequence can successfully image the rotator cuff, but there are some limitations. The absence of the 180-degree refocusing pulse results in more artifact, and image quality decreases as one tries to obtain more heavily T2-weighted images. Finally, signal in the tendons often is relatively greater, confusing the interpretation of these images with regard to tears.[2]

MRI ANATOMY

MRI anatomy of the shoulder is well displayed in the axial, coronal oblique, and sagittal oblique planes (Figs. 5–2, 5–3, 5–4, and 5–5).

The scapula is a flat, triangular bone. The superior and inferior angles are at the medial and inferior apices of the bone, respectively. The glenoid fossa is at the remaining apex. The coracoid process is an anterior hook of bone arising near the anterior corner of the glenoid. The scapular notch is a small groove in the superior border of the scapula at the medial base of the coracoid. The suprascapular nerve wraps around the scapular notch, innervating the supraspinatus muscle, and continues inferiorly through the spinoglenoid notch to innervate the infraspinatus muscle. Local cysts or ganglions in this location can compress the nerve and cause shoulder pain and atrophy of one or both muscles.[8] The acromion arises from the spine of the scapula and continues laterally to form a posterior hook of bone.

The scapula is particularly important in understanding the nomenclature of the rotator cuff. The scapular spine divides the dorsal aspect of the scapula into supraspinous and infraspinous fossae. Two important muscles of the rotator cuff, the supraspinatus and the infraspinatus muscles, are related to the spine. The ventral aspect of the scapula consists of a flat region called the subscapularis fossa. This is the origin of the subscapularis muscle. The fourth and last muscle of the rotator cuff is the teres minor, a small muscle below the infraspinatus muscle (see Fig. 5–5). The tendons of the four muscles of the rotator cuff blend together at the glenohumeral joint and form the conjoint tendon of the rotator cuff. The humeral head articulates with the scapula at the glenoid fossa. The joint would be unstable because the humeral head is much larger than the glenoid fossa, but the rotator cuff muscles, the biceps, and the joint capsule stabilize the joint. The humeral head has a greater and a lesser tuberosity, separated by the bicipital groove. The subscapularis muscle is the only muscle inserting on the lesser tuberosity. It provides internal rotation of the humeral head. The supraspinatus, infraspinatus, and teres minor muscles insert on the greater tuberosity. The supraspinatus muscle allows for abduction of the humerus and assists in external rotation. The infraspinatus and teres minor muscles provide for external rotation of the humeral head. The long head of the biceps muscle slides in the synovia

Text continues on page 146

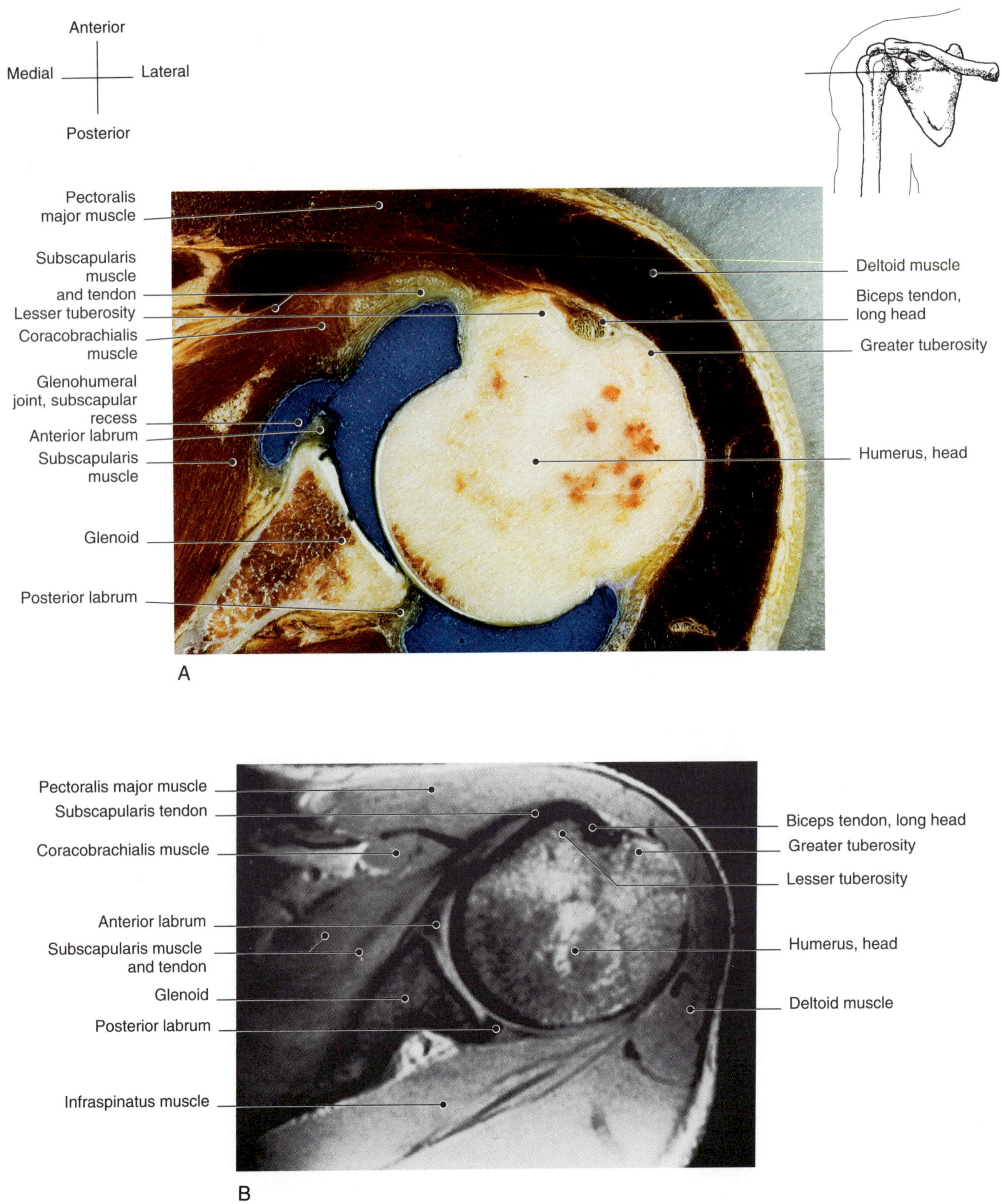

Figure 5–2

Axial cryoplaned section (A) *and MRI* (B) *of the shoulder at the level of the glenohumeral joint. (From Chan WP, Rauschning W, Wu CY, et al. Magnetic resonance imaging anatomy and cryomicrotome atlas.* In *Chan WP, Lang P, Genant HK, eds. MRI of the Musculoskeletal System. Philadelphia: WB Saunders, 1994.)*

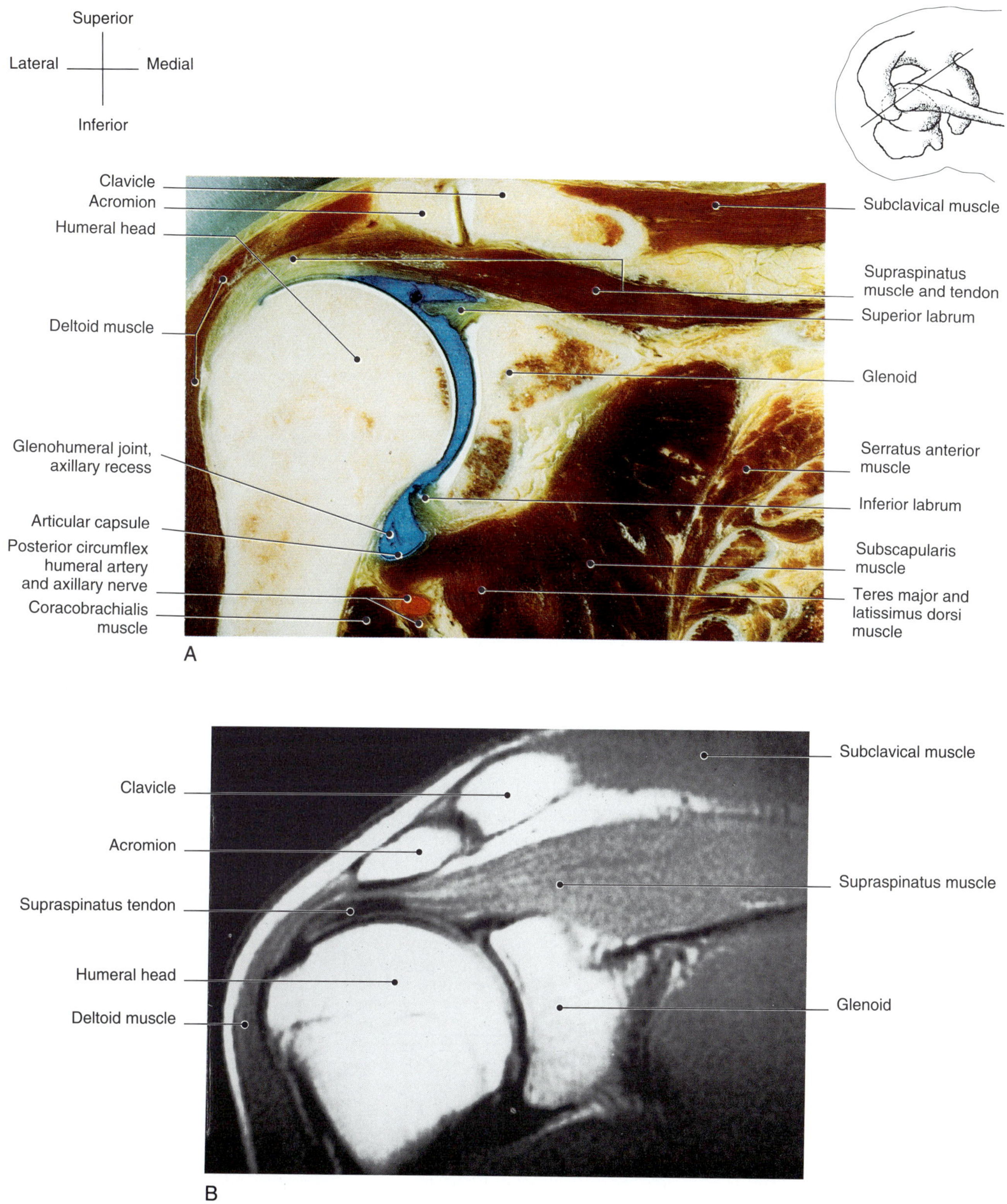

Figure 5–3

Oblique coronal cryoplaned section (A) *and MR image (TR, 1000 ms; TE, 20 ms)* (B) *of the shoulder parallel to the supraspinatus muscle and tendon. (From Chan WP, Rauschning W, Wu CY, et al. Magnetic resonance imaging anatomy and cryomicrotome atlas.* In *Chan WP, Lang P, Genant HK, eds. MRI of the Musculoskeletal System. Philadelphia: WB Saunders, 1994.)*

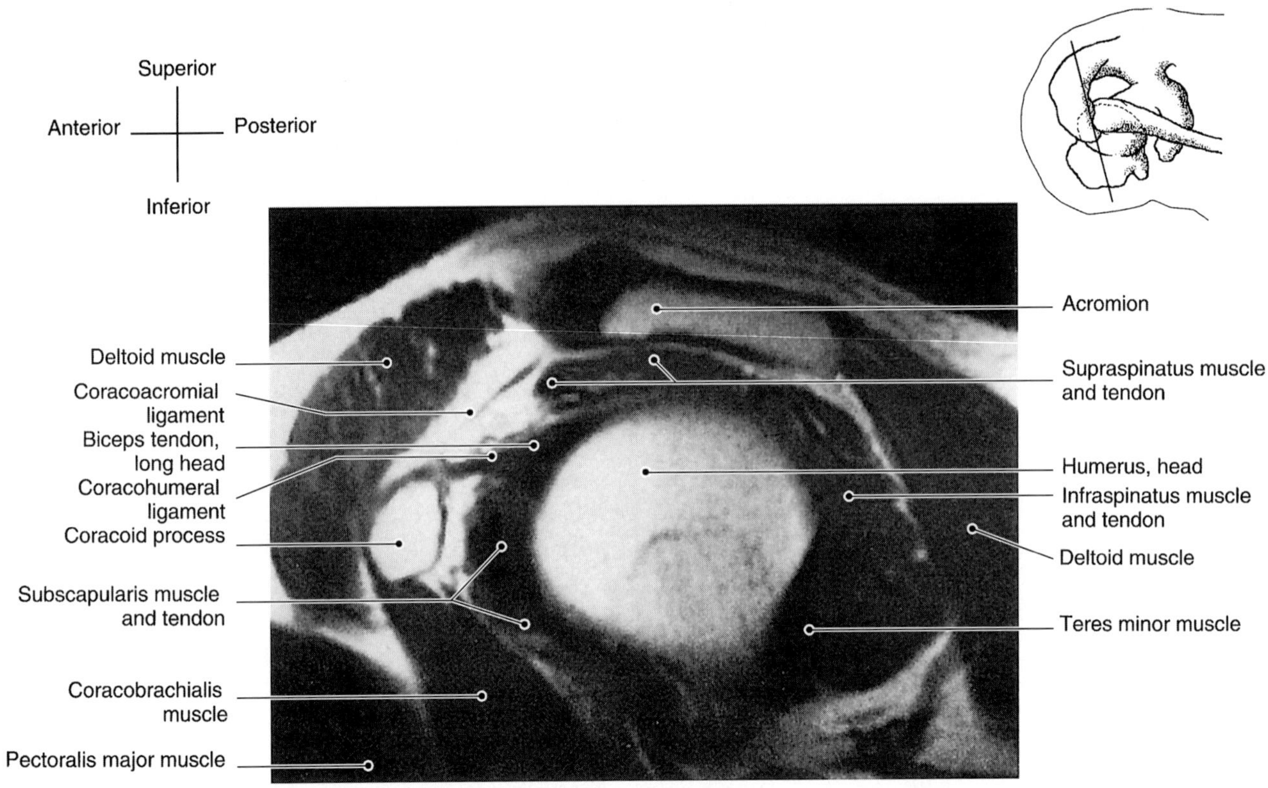

Figure 5–4
Oblique-sagittal MR image (TR, 800 ms; TE 20 ms) of the shoulder at the level of the coracoid process. (From Chan WP, Rauschning W, Wu CY, et al. Magnetic resonance imaging anatomy and cryomicrotome atlas. In *Chan WP, Lang P, Genant HK, eds. MRI of the Musculoskeletal System. Philadelphia: WB Saunders, 1994.)*

lined sheath of the bicipital groove and blends into the superior and anterior margin of the glenoid labrum. The bicipital groove communicates with the shoulder joint and normally may contain a small amount of fluid. The short head of the biceps and the coracobrachialis muscles insert on the tip of the coracoid process.

The shoulder capsule contains the humeral head and inserts onto the bony glenoid. The glenoid labrum is part of the capsule, originating as a redundant thickening of the cap-

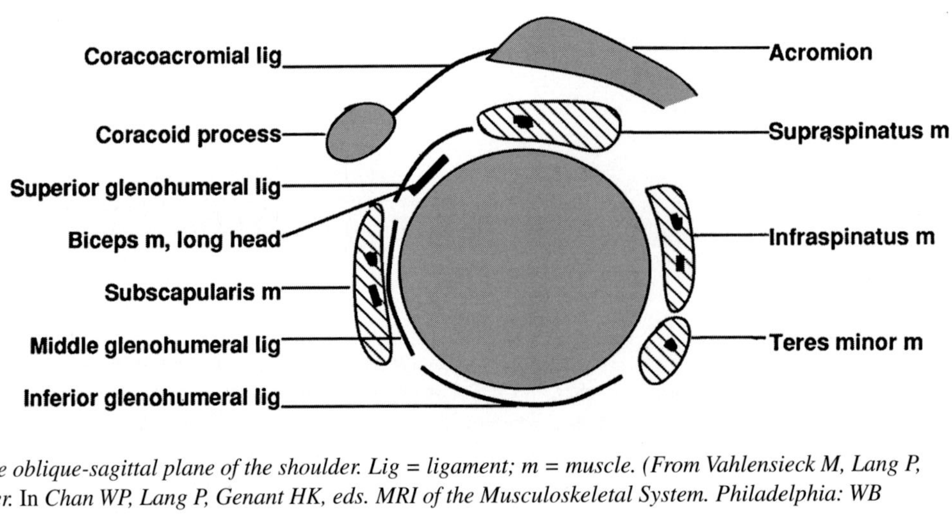

Figure 5–5
Schematic drawing of the oblique-sagittal plane of the shoulder. Lig = ligament; m = muscle. (From Vahlensieck M, Lang P, Genant HK. The shoulder. In *Chan WP, Lang P, Genant HK, eds. MRI of the Musculoskeletal System. Philadelphia: WB Saunders, 1994.)*

sule itself. Three fibrous bands at the anterior portion of the capsule (superior, middle, and inferior glenohumeral ligaments) provide additional stability. The middle glenohumeral ligament is often seen on MRI at or below the level of the coracoid process. Capsular folds create a series of communicating recesses. The axillary recess is a redundancy at the inferior and medial aspect of the glenohumeral joint. The subscapular recess is located between the scapula and subscapularis tendon and muscle. The subscapularis recess is a common site for loose bodies in the joint and may have an anterior extension around the subscapularis tendon. The subdeltoid and subacromial bursae almost always communicate and are located immediately above the rotator cuff tendon. The rotator cuff tendon is a mechanical barrier between the shoulder joint and these bursae. A tear in the rotator cuff tendon allows fluid from the joint to enter the bursae. This is one of the ancillary signs of a complete rotator cuff tear.[2]

PATHOLOGY

Impingement

Impingement syndrome is a term used for a variety of clinical disorders of the shoulder that present as anterior shoulder pain. In the anatomic sense, *impinge* means "to push against." Impingement usually is due to entrapment of the supraspinatus tendon or subacromial bursa between the humeral head and the coracoacromial arch or to impingement of the cuff by a degenerated acromioclavicular joint. Anatomic impingement can be determined by MRI. Impingement syndrome, a painful clinical condition precipitated by anatomic impingement, can only be diagnosed by a clinician who is examining a patient. In MRI, then, "impingement" implies mechanical deformity of tissue by an extrinsic process. One could argue that descriptive interpretation is more appropriate at this point—perhaps one could say an "impression" of one structure on another—so that there is no confusion with the impingement syndrome.

Impingement of the rotator cuff can be primary or secondary. Primary mechanical impingement is due to an abnormal acromioclavicular joint or coracoacromial arch. Secondary mechanical impingement is due to a rotator cuff that impinges against normal structures as a result of abnormal shoulder motion at the glenohumeral or scapulothoracic joint. The pain in primary and secondary mechanical impingement is similar. The common pathway is inflammation and degeneration of the rotator cuff and the surrounding soft tissues.[18]

The diagnosis of impingement is determined by the detection of anatomic alterations that may cause rotator cuff impingement. It should be noted, however, that MRI has a significant limitation at this point: the examination is performed with the patient's arm at his or her side. The pain, however, is typically induced with the patient erect and in a position other than the scanning position—for example, abduction and forward flexion. Nevertheless, MRI findings identified with the impingement syndrome have been classified.[18] Type I describes subacromial bursitis in which there is bursal thickening and normal signal intensity of the supraspinatus tendon. The abnormal bursa may have bright signal on the Tl sequence similar to subcutaneous fat, perhaps from increased fibrofatty tissue due to hypertrophied synovium. Type IIA describes abnormally high signal intensity in the supraspinatus tendon on the T1 but not the T2 sequence. Type IIB describes bright signal in the supraspinatus tendon on the T1 and T2 sequences and no focal disruption of the rotator cuff. There is an increased likelihood of impingement syndrome if the subacromial bursa and rotator cuff tendon are compressed by overlying extrinsic structural abnormalities. Type III describes a complete rotator cuff tear (Fig. 5–6). This classification assumes that any abnormality of the rotator cuff is secondary to extrinsic impingement; however, intrinsic overload, not extrinsic impingement, of the rotator cuff can be related to sports activities, which may be a cause of its failure in younger persons.[9]

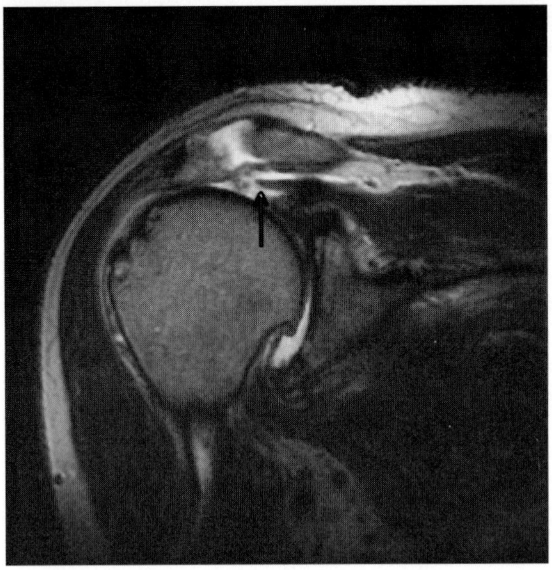

Figure 5–6
Oblique coronal FSE image, supraspinatus tendon tear. *A retracted torn tendon* (arrow) *is highlighted by joint fluid.*

Assessment of the acromioclavicular joint should include the presence and extent of degenerative osseous proliferation, the appearance of the joint capsule, and the size of the clavicular head and adjacent acromion. Assessment of the coracoacromial arch includes the shape and orientation of the acromion (Fig. 5–7), the thickness and orientation of the coracoacromial ligament, and the size and shape of enthesophytes located at the acromial insertion of the coracoacromial ligament. The shape of the acromial process has been classified into three types. Type I is flat. Type II is curved to conform with the humeral head. Type III is hooked (Fig. 5–8). The anterior hook is related to the basic shape of the acromion and not to degenerative osseous proliferation. Clinical studies indicate interobserver variation and distributions of the types, but Types II and III seem to be associated with painful shoulders with impingement and complete rotator cuff tears.[1]

Rotator Cuff Disease

MRI can noninvasively define complete rotator cuff tears with good diagnostic performance.[7] Other abnormalities, such as tendinosis and partial tears, can also be seen but with lesser efficacy. The MRI findings considered indicative of tendinosis include diffuse increase in signal intensity within the supraspinatus tendon on the T1 and proton-density sequences. The T2 sequence reveals fading or absence of this same signal. Arthroscopic

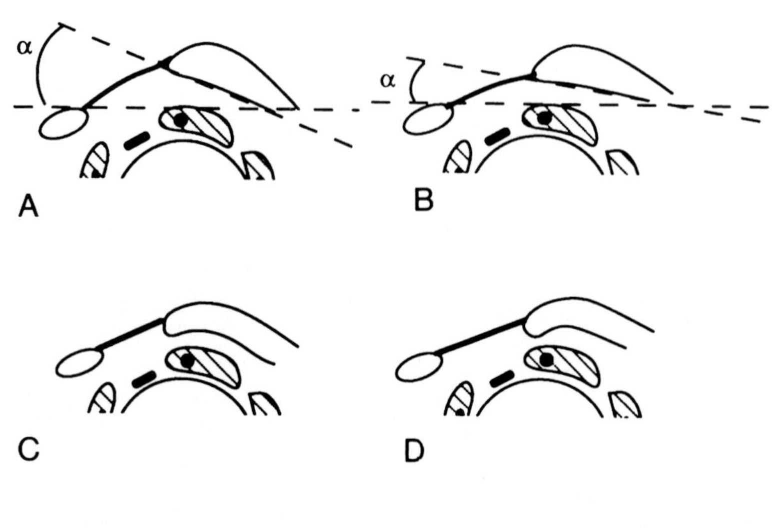

Figure 5–7
Schematic drawing of the oblique-sagittal plane of large (A) *and small* (B) *acromial slope* (A) *and flat* (A, B), *curved* (C), *and hooked* (B) *acromial shape. (From Vahlensieck M, Lang P, Genant HK. The shoulder.* In *Chan WP, Lang P, Genant HK, eds. MRI of the Musculoskeletal System. Philadelphia: WB Saunders, 1994.)*

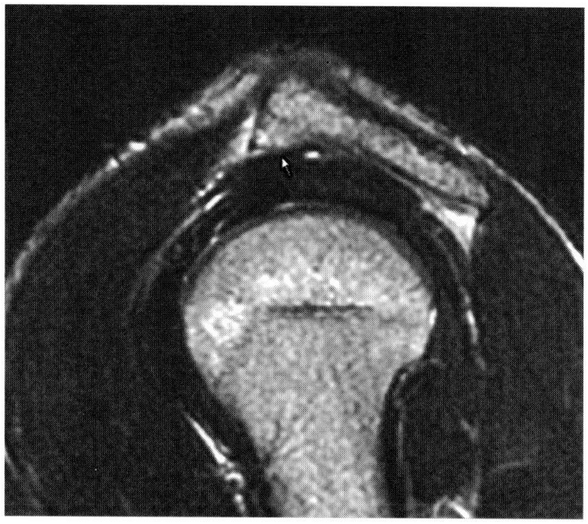

Figure 5–8
Oblique sagittal T2 FSE image, Type-III acromion. *The undersurface of the anterior aspect of the acromion has a "hook"* (arrow).

correlation reveals hyperemia of the tendon surface and bursal inflammation or scarring. Careful clinical correlation is indicated because tendons have had a similar MRI appearance in asymptomatic persons.[18] Tendon surface degeneration is most common on the bursal side. MRI reveals tendon thinning and mild irregularity. Arthroscopically, the tendon appears frayed. The distinction between this stage of disease and early partial thickness tears may be difficult.[19]

Rotator cuff tears can be defined as partial or complete. Partial tears are divided into inferior surface, superior surface, or intra-substance tears.[6] A partial tear can be diagnosed with MRI when a discrete defect in the tendon shows increased signal on the T2 sequence. The T1 sequence with fat saturation after the intra-articular administration of gadolinium may also help diagnose partial tears of the articular surface.[11]

A complete tear has occurred when the entire thickness of the cuff is torn from the bursal to the articular surfaces. Marked increased signal consistent with fluid traverses the full thickness of the tendon (Fig. 5–9). Complete tears can be classified by size or number of tendons involved.[7, 21] MRI can determine the size of the tendon defects. Both the sagittal and coronal oblique images can be used to determine the medial and anteroposterior extent of cuff tears. Secondary signs of rotator cuff tear include diffuse loss of the peribursal fat plane and fluid in the subdeltoid bursa. Acute tears occur suddenly and are less common. Chronic tears are much more common (> 90%) and have existed 3 months or more.

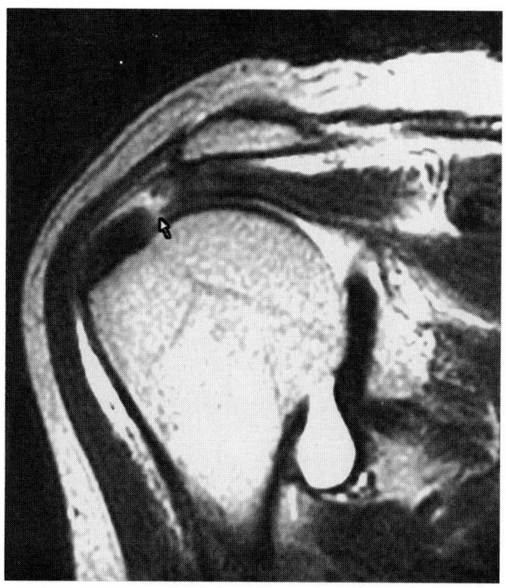

Figure 5–9
Oblique coronal T2 FSE image, supraspinatus tendon tear. *Fluid* (arrow) *completely traverses the distal tendon.*

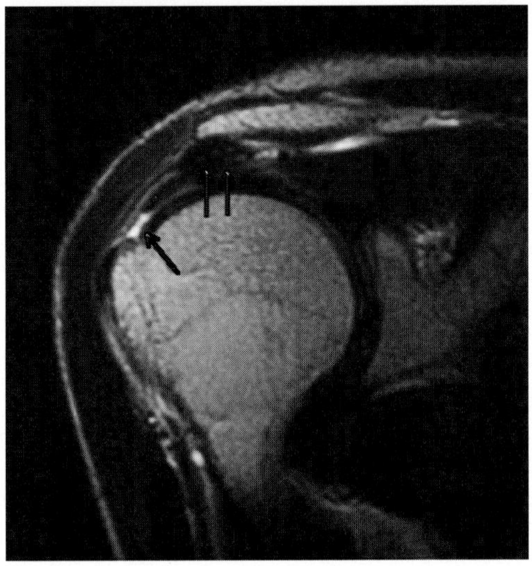

Figure 5–10
Oblique coronal T2 FSE image. *A small, distal tear* (large arrow) *is manifested by bright signal from fluid. Note also a large subacromial spur* (arrows), *seen as a sizable area of dark signal. This was correlated with plain radiography.*

Their onset is insidious. Note, however, that a chronic tear can undergo acute extension. Rotator cuff tears almost always occur at the more distal and anterior portion of the tendon near the tuberosity (Fig. 5–10). Bone changes occur in persons with rotator cuff disease and impingement. Once present, they further exacerbate the problem. The most common bone changes are acromioclavicular osteophytes, subacromial spurring, cysts, and sclerosis in the greater tuberosity.[7, 21]

Postoperative evaluation is much more difficult. Assessment of the symptomatic postoperative rotator cuff can be divided into two categories. A prior acromioplasty without cuff repair is the first category. MRI findings include a flattened acromial undersurface, absence of the anterior one third of the acromion, and decreased marrow signal in the distal acromion. Low-signal artifacts from metal fragments may be evident. Persistent pain may be due to subsequent development of a rotator cuff tear or persistent mechanical impingement. Postoperative alteration of the adjacent soft tissues and signal alteration in the rotator cuff can confuse the interpretation of findings. MRI is sensitive but not specific in this setting. A prior rotator cuff tear is the second category. MRI findings include distortion of adjacent soft tissues, metal artifacts, a surgical trough in the humeral head, and intermediate signal within the rotator cuff. Increased signal from fluid within a gap in the rotator cuff is a reliable indicator of a re-tear. Intra-articular contrast is also useful in the postoperative rotator cuff evaluation.[10]

Biceps tendon lesions include tendonitis (Fig. 5–11), subluxation, dislocation, and rupture. These lesions commonly occur in relation to ongoing impingement and degeneration of the rotator cuff. A small amount of fluid on MRI is common in the biceps tendon sheath. Large amounts of fluid may indicate tendonitis or tenosynovitis. Rupture of the long head of the biceps tendon usually occurs in older patients. Most ruptures occur at the weakest portion of the tendon just distal to its exit from the joint cavity. A large anterior cuff tear is probably the most common setting for medial dislocation of the biceps tendon. MRI reveals a low-signal biceps tendon displaced medially outside the intertubercular groove. The dislocation can be extra-articular or intra-articular. Axial or coronal oblique images are best for this evaluation.[4]

Labral Tears

The appearance of the glenoid labrum varies considerably, which complicates the detection of a true labral tear.[16] The labrum is normally triangle-shaped and low-signal on the axial sequences, but it can be rounded and have clefts. The anterior labrum is usually larger and more commonly torn than the posterior labrum. If no joint effusion is present, a labral

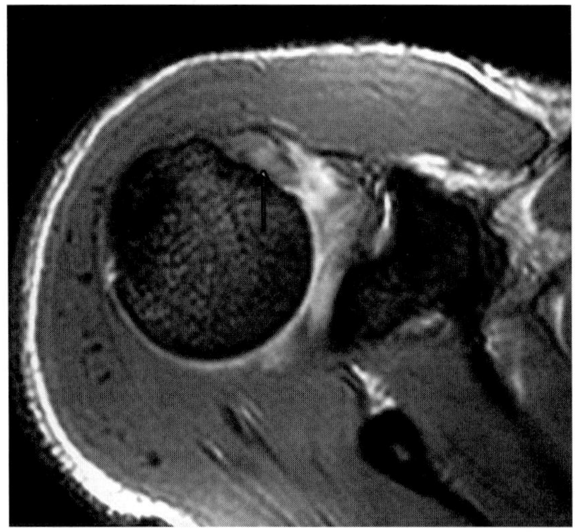

Figure 5–11
Axial GRE image, biceps tendonitis. *The biceps tendon* (arrow) *shows thickening and increased signal indicative of tendonitis.*

tear can be difficult to see unless it is severe, although linear increased signal through the labral base, significant deformity, or complete absence of the labrum make a tear likely. Insertion of the middle glenohumeral ligament may mimic a tear of the anterior labrum. Several ancillary findings aid the interpretation. The insertion site of the anterior capsule on the glenoid can indicate joint laxity. The capsular insertion has been divided into three types (Fig. 5–12). Type I inserts onto the anterior labrum. Type II inserts into the bony glenoid at the base of the labrum. Type III inserts into the bony glenoid more than 1 cm prox-

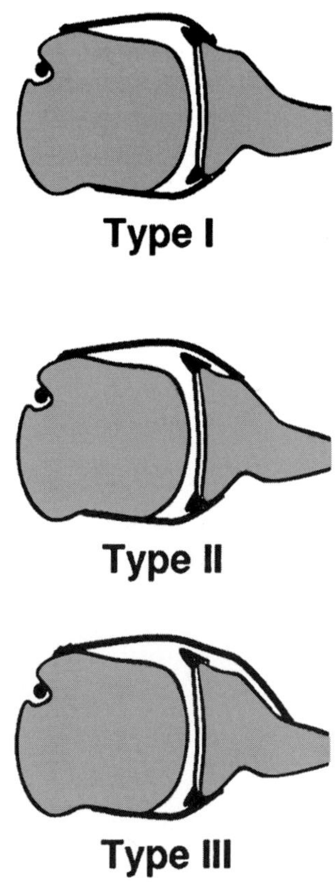

Figure 5–12
Schematic drawings of the axial plane of the variable anterior insertion of the shoulder capsule (Types I–III). (From Vahlensieck M, Lang P, Genant HK. The shoulder. In *Chan WP, Lang P, Genant HK, eds. MRI of the Musculoskeletal System. Philadelphia: WB Saunders, 1994.)*

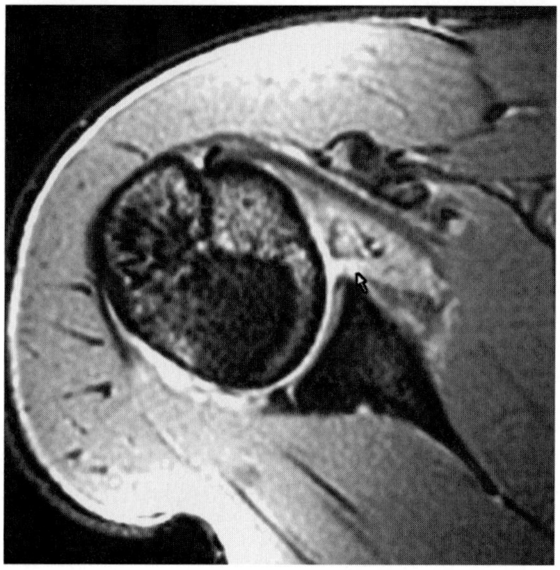

Figure 5–13
Axial GRE image, anterior labral tear. *Fluid filling the tear significantly displaces the anterior labrum from the glenoid* (arrow).

imal to the tip of the labrum. The latter can indicate anterior instability. A Hill-Sachs deformity of the humeral head certainly indicates some degree of laxity. The corresponding bony abnormality of the glenoid is the Bankart lesion, the significance of which is similar (Fig. 5–13).[5, 14]

The superior anterior labrum is best evaluated on the coronal oblique sequence. This particular imaging plane would, therefore, be relevant in a suspected superior labrum, anterior and posterior (SLAP) lesion.

SLAP lesions are well described.[3, 19] In a Type-I lesion, the superior labrum appears roughened and degenerative, with an intact labral edge and biceps tendon anchor. In a Type-II lesion, the roughened superior labrum detaches from its insertion. With traction, this labrum along with its biceps tendon anchor arches away from the bone, rendering the biceps labral complex unstable. In a Type-III lesion, the superior labrum has a bucket-handle tear, and there is a split tear of the biceps tendon, which is displaced with the labral flap into the joint. A Type-IV lesion involves a bucket-handle tear and a split tear of the biceps tendon, which is displaced with the labral flap into the joint. A complex tear is any combination of these types. Not all superior labrum abnormalities fit into this classification. Such unclassifiable lesions have been fitted into three distinct categories.[13] Therefore, in a Type-V lesion, an anteroinferior Bankart lesion continues superiorly to include separation of the biceps tendon. In a Type-VI lesion, an unstable flap tear of the labrum is present in addition to biceps tendon separation. In a Type-VII lesion, the superior labrum-biceps tendon separation extends anteriorly beneath the middle glenohumeral ligament.

Suprascapular Nerve Entrapment

The suprascapular nerve is made up of branches from the C4, C5, and C6 roots of the brachial plexus. It courses anteriorly to posteriorly through the suprascapular notch and spinoglenoid notch on the superior aspect of the scapula just medial to the coracoid process. Branches of the nerve innervate the supraspinatus and infraspinatus muscles. A tumor or ganglion cyst (Fig. 5–14) can easily entrap the nerve at this location because it is relatively fixed in position by a transverse ligament. Muscular pain and atrophy can result.[8]

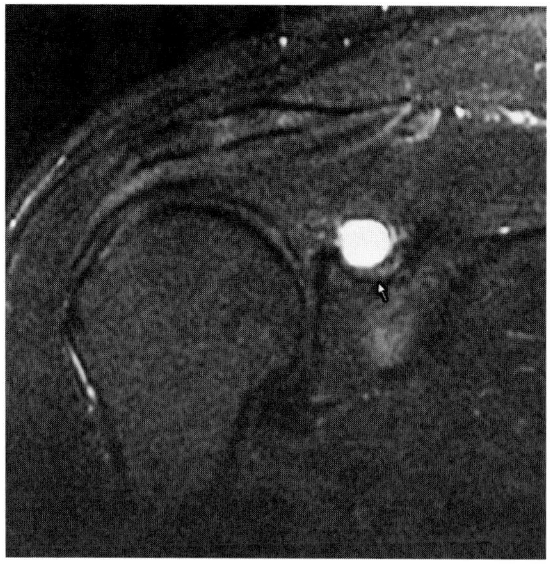

Figure 5–14
Oblique coronal T2 FSE image with fat suppression, suprascapular notch ganglion. *A round cystic mass* (arrow) *is seen as tremendously bright signal against the fat-suppressed background.*

Miscellaneous Conditions

Inflammatory conditions of the synovial tissue of the joint capsule include pigmented villonodular synovitis. The MRI findings are characteristic in that areas of low signal on both the T1 and T2 sequences are nicely demonstrated because of the superparamagnetic effect from nodular deposition of hemosiderin.

Synovial osteochondromatosis manifests as numerous low-signal areas within the joint capsule due to calcified and ossified intra-articular loose bodies (Fig. 5–15).

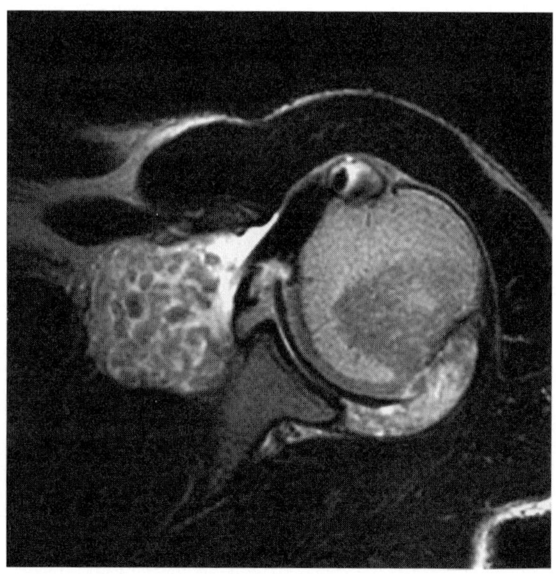

Figure 5–15
Axial T2 FSE image, osteochondromatosis. *The joint is markedly distended with fluid and multiple low-density osteochondral bodies.*

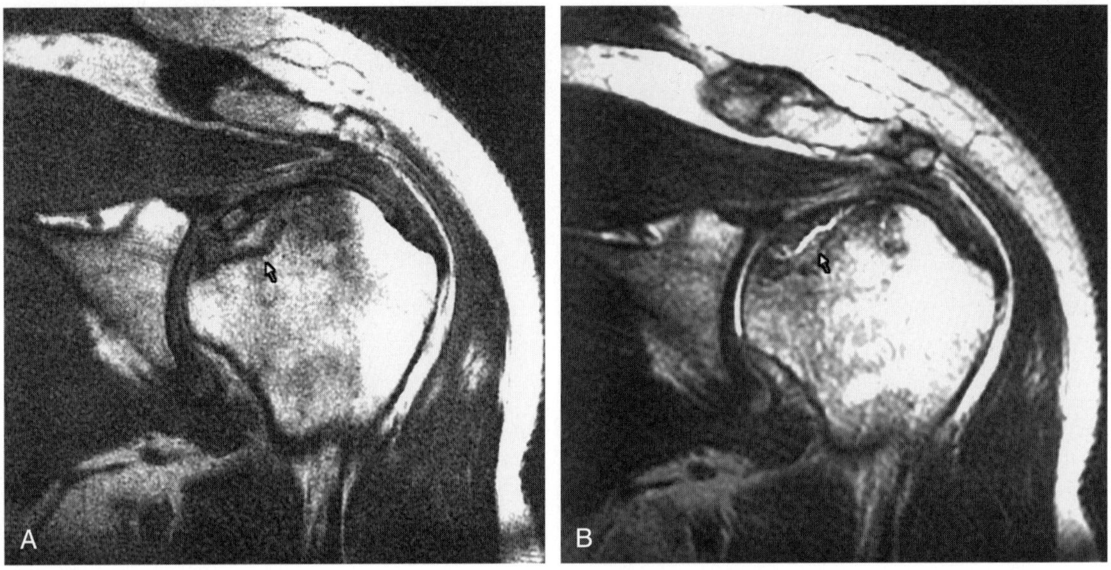

Figure 5–16
A, ***Oblique coronal T1 SE image.*** *Subchondral focus of avascular necrosis with a characteristic maintenance of bone-marrow signal marginated by a band of low signal* (arrow). B, ***Oblique coronal T2 FSE image.*** *Findings are similar to those in* A *except a bright band of signal also marginates the lesion.*

Rheumatoid arthritis commonly involves the shoulder joint. Soft tissue edema from synovitis and an effusion are common early findings. A more proliferative synovitis can ensue and destroy articular cartilage, erode bone, and disrupt ligaments, tendons, and joint capsule. MRI can demonstrate all these findings noninvasively.

Finally, although MRI does not play a distinct role in evaluation of fractures, it can nicely demonstrate bone bruises, stress fractures, avascular necrosis (Fig. 5–16), or occult bone injury (Fig. 5–17) to the shoulder region because of the sensitivity of the T1 sequence to bone marrow alterations.

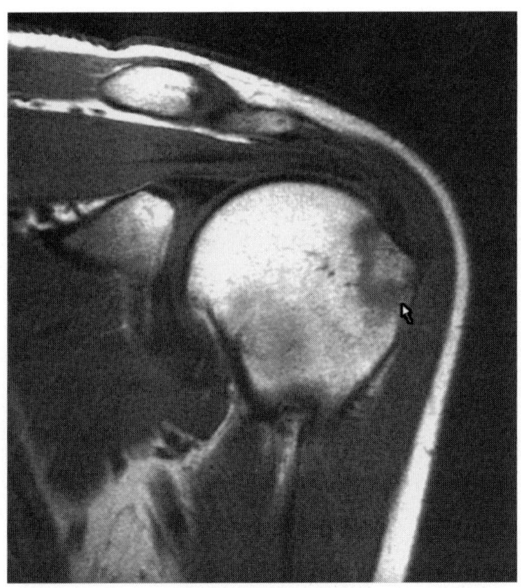

Figure 5–17
Occult bone injury. *A band of intermediate signal at the greater tuberosity* (arrow) *is distinctly different from normal bone marrow.*

References

1. Bigliani LU, Morrison DS, April EW. The morphology of the acromion and its relationship to rotator cuff tears. Orthop Trans 1986; 10:216.
2. Buckwalter KA. Magnetic resonance imaging of the shoulder. Radiologist 1994; 1:55-71.
3. Cartland JP, Crues JV III, Stauffer A, et al. MR imaging in the evaluation of SLAP injuries of the shoulder: Findings in 10 patients. AJR 1992; 159:787-792.
4. Chan TW, Dalinka MK, Kneeland JB, et al. MR imaging of the biceps tendon dislocation. Radiology 1991; 179:649-652.
5. Coumas JM, Waite RJ, Goss TP, et al. CT and MR evaluation of the labral capsular ligamentous complex of the shoulder. AJR 1992; 158:591-597.
6. Ellman H. Diagnosis and treatment of incomplete rotator cuff tears. Clin Orthop 1990; 254:64-74.
7. Farley TE, Neumann CH, Steinbach LS, et al. Full-thickness tears of the rotator cuff of the shoulder: Diagnosis with MR imaging. Am J Roentgenol 1992; 158:347-351.
8. Fritz RC, Helms CA, Steinbach LS, et al. Suprascapular nerve entrapment: Evaluation with MR imaging. Radiology 1992; 184:437-444.
9. Fu FH, Harner CD, Klein AH. Shoulder impingement syndrome: A critical review. Clin Orthop Rel Res 1991; 269:162-173.
10. Haygood TM, Oxner KG, Kneeland JB, et al. MR imaging of the postoperative shoulder. MRI Clin North Am 1993; 1:143-157.
11. Karzel RP, Snyder SJ. Magnetic resonance arthrography of the shoulder. Clin Sports Med 1993; 12:123.
12. Legan JM, Burkhard TK, Goff WB II, et al. Tears of the glenoid labrum: MR imaging of 88 arthroscopically confirmed cases. Radiology 1991; 179:241-246.
13. Maffet MW, Gartsman GM, Moseley B. Superior labrum-biceps tendon complex lesions of the shoulder. Am J Sports Med 1995; 23:93-98.
14. McCauley TR, Pope CF, Jokl P. Normal and abnormal glenoid labrum: Assessment with multiplanar gradient-echo MR imaging. Radiology 1992; 183:35-37.
15. Neumann CH, Holt RG, Steinbach LS, et al. MR imaging of the shoulder: Appearance of the supraspinatus tendon in asymptomatic volunteers. AJR 1992; 158:1281-1287.
16. Neumann CH, Petersen SA, Jahnke AH. MR imaging of the labral capsular complex: Normal variations. AJR 1991; 157:1015-1021.
17. Rafii M, Firooznia H, Sherman O, et al. Rotator cuff lesions: Signal patterns at MR imaging. Radiology 1990; 177:817-823.
18. Seeger LL, Gold RH, Bassett LW, et al. Shoulder impingement syndrome: MR findings in 53 shoulders. AJR 1988; 150:343-347.
19. Snyder SJ, Karzel RP, Delpizzo W, et al. SLAP lesions of the shoulder. Arthroscopy 1990; 6:274-279.
20. Zlatkin MB, Iannotti JP, Roberts MC, et al. Rotator cuff tears: Diagnostic performance of MR imaging. Radiology 1989; 172:22-29.
21. Zlatkin MB. Rotator cuff disease. *In* Zlatkin MB, ed. MRI of the Shoulder. New York: Raven Press, 1991, pp 55-98.

Shoulder Arthroscopy

Shoulder arthroscopy was first attempted in 1931,[7] but it has only become popular since the 1980s following successful use of the arthroscope in the knee. In recent years, shoulder arthroscopy has blossomed, and its use as both a diagnostic and therapeutic tool has dramatically increased.

INDICATIONS

Indications for shoulder arthroscopy are still evolving, but there are proponents and opponents for each proposed application, and the controversy continues. Much like the early days of knee arthroscopy, many of the early indications for shoulder arthroscopy were simply for diagnostic purposes. Shoulder arthroscopy has been applied in the diagnosis and treatment of shoulder instability, impingement syndrome, distal clavicle problems, rotator cuff disease, inflammatory and degenerative diseases of the shoulder, adhesive capsulitis, sepsis, and other diagnoses.

In the setting of shoulder instability, arthroscopy can help to identify the pathology.[5] Labral tears, Hill-Sachs defects, loose bodies, and glenohumeral ligament detachment can be easily identified with arthroscopic examination.[2] Arthroscopic correction of instability yields mixed results and is technique-dependent; it is perhaps best applied to the traumatic, first-time dislocation.[3, 4, 22–24]

Superior labral and biceps injuries (the SLAP lesions described earlier) have only been recognized recently.[20] Patients may have a history of a sudden traction force or compression and complain of "clicking" in the affected shoulder. The original classification scheme for these injuries[20] has recently been expanded to include seven varieties (Fig. 5–18).[15] Types V, VI, and VII may be associated with anterior shoulder instability. Arthroscopic evaluation and treatment of these lesions has been advocated.[18]

Arthroscopic treatment of impingement syndrome offers several advantages over traditional open procedures. The surgery can be done as an outpatient procedure through small incisions without disrupting the insertion of the deltoid muscle, and the rehabilitation and recovery time is shorter. Additionally, the glenohumeral joint can be evaluated for other forms of pathology (e.g., SLAP lesions, rotator cuff tears, degenerative joint disease) during the procedure. Decompression is accomplished by placing the arthroscope above the rotator cuff and below the acromion, in the subacromial bursa. "Bursoscopy" is then undertaken,[16] bursectomy and coracoacromial ligament resection is completed, and the "roof" of the acromion is raised with a combination of arthroscopic shavers and burrs. The goal is to convert a Type-III, or "hooked," acromion[6] into a Type-I, or flat, acromion (Fig. 5–19).

Distal clavicle resection can also be accomplished arthroscopically.[12, 19] This procedure is indicated for acromioclavicular degenerative joint disease or distal clavicle osteolysis. Arthroscopic techniques have been advocated to avoid problems associated with open techniques such as a painful noncosmetic scar, residual acromioclavicular joint instability, and postoperative shoulder weakness.[19]

Arthroscopic treatment of rotator cuff tears has been proposed. Early reports demonstrated the efficacy of arthroscopically assisted repairs with a "mini-incision."[11] More recently, some surgeons have repaired rotator cuff tears with suture anchors with no

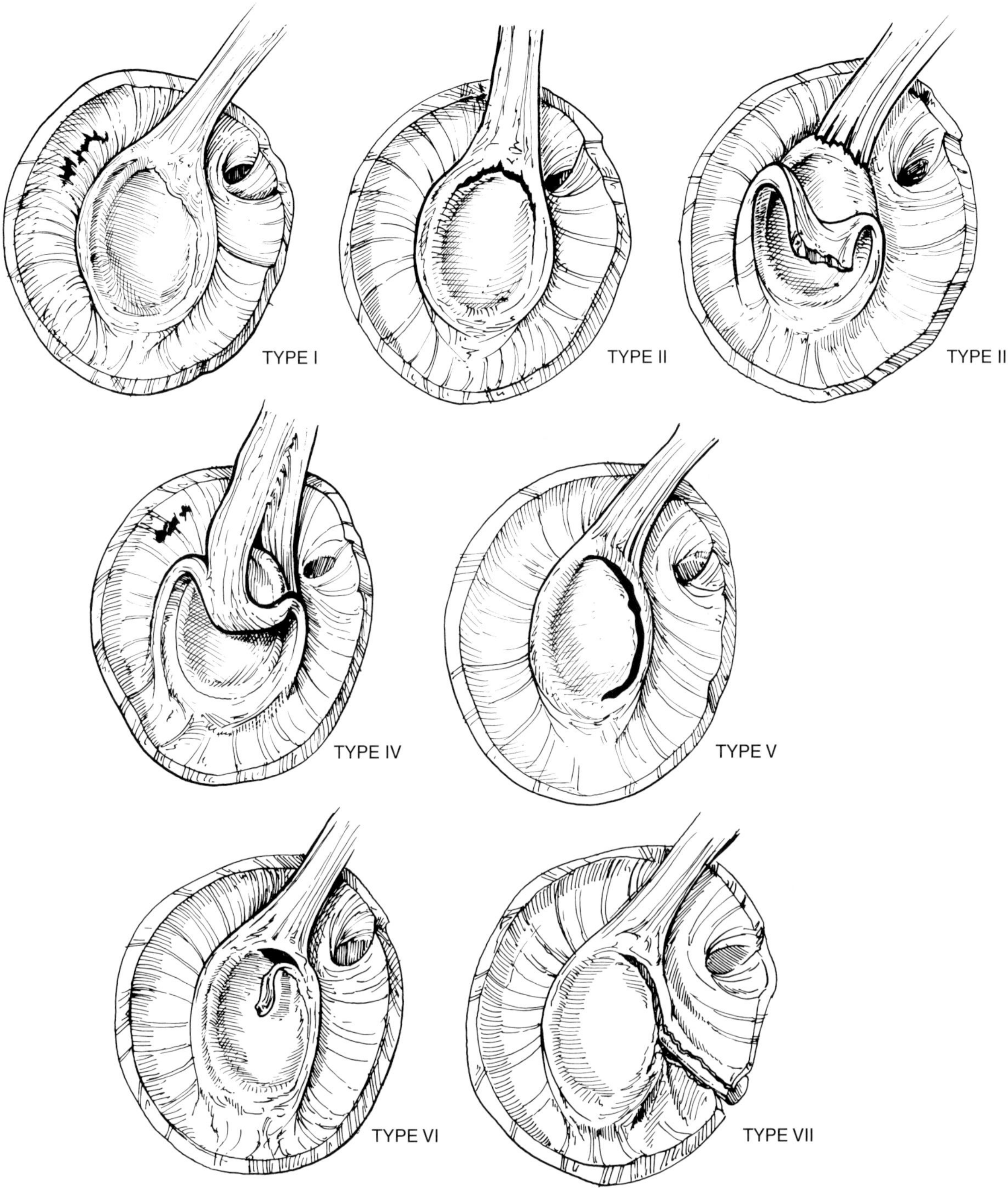

Figure 5–18
Superior labral anterior posterior lesions Types I–IV (described by Snyder, et al[20]) and Types V–VII (described by Maffet, et al[15]).

additional incisions. Certainly, larger, chronic tears may not be repairable with these techniques, but smaller, less chronic tears may be treatable arthroscopically.

Arthroscopy has also been advocated for debridement of loose tissue and "wash out" of degenerative arthritis,[9] treatment of adhesive capsulitis,[1, 13] irrigation and debridement of a septic joint,[17] removal of foreign bodies, and a variety of other procedures.

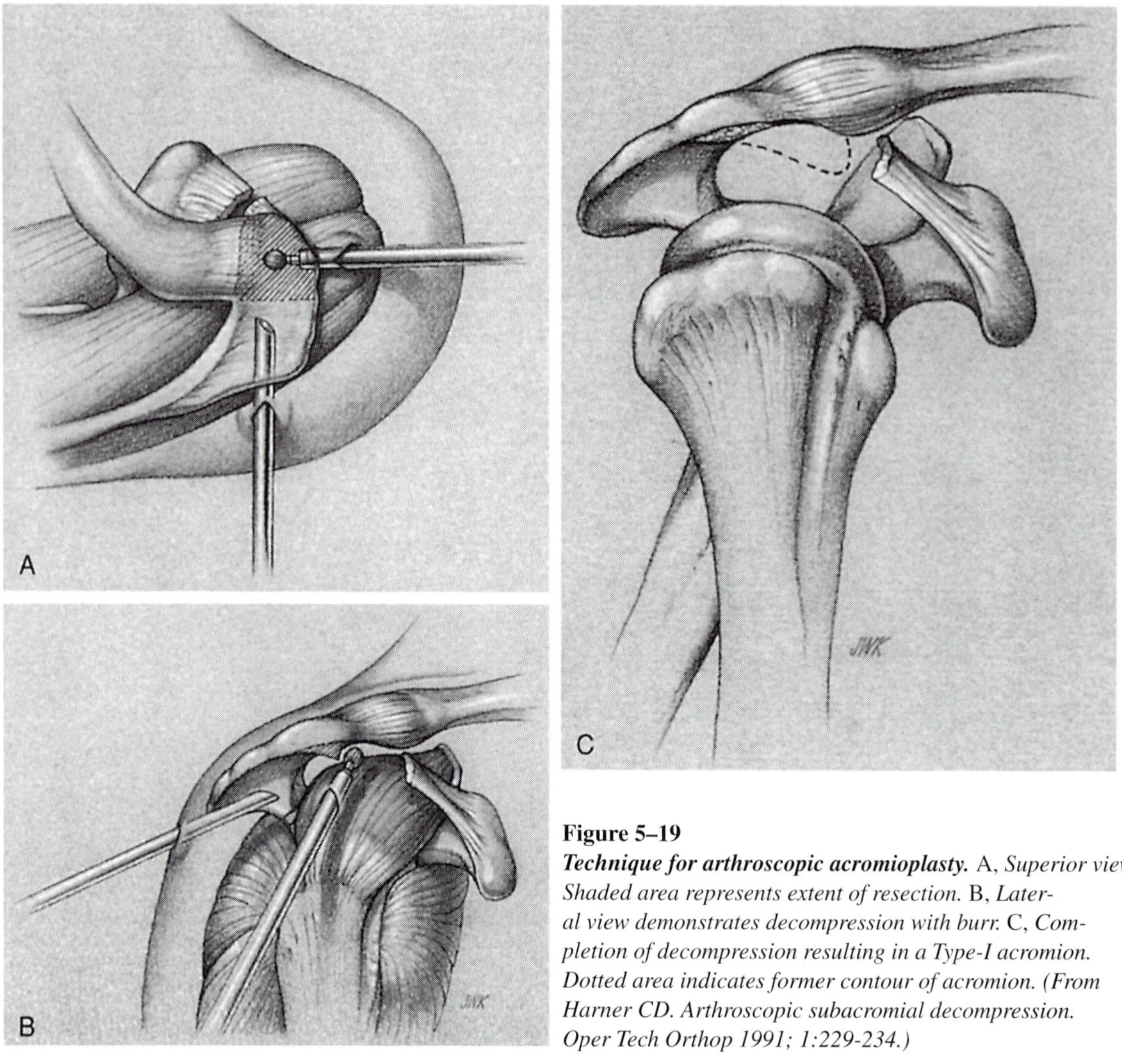

Figure 5–19
Technique for arthroscopic acromioplasty. A, *Superior view. Shaded area represents extent of resection.* B, *Lateral view demonstrates decompression with burr.* C, *Completion of decompression resulting in a Type-I acromion. Dotted area indicates former contour of acromion. (From Harner CD. Arthroscopic subacromial decompression. Oper Tech Orthop 1991; 1:229-234.)*

POSITIONING AND PORTAL PLACEMENT

Two methods of positioning are popular, the lateral decubitus position and the "beach-chair" position. The lateral decubitus position involves placement of the patient with the affected arm up; traction is used to suspend the arm. Transient neuropraxia can be a common problem with this positioning.[14] Other disadvantages of this position are that regional anesthesia is poorly tolerated, conversion to an open procedure is difficult, the capsular anatomy is distorted, and arm positioning can be more difficult (Table 5–1).[2] Because of these problems, the beach-chair position was developed by Warren in 1986.[21] This positioning allows easy access for arthroscopy without the disadvantages of other positions (Fig. 5–20).

The most commonly used arthroscopic shoulder portals are the posterior, anterosuperior, anteroinferior, and lateral portals. The superior, or Neviaser portal, is used by some surgeons as an accessory portal (Fig. 5–21). The posterior portal, placed 2 cm medial and 2 to 3 cm inferior to the posterolateral corner of the acromion, is used primarily for arthroscopic visualization. The anterosuperior portal, located lateral to the coracoid and just distal to the anterior edge of the acromion, is used most commonly for instrumentation. The anteroinferior portal, located approximately 2 cm below the anterosuperior portal just above the subscapularis tendon (visualized arthroscopically), is used primarily for arthroscopic Bankart repair. The lateral portal is used for instrumentation during bursoscopy. The superior (or supraspinatus or Neviaser) portal is located at the corner of the

Table 5–1 • Comparison of Advantages and Disadvantages of Shoulder Arthroscopy Performed in the Lateral Decubitus and Beach-Chair Positions

Lateral Decubitus	Beach Chair
Requires weights for traction	Arm hangs free with gravity traction
Risk of traction neuropraxia	No risk of traction neuropraxia
Risk of plexus injury with anterior-inferior portals	Less risk of plexus injury with anterior-inferior portals
Limited ability to move shoulder during arthroscopy	Full freedom of shoulder motion during arthroscopy
Capsuloligamentous anatomy placed in a stretched and distorted position	Capsuloligamentous anatomy placed in situ, "normal" orientation with different shoulder positions
Access to anterior glenoid cavity may be difficult	Easy access to anterior glenoid cavity
Requires patient repositioning and re-preparation for open procedure	Allows direct conversion to open procedure without position change or need to redrape
Interscalene block not as well tolerated	Interscalene block well tolerated
Minimal risk of camera fogging	Risk of camera fogging
Minimal risk of orthostatic hypotension	Risk of orthostatic hypotension

From Warner JJP. Shoulder arthroscopy in the beach-chair position. Op Tech Orthop 1:147–154, 1991.

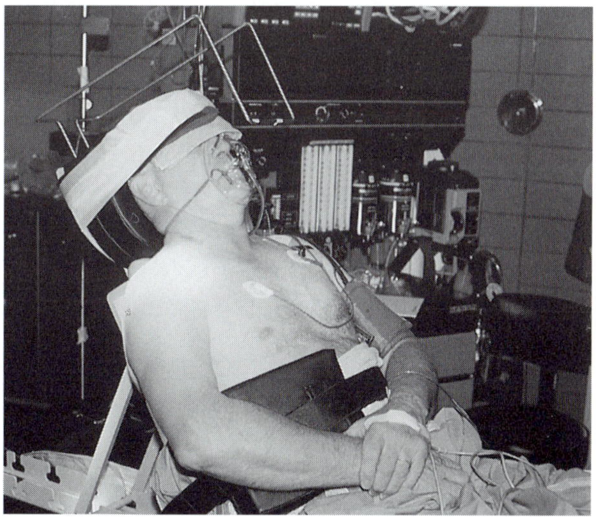

Figure 5–20
Beach-chair position with the head elevated and the shoulder free. *(From Warner JJP. Shoulder arthroscopy in the beach-chair position: Basic setup. Oper Tech Orthop 1991; 1:147-154).*

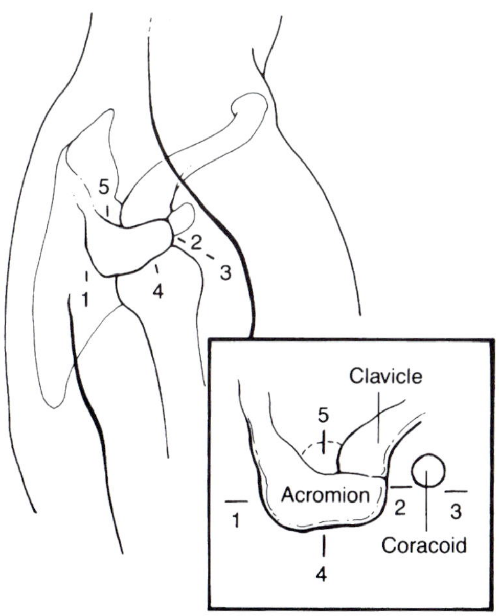

Figure 5–21
Arthroscopic portals for shoulder arthroscopy. *1, Posterior; 2, anterosuperior; 3, anteroinferior; 4, lateral; 5, superior or Neviaser portal. (From Miller MD, Cooper DE, Warner JJP. Review of Sports Medicine and Arthroscopy. Philadelphia: WB Saunders, 1995.)*

supraspinatus fossa and is oriented slightly anteriorly and laterally. It is used for visualization of the anterior glenoid and may be helpful in addressing superior labral and biceps injuries.

ARTHROSCOPIC ANATOMY

Although many sequences are recommended for arthroscopic evaluation of the shoulder, it is important to visualize and palpate the biceps tendon, labrum, glenohumeral articular surfaces, glenohumeral ligaments, and rotator cuff as a minimum (Fig. 5–22).[8] During

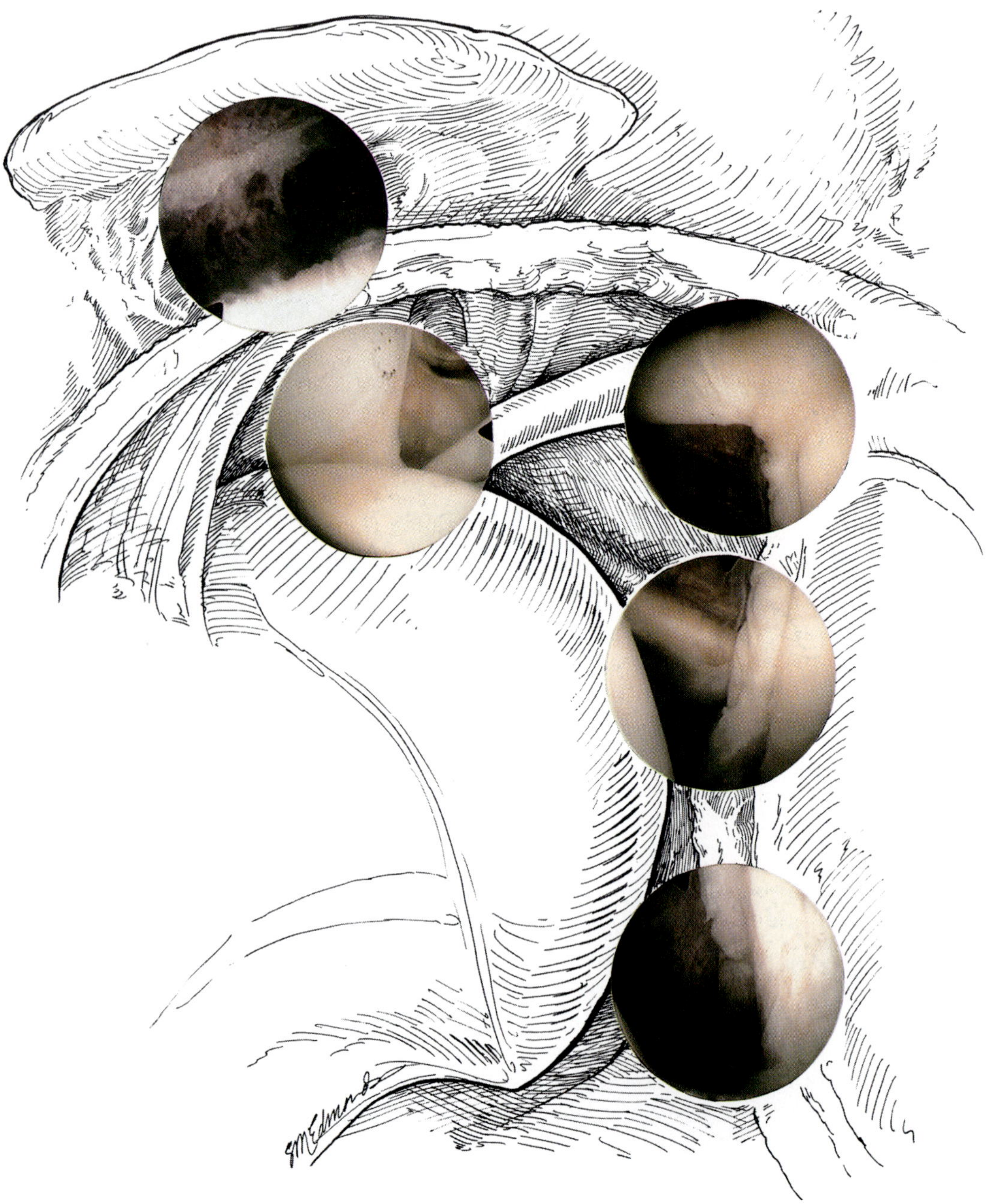

Figure 5–22
Arthroscopic anatomy of the shoulder.

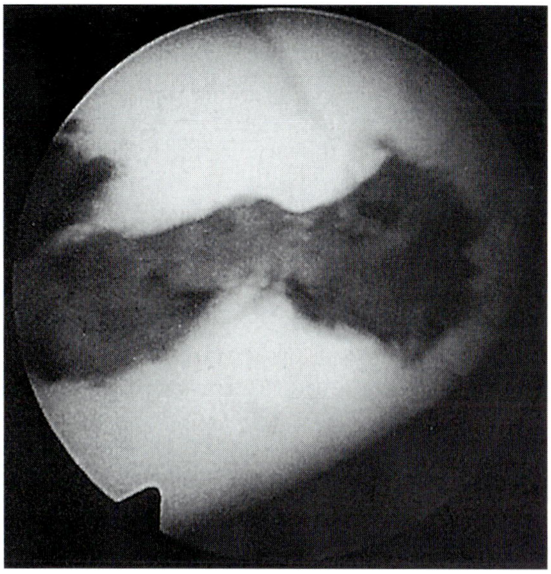

Figure 5–23
Hill-Sachs defect (posterior humeral head impression fracture) as seen arthroscopically. (From Miller MD, Cooper DE, Warner JJP. Review of Sports Medicine and Arthroscopy. Philadelphia: WB Saunders, 1995.)

bursoscopy, the superior surface of the rotator cuff, the inferior acromion, and the acromioclavicular joint should be evaluated. The interface of the biceps tendon and superior labrum is most commonly visualized first to allow the surgeon to become oriented; the surgeon can then address the possibility of a SLAP lesion. The labrum is inspected and probed to detect any labral injury (Bankart tear), especially in a patient with anterior instability. Separation of the superior labrum from the glenoid may be normal.[10] The articular surfaces of the glenoid and humerus are then examined for any articular injuries or degenerative joint disease. By rotating the arm, one can visualize most of the proximal humerus. With the arthroscope positioned posterior and inferior to the superior surface of the glenoid, internal rotation of the humerus allows visualization of a Hill-Sachs defect, or impression fracture, associated with anterior instability (Fig. 5–23). The glenohumeral ligaments can then be evaluated. The superior glenohumeral ligament is located between the biceps tendon and subscapularis. The middle glenohumeral ligament drapes over the subscapularis tendon. The inferior glenohumeral ligament complex is composed of two bands, anterior and posterior, and attaches to the inferior labrum (Fig. 5–24). Arthroscopy of the inferior axillary pouch, the rotator cuff insertion (superiorly), and the subacromial bursa completes the examination.

COMPLICATIONS

In addition to transient neuropraxia associated with traction (discussed earlier) and the complications associated with all arthroscopic procedures (e.g., articular cartilage injury, instrument breakage, bleeding, infection), most of the complications of shoulder arthroscopy are related to the procedure being performed. Recurrent shoulder instability can occur following arthroscopic Bankart repair. This may be related to the chronicity of the injury, underlying laxity of the patient, quality of the tissue, and activity level of the patient. Patient selection may be the critical factor in reducing this problem, and the arthroscopist should always be prepared to convert to an open procedure whenever necessary. Transglenoid suture techniques have the attendant risk of suprascapular nerve injury. Arthroscopic acromioplasty is technique-dependent, and insufficient or excessive removal of bone can result in complications (recurrence or fracture, respectively). As new procedures are developed, unfortunately, new complications will appear; however, arthroscopy has proven itself a useful tool for surgery about the shoulder.

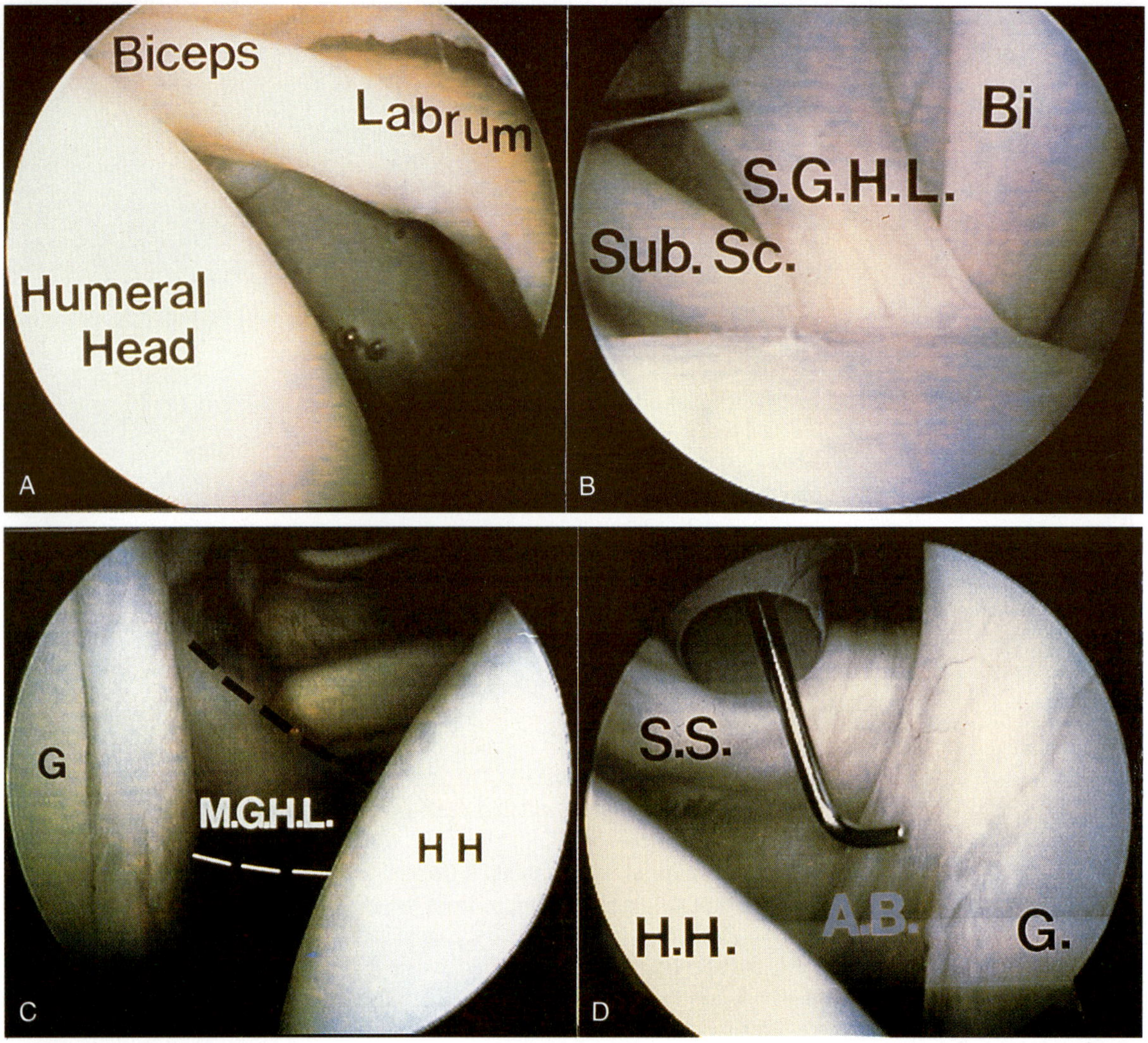

Figure 5–24
A *and* B, *Arthroscopic view of the superior aspect of the glenohumeral joint. Note the normal relationship of the biceps tendon and labrum* (A) *and the position of the superior glenohumeral ligament (SGHL) between the biceps tendon (Bi) and the subscapularis tendon (Sub Sc)* (B). C, *The middle glenohumeral ligament (MGHL) drapes over the subscapularis tendon between the glenoid (G) and the humeral head (HH).* D, *The anterior band (AB) of the inferior glenohumeral ligament complex attaches to the labrum and glenoid (G). (From Miller MD, Cooper DE, Warner JJP. Review of Sports Medicine and Arthroscopy. Philadelphia: WB Saunders, 1995.)*

References

1. Allen AA, Warner JJP. Management of the stiff shoulder. Op Tech Orthop 1995; 5(3):238-247.
2. Altchek DW, Warren RF, Skyhar MJ. Shoulder arthroscopy. *In* Rockwood CA Jr, Matsen FA III, eds. The Shoulder. Philadelphia: WB Saunders, 1990, pp 258-277.
3. Arciero RA, Taylor DC, Snyder RJ, Uhorchak JM. Arthroscopic bioabsorbable tack stabilization of initial anterior shoulder dislocations: A preliminary report. Arthroscopy 1995; 11(4):410-417.
4. Arciero RA, Wheeler JH, Ryan JB, McBride JT. Arthroscopic bankart repair vs nonoperative treatment for acute, initial, anterior shoulder dislocations. Am J Sports Med 1994; 22:589-594.
5. Baker CL, Uribe JW, Whitman C. Arthroscopic evaluation of acute initial anterior shoulder dislocations. Am J Sports Med 1990; 18:25-28.
6. Bigliani LU, Morrison D, April EW. The morphology of the acromion and its relationship to rotator cuff tears. Orthop Trans 1986; 10:228.
7. Burman MS. Arthroscopy or the direct visualization of joints. An experimental cadaver study. J Bone Joint Surg [Am] 1931; 13:669.

8. Caborn DNM, Fu FH. Arthroscopic approach and anatomy of the shoulder. Op Tech Orthop 1991; 1:126-133.
9. Cofield RH. Arthroscopy of the shoulder. Mayo Clin Proc 1983; 58:501-508.
10. Cooper DE, Arnoczky SP, O'Brien SJ, et al. Anatomy, histology, and vascularity of the glenoid labrum. J Bone Joint Surg [Am] 1992; 74:46-52.
11. Ellman H, Kay SP, Worth M. Arthroscopic treatment of full thickness rotator cuff tears: Two to seven year follow-up study. Arthroscopy 1993; 9:301-314.
12. Gartsman GM. Arthroscopic resection of the acromioclavicular joint. Am J Sports Med 1993; 21:71-77.
13. Harryman DT II. Shoulders: Frozen and stiff. Inst Course Lect 1993; 42:247-257.
14. Klein AH, France JC, Mutschler TA, Fu FH. Measurement of brachial plexus strain in arthroscopy of the shoulder. Arthroscopy 1987; 3:45-52.
15. Maffett MW, Gartsman GM, Moseley B. Superior labrum-biceps tendon complex lesions of the shoulder. Am J Sports Med 1995; 23:93-98.
16. Nisbet JK, Paulos LE. Subacromial bursoscopy. Op Tech Orthop 1991; 1:221-228.
17. Olgilvie-Harris DJ, Wiley AM. Arthroscopic surgery of the shoulder: A general appraisal. J Bone Joint Surg [Br] 1986; 68:201-207.
18. Pagnani MJ, Speer KP, Altchek DW, et al. Arthroscopic fixation of superior labral lesions using a biodegradable implant: A preliminary report. Arthroscopy 1995; 11:194-195.
19. Snyder SJ, Banas MP, Karzel RP. The arthroscopic Mumford procedure: An analysis of results. Arthroscopy 1995; 11:157-164.
20. Snyder SJ, Karzel RP, Del Pizzo W, et al. SLAP lesions of the shoulder. Arthroscopy 1990; 6:274-279.
21. Warner JJP. Shoulder arthroscopy in the beach-chair position: Basic setup. Op Tech Orthop 1991; 1:147-154.
22. Warner JJP, Miller MD, Marks P, Fu FH. Arthroscopic Bankart repair with the Suretac device. Part I: Clinical observations. Arthroscopy 1995; 11:2-13.
23. Warner JJP, Miller MD, Marks P, Fu FH. Arthroscopic Bankart repair with the Suretac device. Part II: Experimental observations. Arthroscopy 1995; 11:14-20.
24. Wheeler JH, Ryan JB, Arciero RA, Molinari RN. Arthroscopic versus nonoperative treatment of acute shoulder dislocations in young athletes. Arthroscopy 1989; 5:213-217.

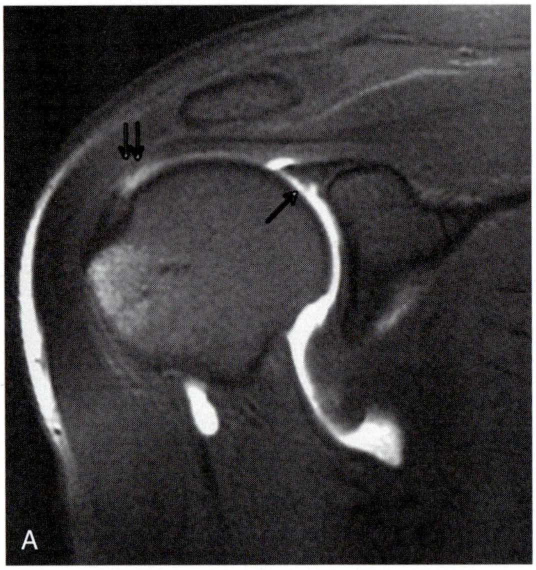

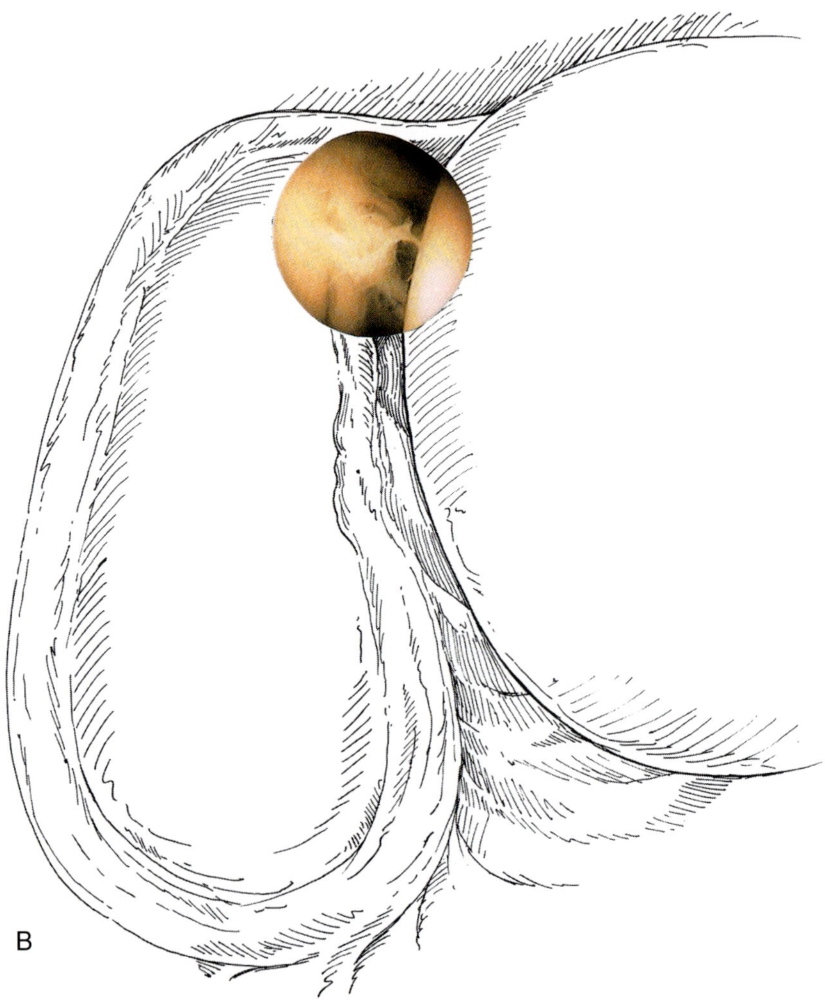

B

Figure 5–25. **Type-I SLAP Lesion, Right Shoulder**
A, *Oblique coronal T1-weighted fat-suppressed image following intra-articular administration of gadolinium demonstrates mild irregularity of the superior anterior labrum* (arrow). *Note also the partial-thickness rotator cuff tear* (arrows). B, *Arthroscopic view demonstrates fraying of the biceps tendon near its attachment to the superior labrum and glenoid.*

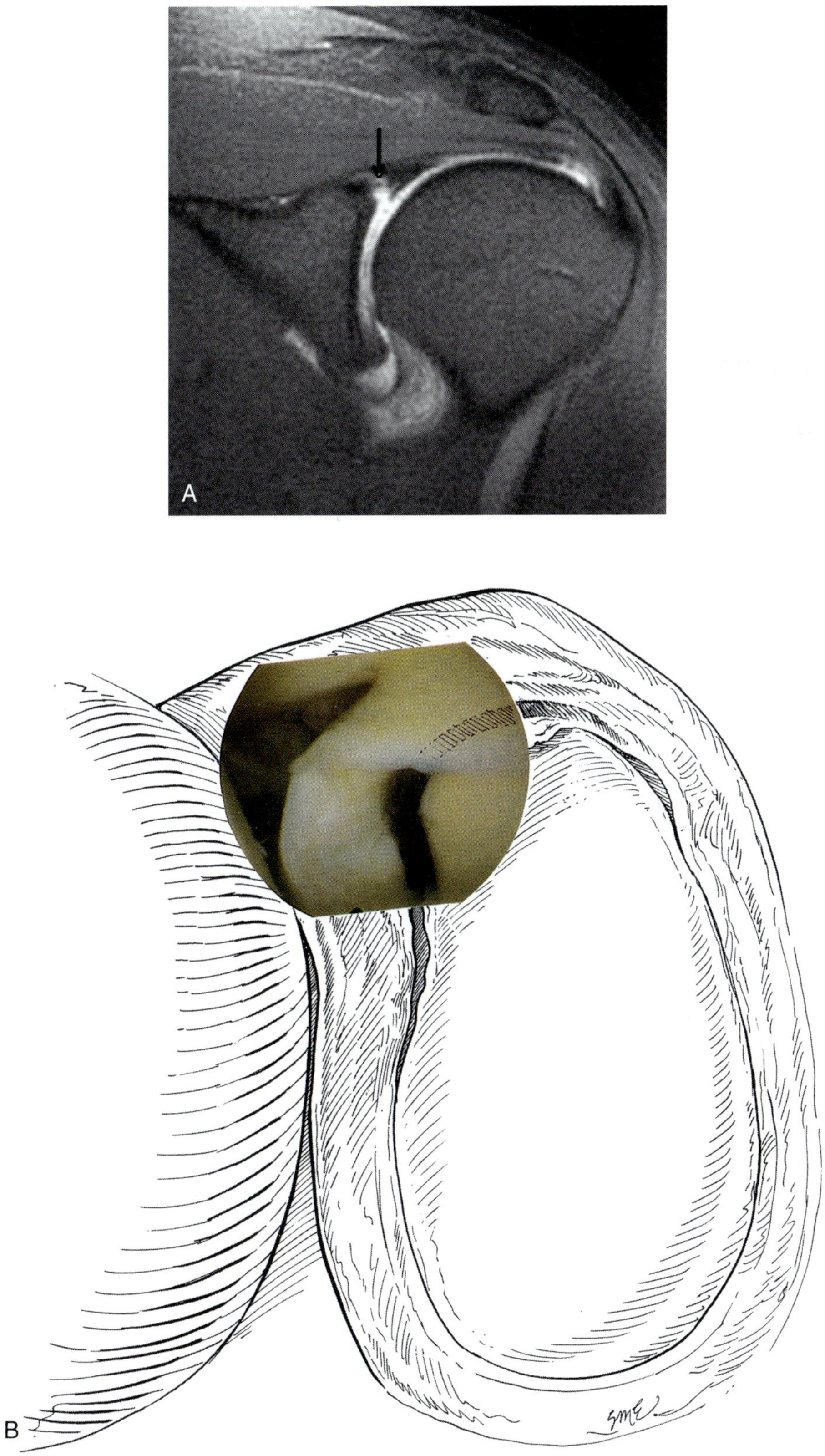

Figure 5–26. **Type-II SLAP Lesion, Left Shoulder**
A, *Oblique coronal T1-weighted SE fat-suppressed image with intra-articular administration of gadolinium. Note superior displacement of the anterosuperior labrum* (arrow). B, *Arthroscopic view demonstrates detachment of the anterosuperior labrum and biceps anchor.*

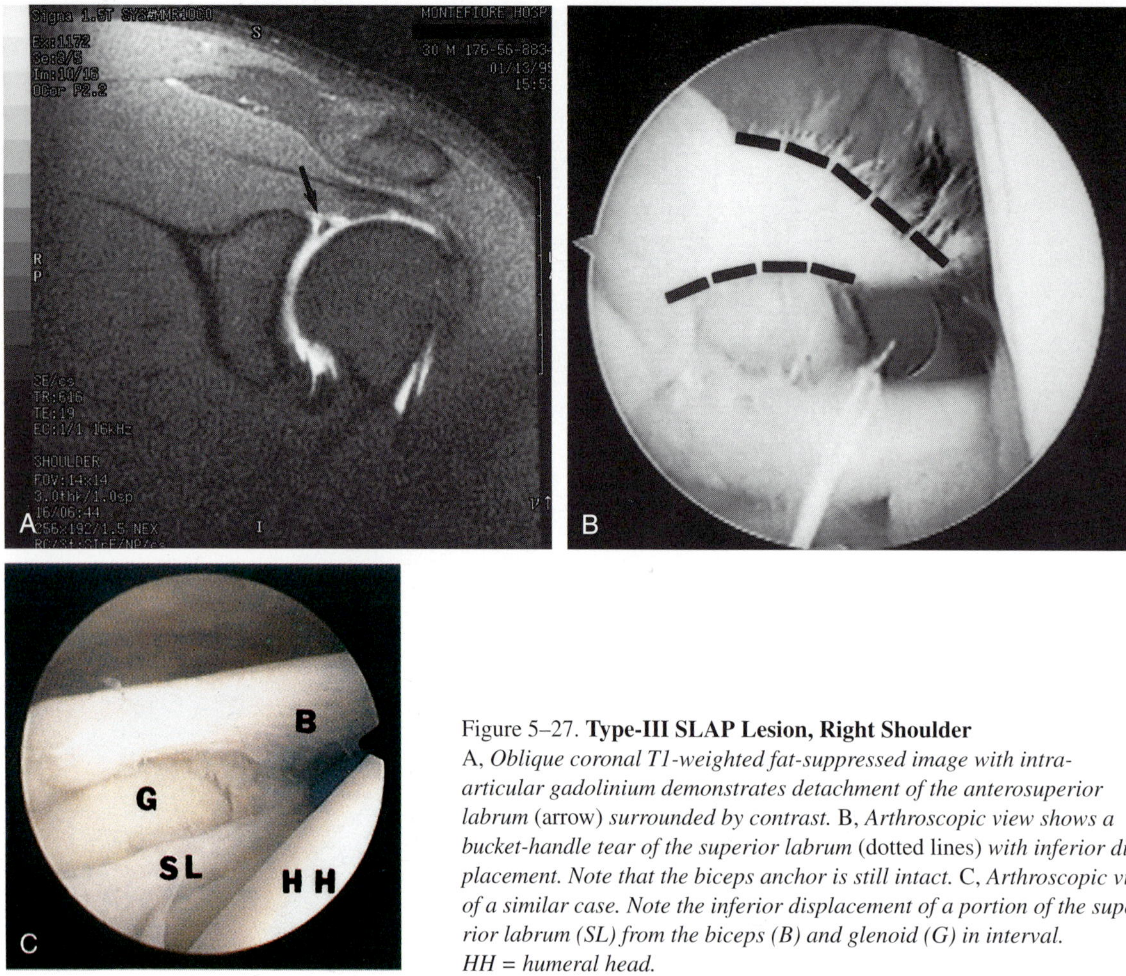

Figure 5–27. **Type-III SLAP Lesion, Right Shoulder**
A, *Oblique coronal T1-weighted fat-suppressed image with intra-articular gadolinium demonstrates detachment of the anterosuperior labrum* (arrow) *surrounded by contrast.* B, *Arthroscopic view shows a bucket-handle tear of the superior labrum* (dotted lines) *with inferior displacement. Note that the biceps anchor is still intact.* C, *Arthroscopic view of a similar case. Note the inferior displacement of a portion of the superior labrum (SL) from the biceps (B) and glenoid (G) in interval. HH = humeral head.*

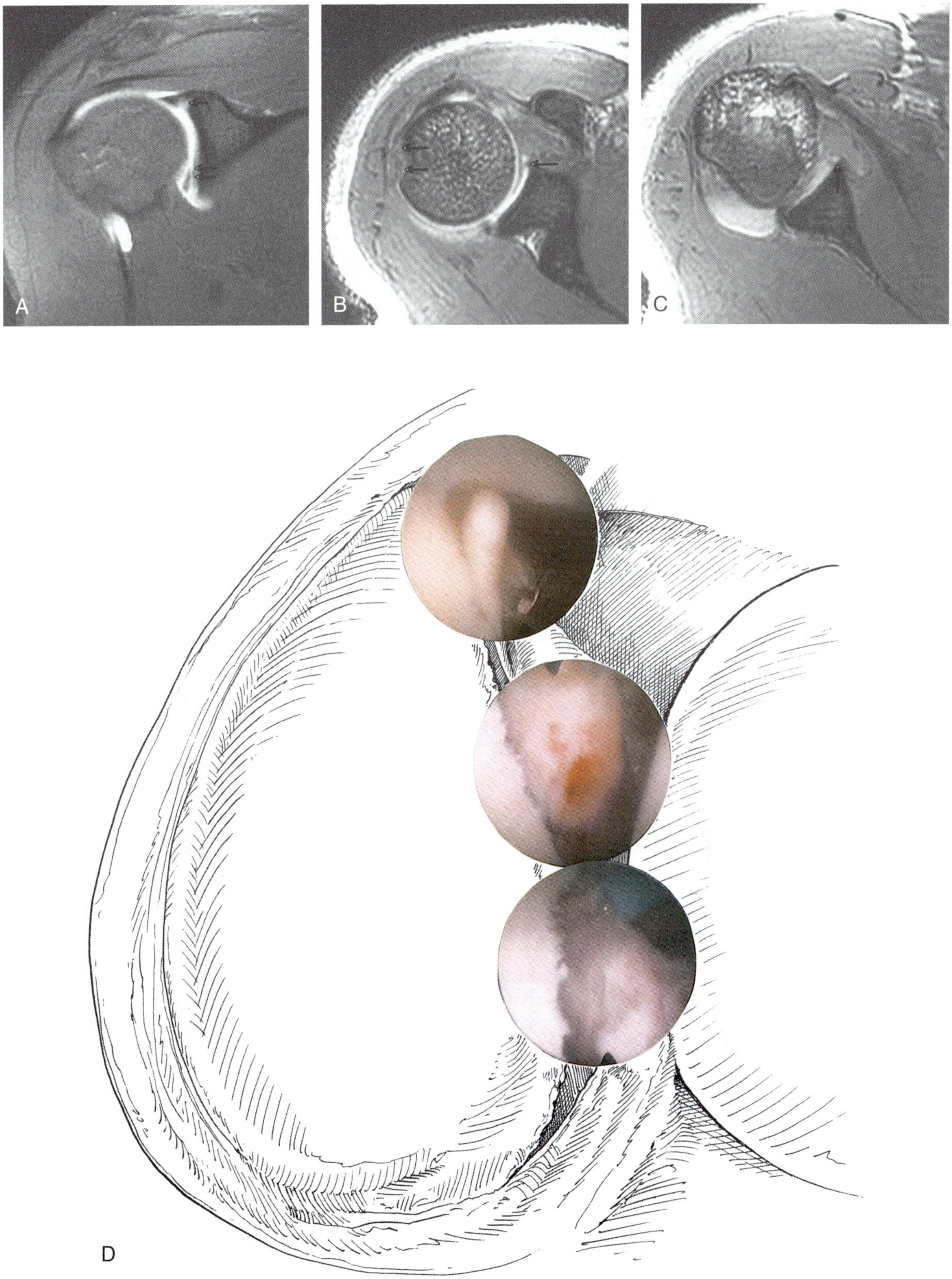

Figure 5–28. **Type-V SLAP Lesion, Right Shoulder**
A, *Oblique coronal T1-weighted SE fat-suppressed image with intra-articular administration of gadolinium shows a broad area of bright signal* (arrow) *undermining the attachment of the superior labrum and biceps tendon as well as blunting of the anterior inferior labrum* (double arrows). B, *Axial GRE volume acquisition image with intra-articular gadolinium demonstrates the diminutive appearance of the superior labrum* (arrow). *Note also a Hill-Sachs deformity* (double arrow). C, *Axial GRE volume acquisition image with intra-articular gadolinium shows blunting of the anteroinferior labrum* (arrow).
D, *Arthroscopic view demonstrates detachment of the superior labrum/biceps and a large Bankart lesion extending from the superior to the inferior labrum.*

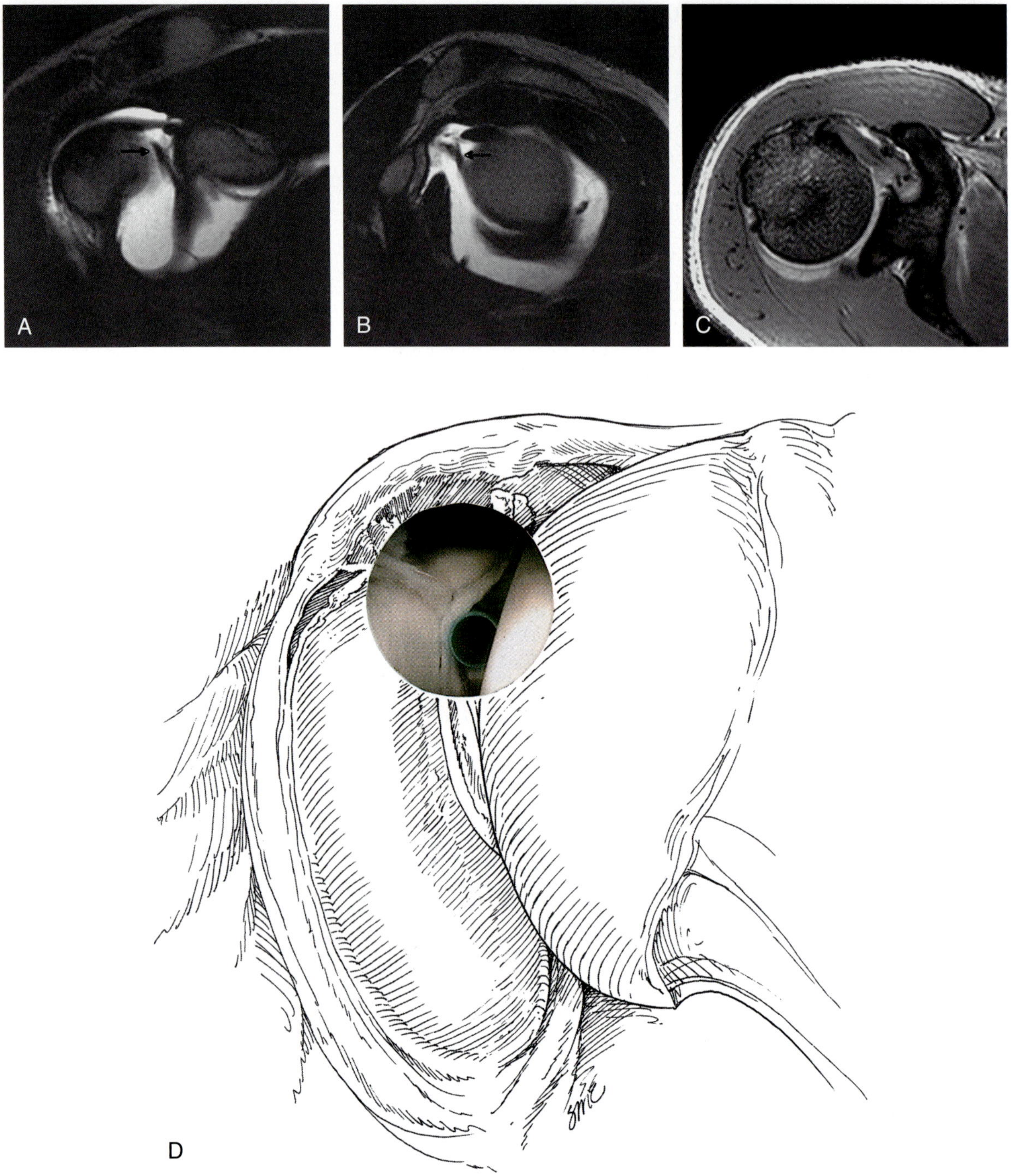

Figure 5–29. **Type-VI SLAP Lesion, Right Shoulder**
A, *Oblique coronal FSE T2-weighted image following intra-articular gadolinium administration shows a large superior labral flap* (arrow) *surrounded by fluid.* B, *Oblique sagittal FSE T2-weighted image following gadolinium administration reveals the same labral flap* (arrow) *anteriorly.* C, *Axial GRE image at the level of the coracoid process superiorly shows a large cleft* (arrow) *in the anterosuperior labrum manifested by bright signal dividing the labrum.* D, *Arthroscopic view demonstrates superior labral detachment and anterosuperior flap.*
Case courtesy of G. Bradford Wright, M.D.

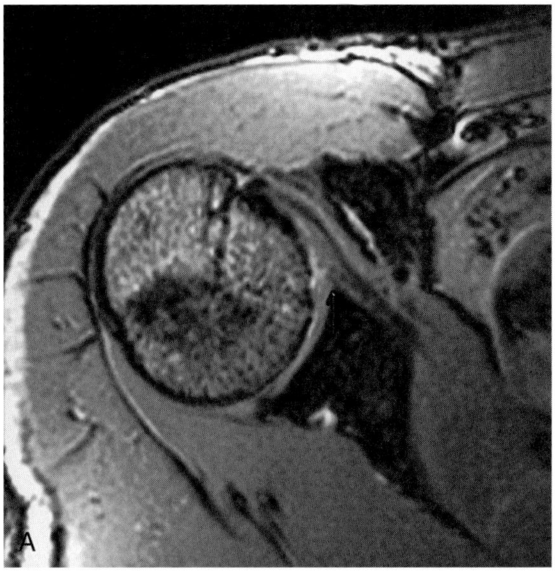

Figure 5–30. **Anterosuperior Labral Flap Tear, Right Shoulder**
A, *Axial GRE image at the level of the coracoid process and subscapularis tendon depicts absence of the anterosuperior labrum* (arrow). B, *Arthroscopic view demonstrates anterosuperior labral tear that was debrided arthroscopically.* Case courtesy of Daniel T. Hinkin, M.D.

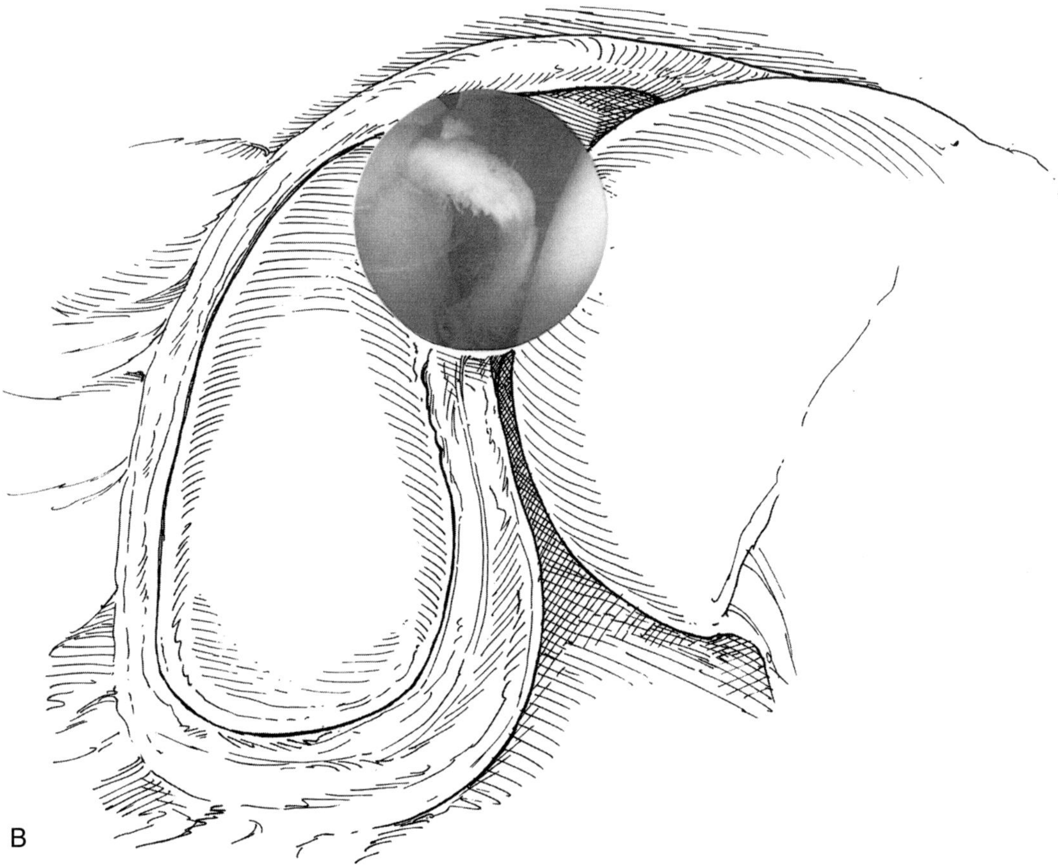

B

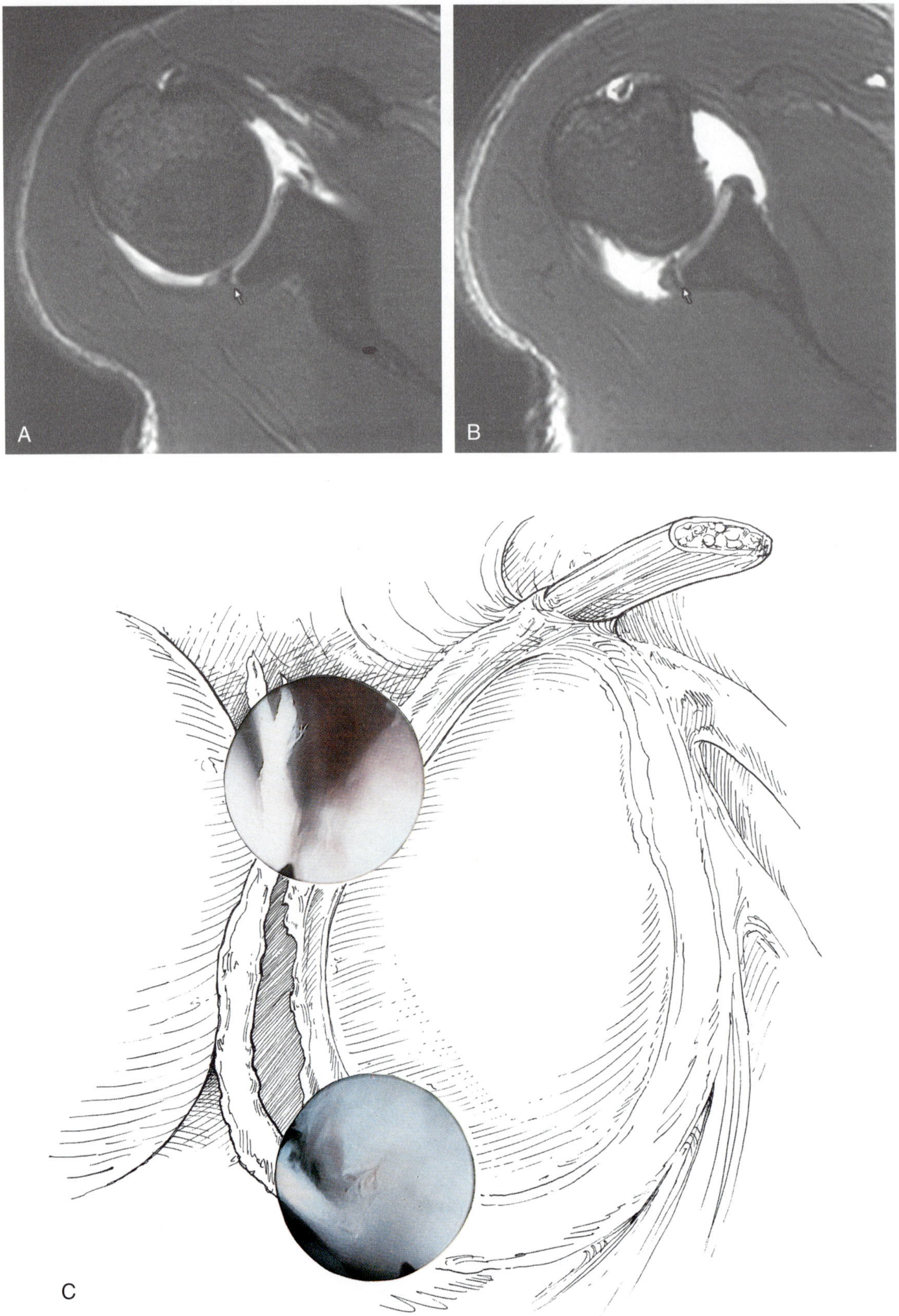

Figure 5–31. **Posterior Labral Flap Tear, Right Shoulder**
A, *Axial GRE image with intra-articular administration of gadolinium shows linear bright signal* (arrow) *between the glenoid margin and posterosuperior labrum.* B, *Axial GRE image with intra-articular administration of gadolinium demonstrates linear bright signal* (arrow) *between the glenoid and the posteroinferior labrum.* C, *Arthroscopic view demonstrates posterior labral tear with inferior and superior components.*

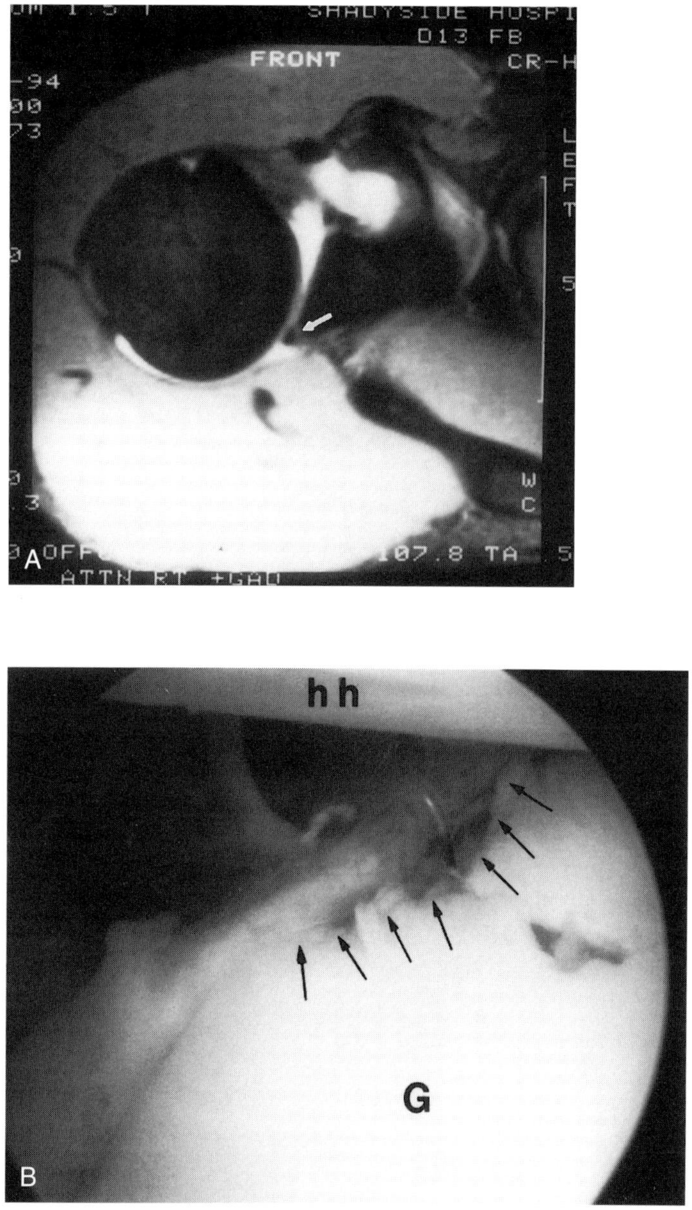

Figure 5–32. **Posterior Labral Tear, Right Shoulder**
A, *Axial GRE image with intra-articular administration of gadolinium demonstrates linear bright signal (arrow) between the posterosuperior labrum and glenoid margin.* B, *Arthroscopic view, from the anterosuperior portal, demonstrates a posterosuperior labral tear from the glenoid margin* (arrows). *G, glenoid; hh, humeral head.*

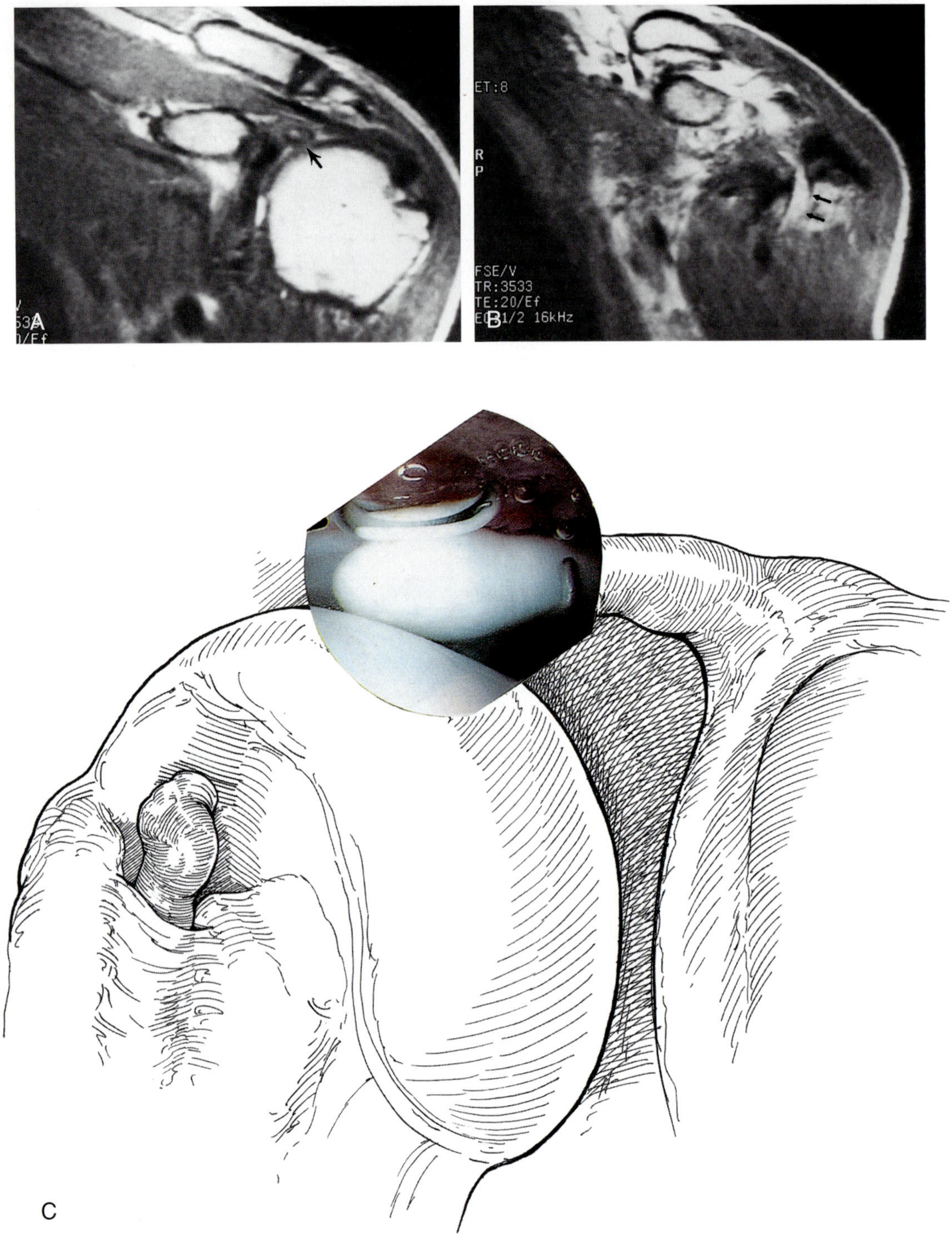

Figure 5–33. **Proximal Biceps Avulsion, Left Shoulder**

A, *Oblique coronal FSE proton-density image shows the proximal stump of torn biceps tendon* (arrow). B, *Oblique coronal FSE proton-density image, anterior to* A, *shows a fluid-filled bicipital groove devoid of biceps tendon* (arrows).
C, *Arthroscopic photo depicts the residual stump of biceps tendon and absent distal portion of this structure.*
Case courtesy of John McBryde, M.D.

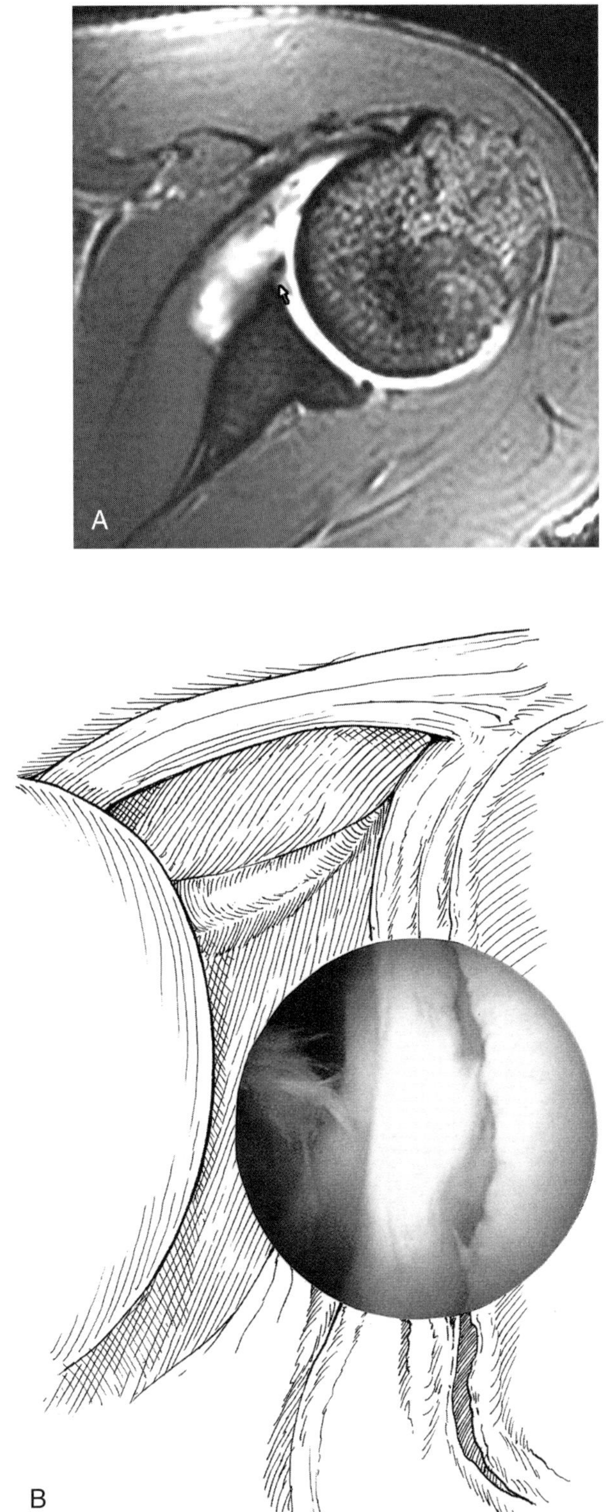

Figure 5–34. **Bankart Tear, Left Shoulder**
A, *Axial T-weighted SE fat-suppressed image with intra-articular administration of gadolinium demonstrates a focal area of bright signal* (arrow) *between the anteroinferior labrum and glenoid.* B, *Arthroscopic image demonstrates a large anterior Bankart lesion with displacement of the inferior labrum and inferior glenohumeral ligament complex from the labrum.*

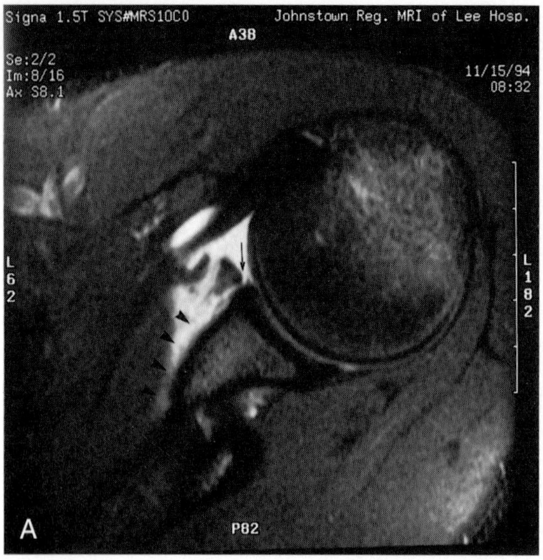

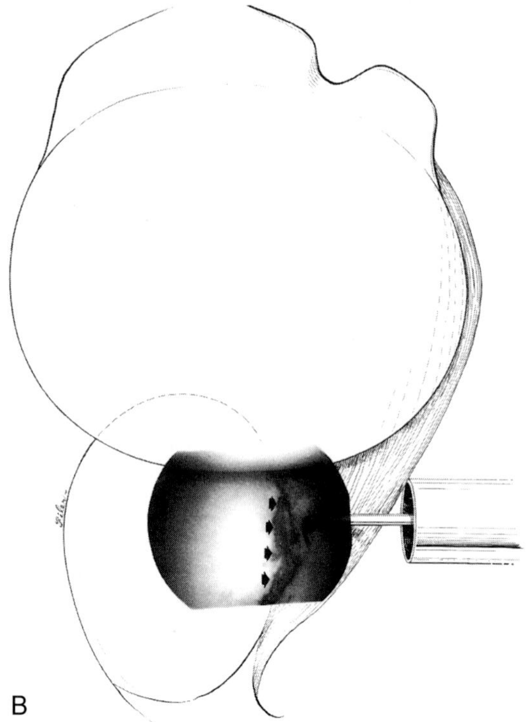

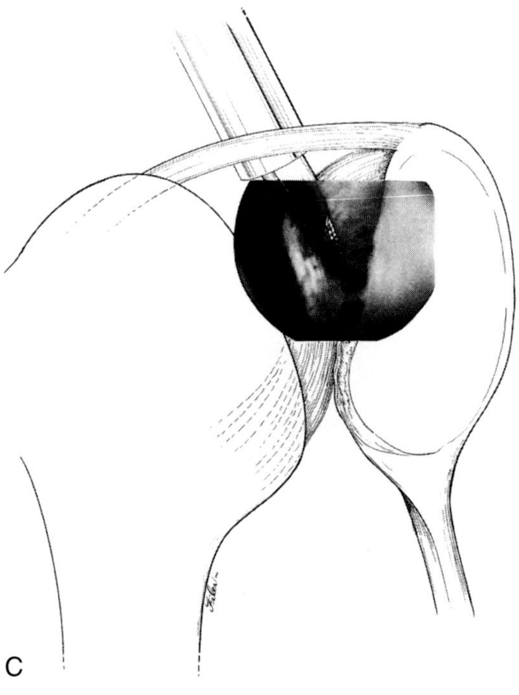

Figure 5–35. **Bankart Tear with Capsular Stripping, Left Shoulder**

A, *Axial T1-weighted SE fat-suppressed image with intra-articular administration of gadolinium demonstrates a linear area of bright signal* (arrow) *between the anteroinferior labrum and glenoid. Note the anterior capsular stripping* (arrowheads). B, *Arthroscopic photo demonstrates a large Bankart tear* (arrows) *displaced by the probe.* C, *Note the degree of anterior capsular stripping in this view. File is placed between the glenoid margin and the anterior labrum/capsule.*

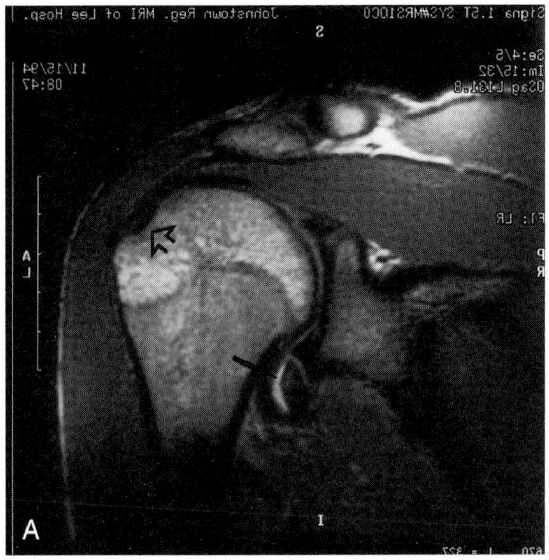

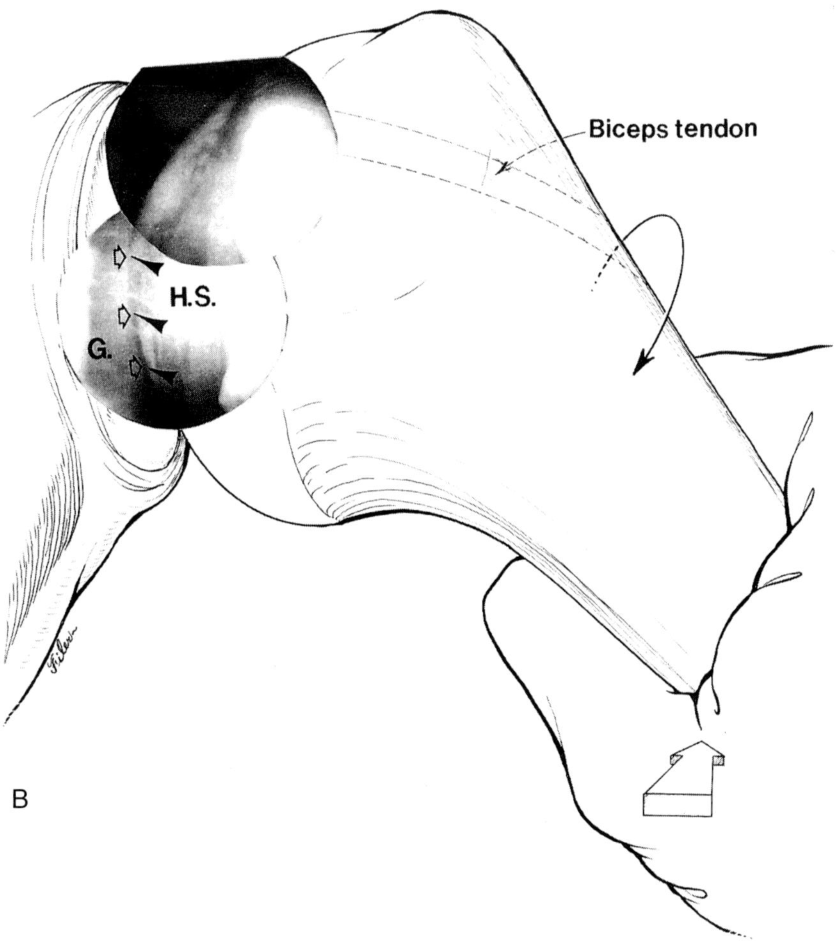

Figure 5–36. **Bankart Tear and Hill-Sachs Defect, Right Shoulder**
A, *Oblique coronal T1-weighted image reveals an inferior Bankart lesion* (arrow) *and a small osseous deformity* (open arrow). B, *Arthroscopic view demonstrates soft tissue Bankart lesion* (arrows) *and Hill-Sachs (H.S.) osteochondral impression fracture* (superior image). *G = glenoid. Note the anteriorly directed external force* (anterior drawer) *causing subluxation.*

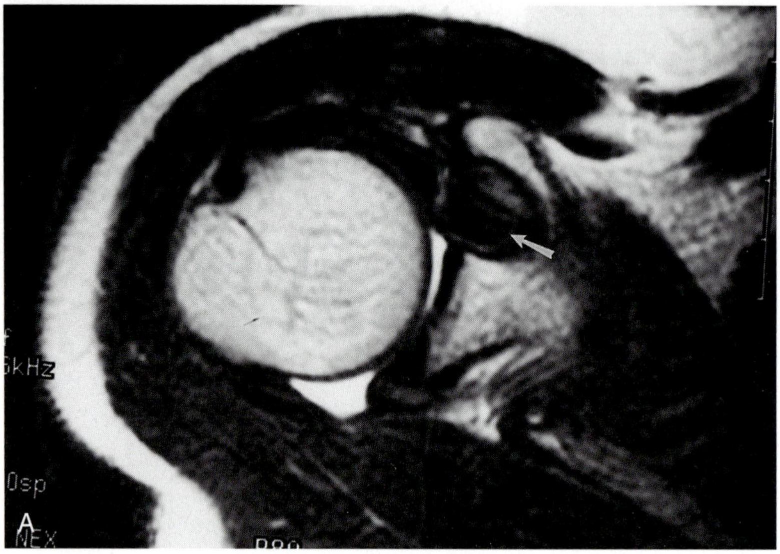

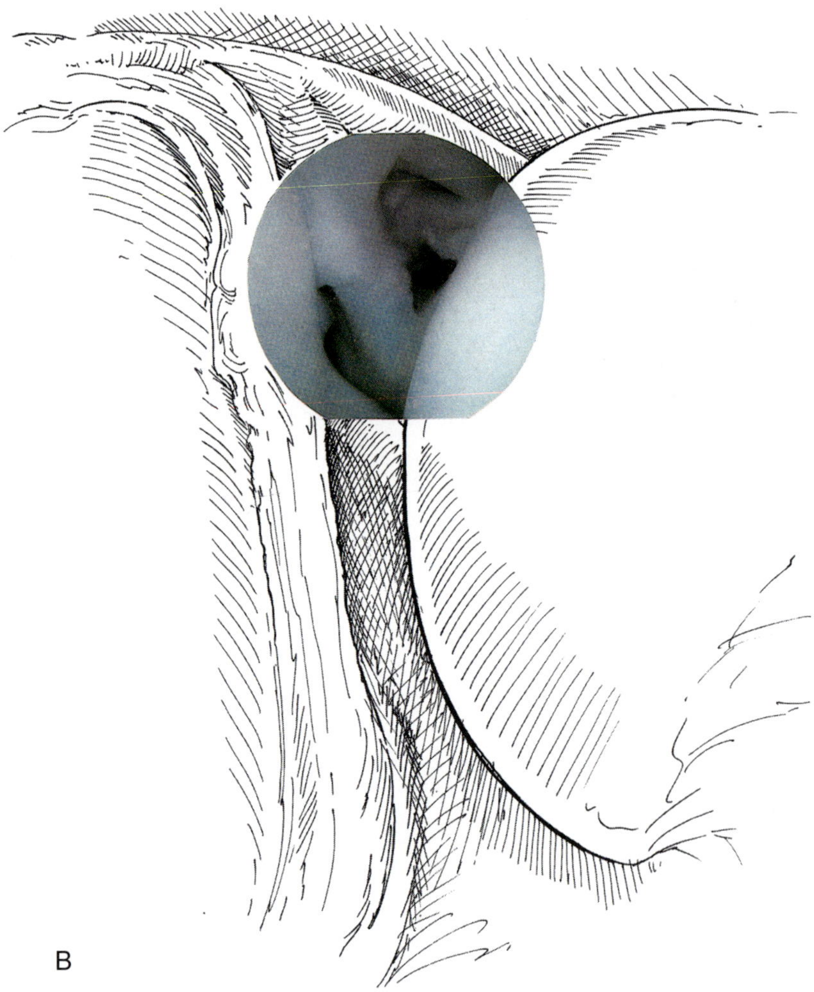

B

Figure 5–37. **Buford Complex, Right Shoulder**
A, *Axial FSE T2-weighted image at the level of the coracoid process shows an extraordinarily thick middle glenohumeral ligament* (arrow). B, *Arthroscopic view shows marked thickening of the middle glenohumeral ligament.*

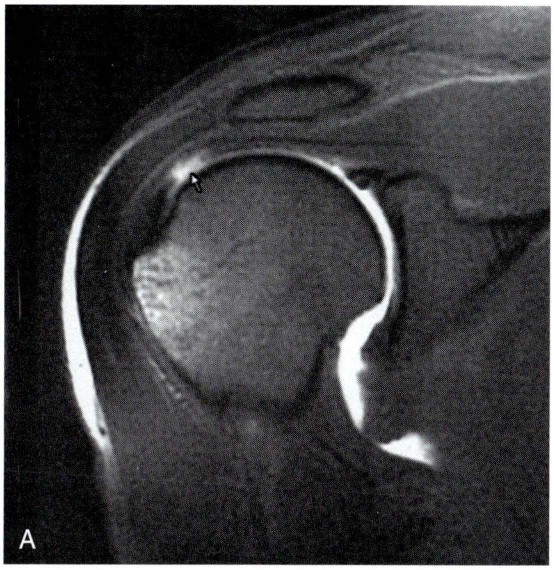

Figure 5–38. **Partial-Thickness Rotator Cuff Tear, Right Shoulder**
A, *Oblique coronal fat-saturated T1-weighted image following intra-articular administration of gadolinium shows marked irregularity* (arrow) *of the articular surface of the supraspinatus tendon near its insertion, highlighted by contrast.* B, *Arthroscopic figure reveals fraying and partial-thickness injury of the supraspinatus tendon.*

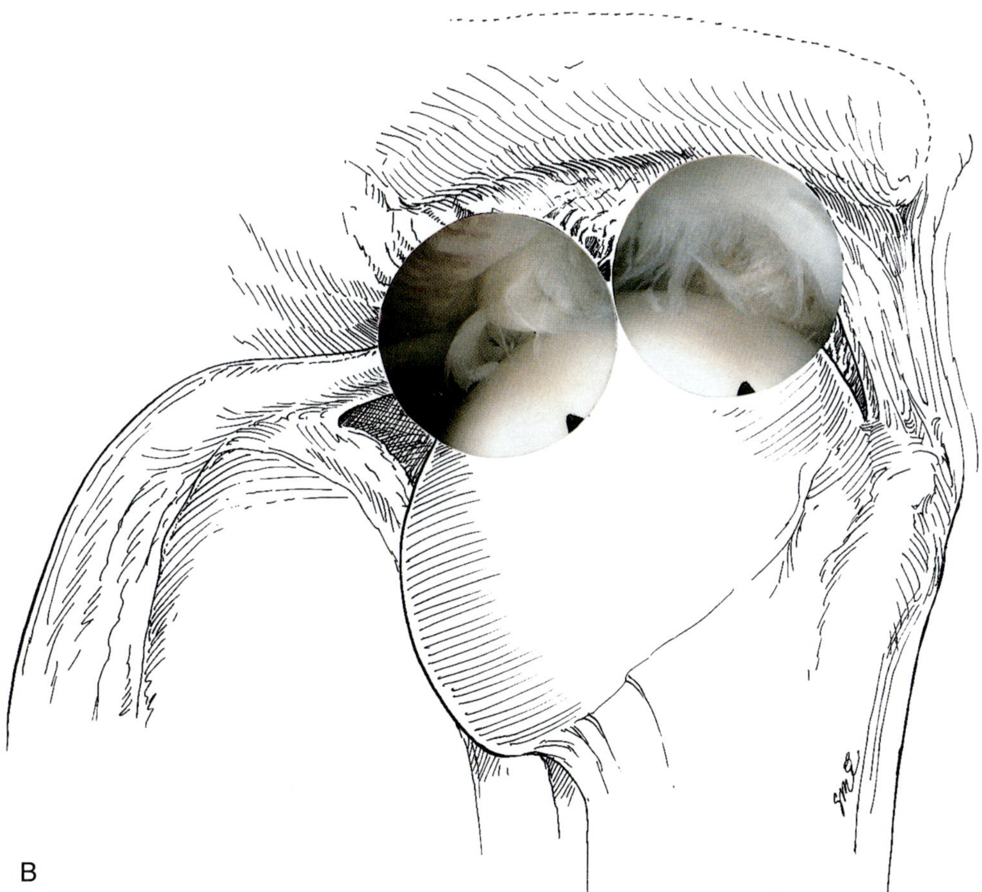

B

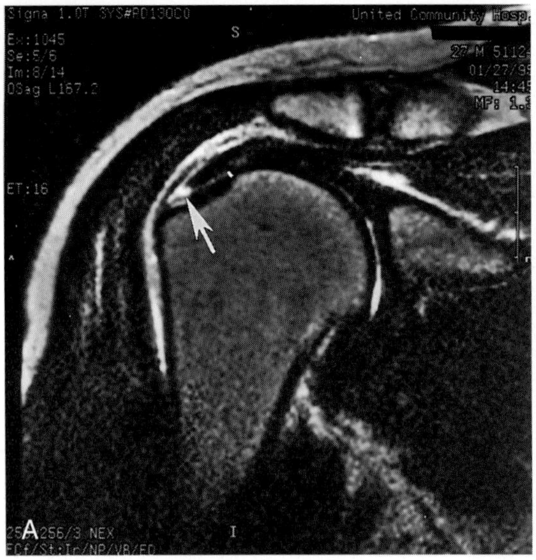

Figure 5–39. **Rotator Cuff Avulsion, Right Shoulder**
A, *Oblique sagittal FSE T2-weighted image reveals a focus of bright signal completely traversing the distal supraspinatus tendon at its insertion into the greater tuberosity* (arrow). B, *Arthroscopic figure shows a small rotator cuff tear near its insertion.*

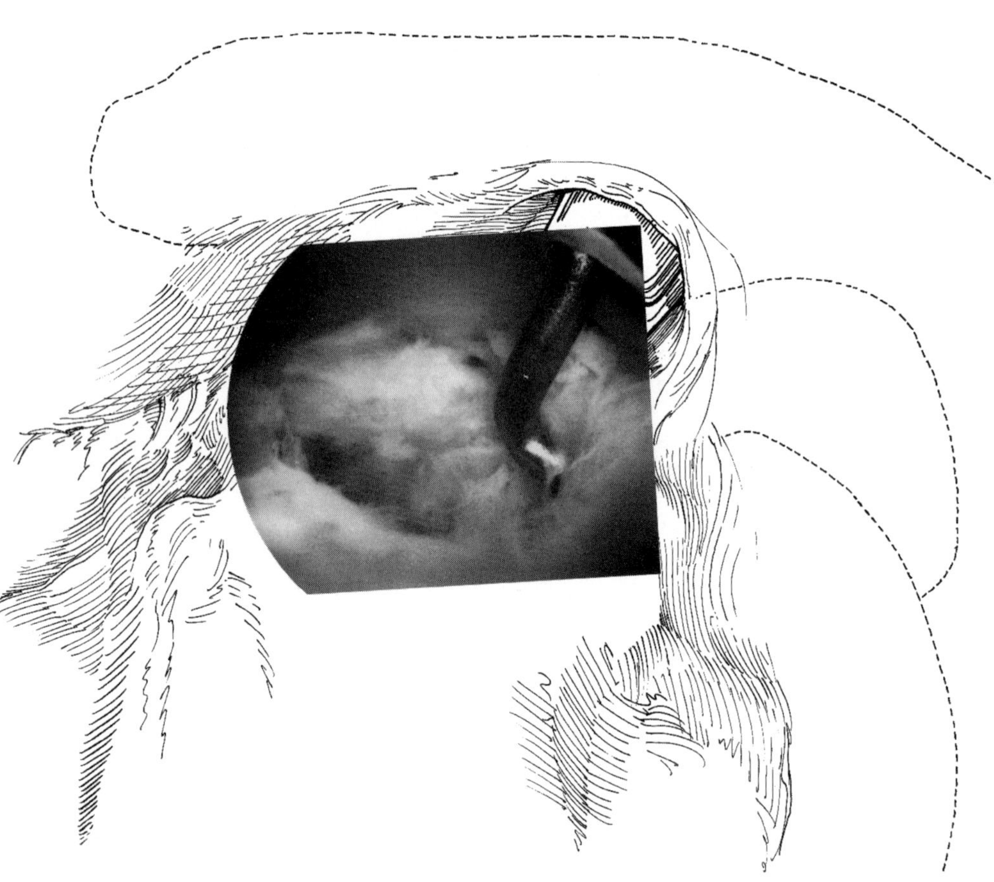

B

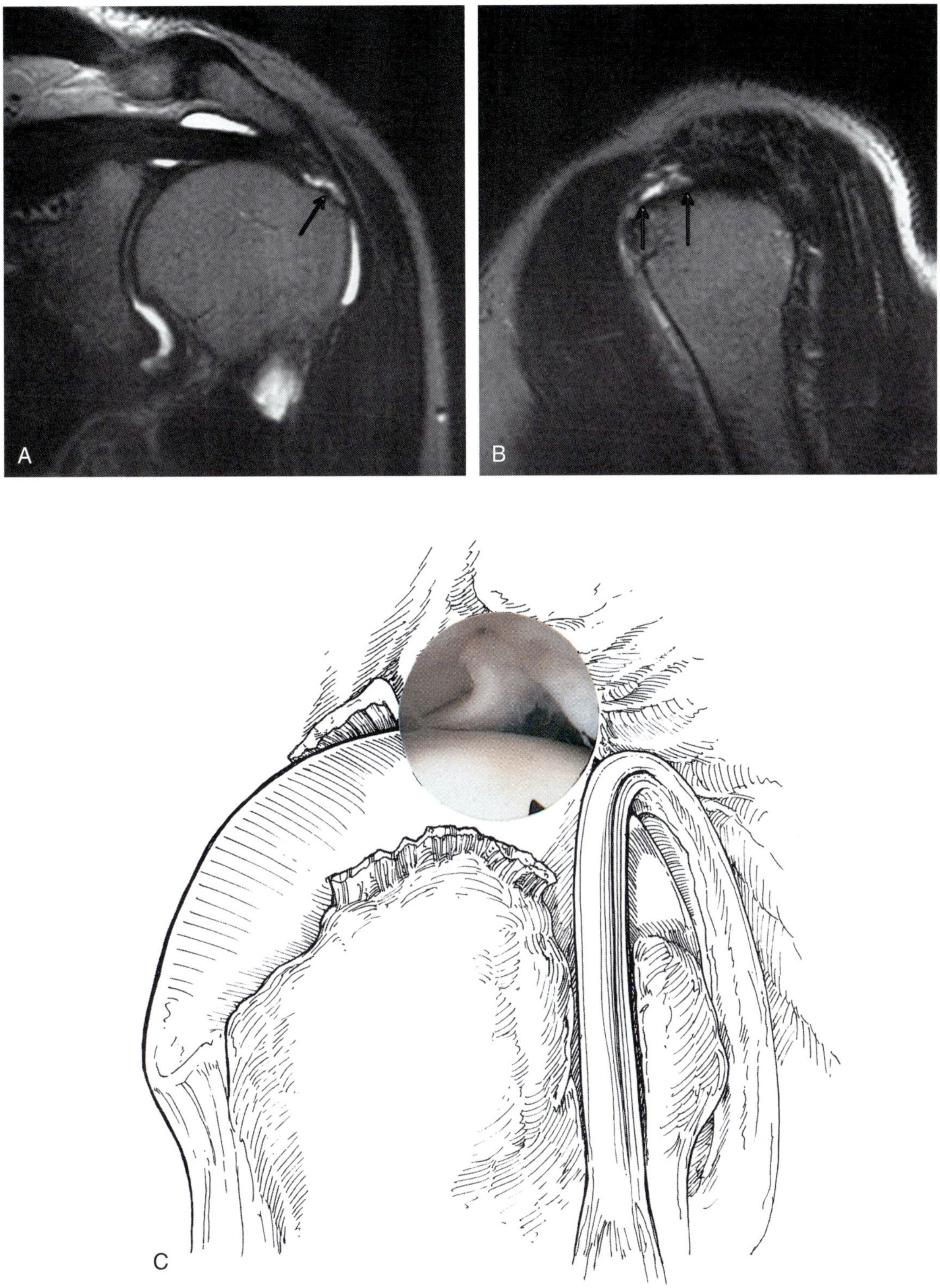

Figure 5–40. **Rotator Cuff Tear, Left Shoulder**
A, *Oblique coronal FSE T2-weighted image demonstrates bright signal* (arrow) *consistent with fluid traversing the supraspinatus tendon near its insertion. Note that fluid also is in the subacromial bursa.* B, *Sagittal oblique FSE T2-weighted image reveals disruption of the tendon manifested by "full-thickness" bright signal from fluid* (arrows). C, *Arthroscopic view shows a complete rotator cuff tear.*

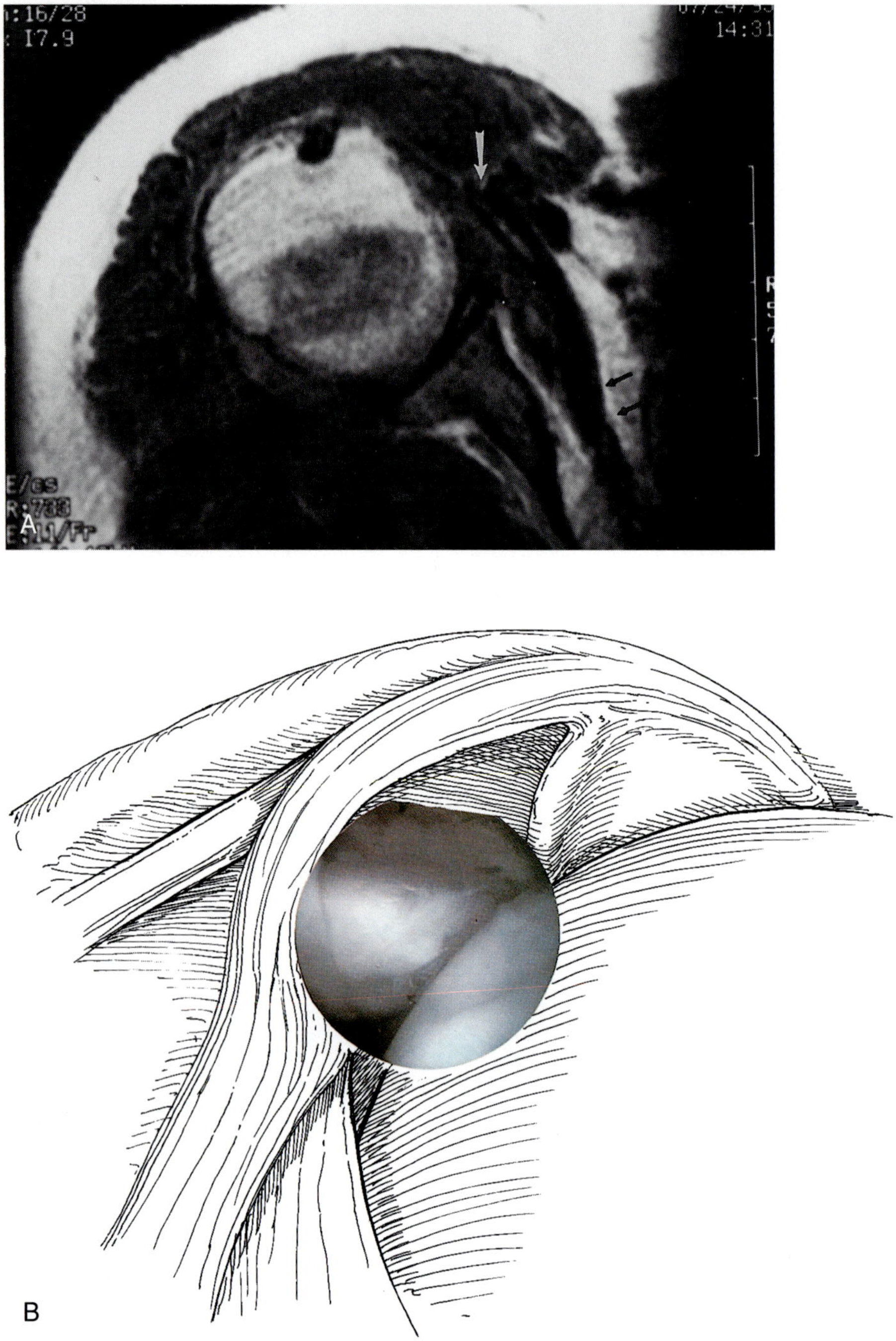

Figure 5–41. **Subscapularis Tear, Right Shoulder**
A, *Axial T1-weighted image demonstrates disruption of the subscapularis tendon* (arrow) *with proximal muscular atrophy* (arrows). B, *Arthroscopic view reveals a tear of the subscapularis tendon from its insertion.*

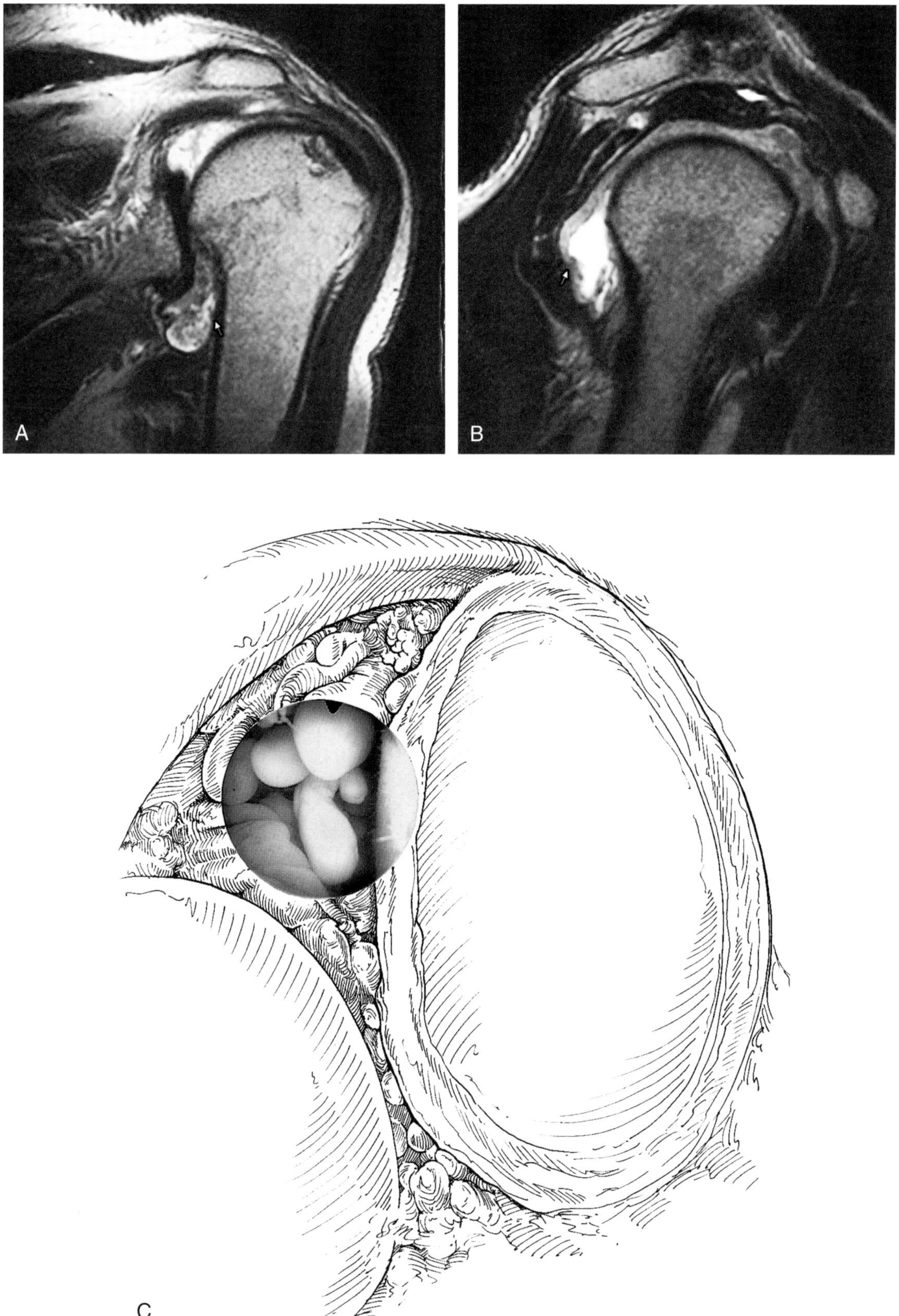

Figure 5–42. **Villonodular Synovitis, Left Shoulder**

A, *Oblique coronal FSE T2-weighted image shows nodular, intermediate-signal soft tissue in the axillary recess* (arrow). B, *Oblique sagittal FSE T2-weighted image reveals intermediate-signal synovial thickening* (arrow) *highlighted by adjacent synovial fluid.* C, *Arthroscopic view shows "fingers" of hypertrophic synovium extending into the joint.*

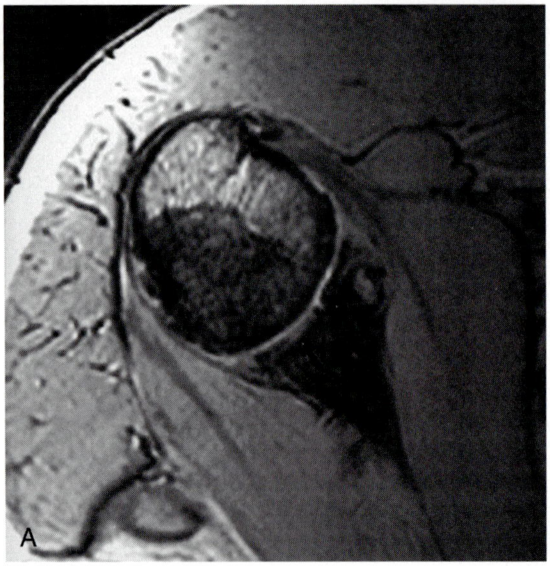

Figure 5–43. **Glenoid Degenerative Joint Disease, Right Shoulder**
A, *Axial GRE image reveals multiple irregularities manifested by bright and dark signal in the region of the hyaline cartilage* (arrows). B, *Arthroscopic view demonstrates advanced chondrosis of the glenoid with normal "islands" of articular cartilage in a "sea" of exposed bone.*

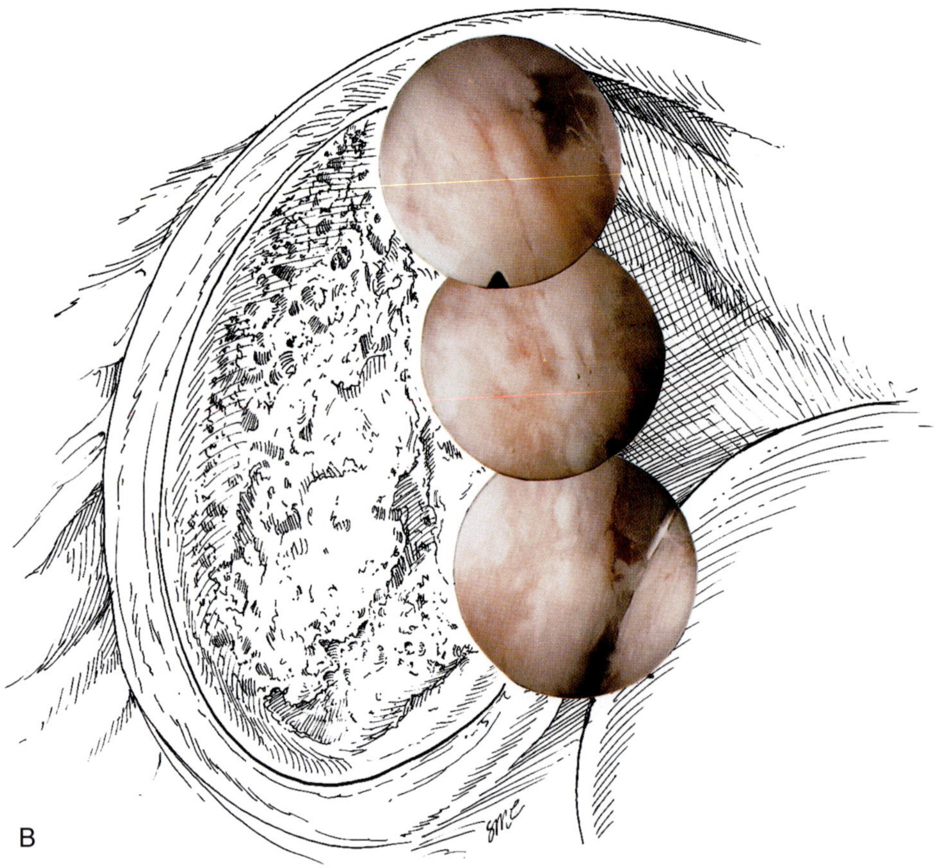

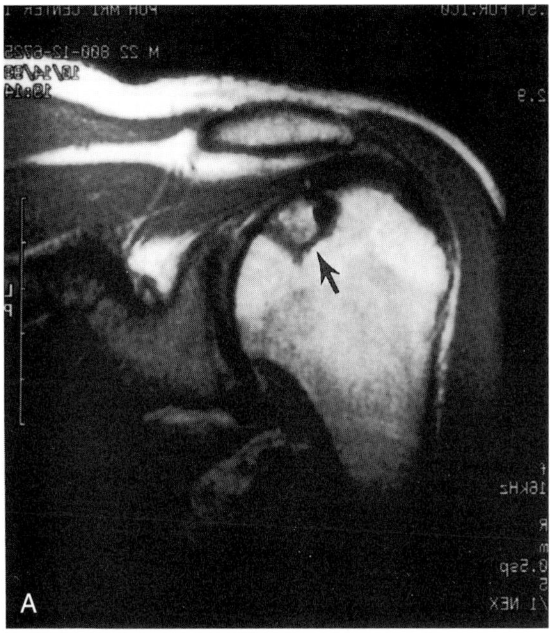

Figure 5–44. **Osteochondral Defect, Humeral Head, Left Shoulder**
A, *Oblique coronal FSE proton density–weighted image reveals a 1.5-cm, well-delineated osteochondral lesion* (arrow). B, *Arthroscopic figure shows the osteochondral defect in the humeral head.*

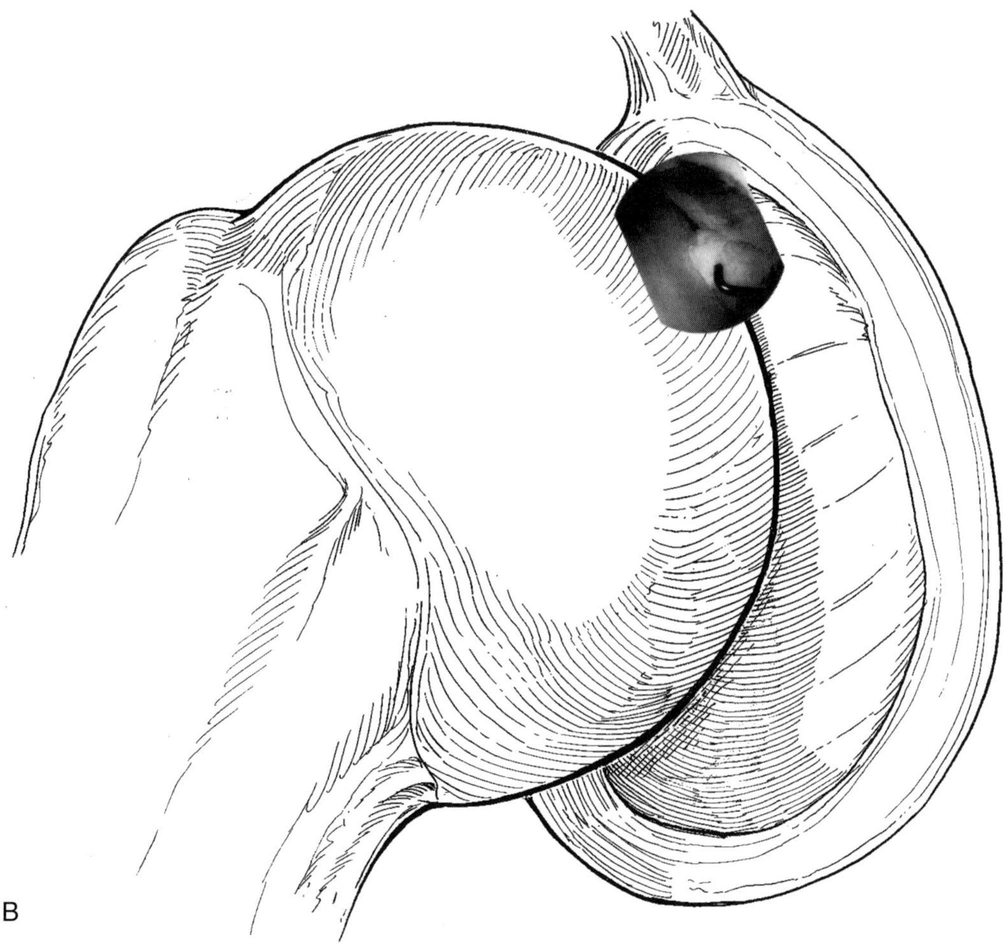

B

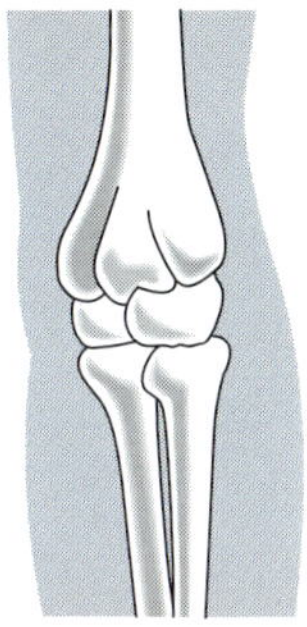

CHAPTER

6

Elbow

MRI of the Elbow

MRI of the elbow can enable visualization of epicondylitis, pediatric fractures, osteochondral defects, osteonecrosis, biceps and triceps tendon injuries, ulnar collateral ligament (UCL) injury, loose bodies, and osteophytes.[12] At the Mayo Clinic, 85% of non-neurologic MRI examinations are for musculoskeletal indications, and 15% of these are for examinations of the elbow and wrist.[2] Although MRI has not yet been proven the modality of choice in many clinical settings, its use is increasing. It has enormous potential and can surely be a useful adjunct to the arthroscopist.

TECHNIQUE

The most comfortable position for examining the elbow is the supine position with the arm at the side. Although indications may vary the position, most patients are evaluated with the elbow in extension and hand palm-up. Certain structures such as the biceps tendon may need to be studied with the elbow in flexion.

Surface coils significantly improve the signal-to-noise ratio (Fig. 6–1). The depth of view is limited with flat coils to approximately one half the radius of the coil. The elbow, however, fits well within the range of such a coil.[3, 5] We have even used an anterior neck coil successfully and currently use a flexible coil with excellent results.

Surface coils, then, with a small field of view (10 to 12 cm), a matrix of 256 × 256, and a 4-mm slice thickness with a 0.5- to 1-mm inter-slice gap are recommended. One or even two signal averages (number of excitations) may be needed for an acceptable signal-to-noise ratio, depending on the type of pulse sequence and pixel size. More signal averages are needed for a smaller pixel size.

Optimally, MRI sequences should be tailored. A vitamin-E capsule can mark an area of concern. Intravenous or intra-articular contrast may elucidate certain pathologic conditions.[5] In general, three anatomic planes are obtained. The sagittal and coronal imaging planes are useful for analyzing the joint, including the capsule, articulations, and articular

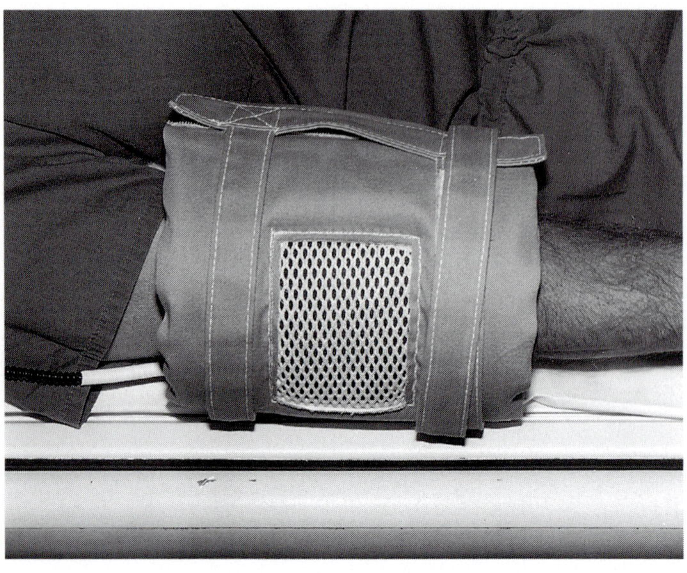

Figure 6–1
A 5- × 7-in. flexible coil used to image the elbow.

hyaline cartilage. Bone marrow and soft tissue processes are well demonstrated in these planes. Axial imaging identifies specific structures and demonstrates anatomic relationships, especially muscle groups, fascial planes, and neurovascular bundles. The pulse sequences used for the elbow examination vary with clinical indications. As a rule, both T1-weighted and T2-weighted sequences are performed, although fast spin-echo, gradient-recalled echo, and short tau inversion recovery (STIR) sequences can provide additional information.

MRI ANATOMY

MRI anatomy of the elbow is viewed adequately in the axial, coronal, and sagittal anatomic planes (Figs. 6–2, 6–3, 6–4).

The elbow joint is composed of three bones: the humerus, ulna, and radius. It consists of three articulations: a lateral articulation between the capitellum and the radius, a medial articulation between the trochlea and the trochlear notch of the ulna, and the radioulnar articulation. The first two articulations form a hinge joint and allow flexion and extension. The third articulation permits supination and pronation.[3, 13, 19]

A common capsule surrounds the three articulations. Medial and lateral capsular thickening constitute the supporting collateral ligaments. The medial and lateral collateral ligaments and the annular ligament are the major ligaments of the elbow joint. The medial (ulnar) collateral ligament originates from the inferior surface of the medial epicondyle

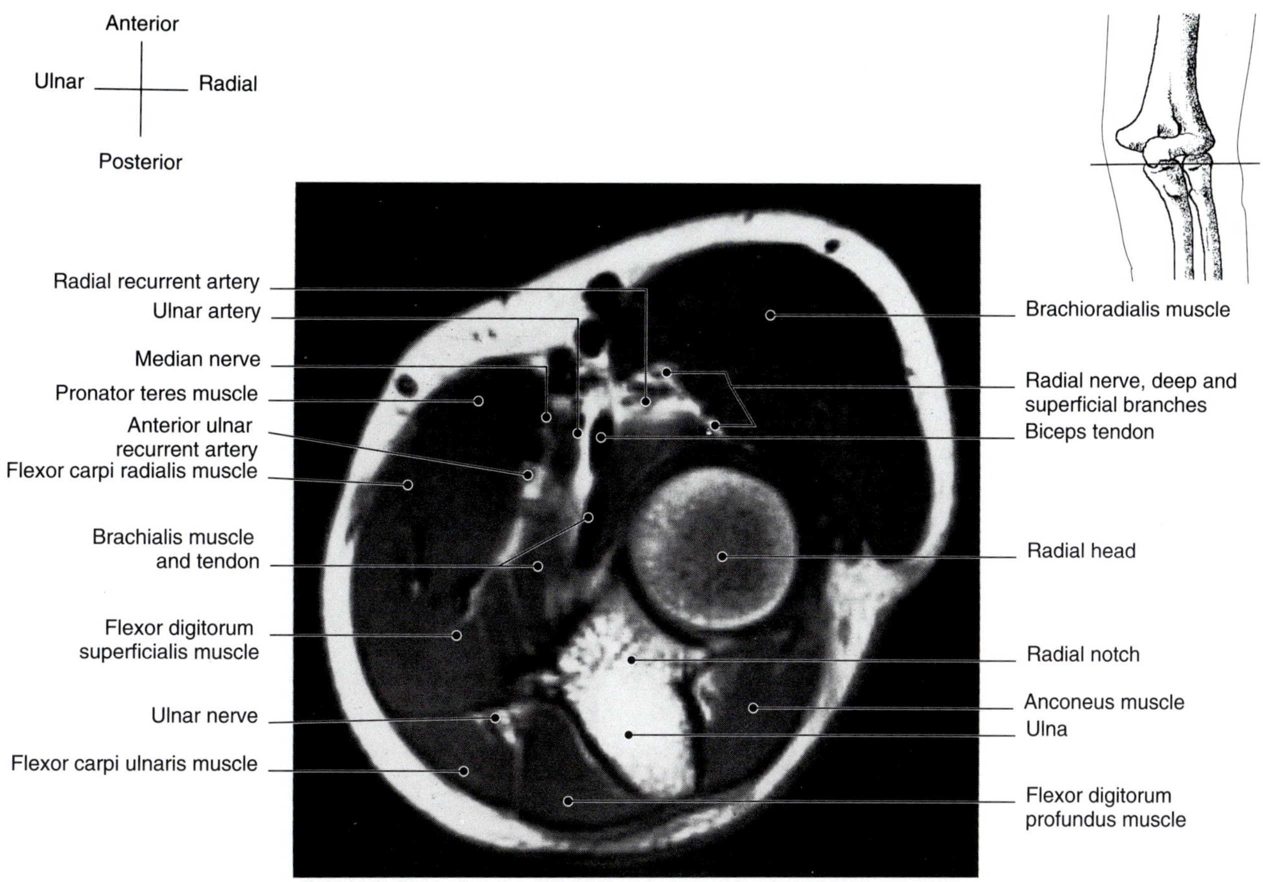

Figure 6–2

Axial magnetic-resonance image (TR, 600 ms; TE, 20 ms) of the elbow at the level of the proximal radioulnar joint. (From Chan WP, Rauschning W, Wu CY, et al. Magnetic resonance imaging anatomy and cryomicrotome atlas. In *Chan WP, Lang P, Genant HK, eds. MRI of the Musculoskeletal System. Philadelphia: WB Saunders, 1994.)*

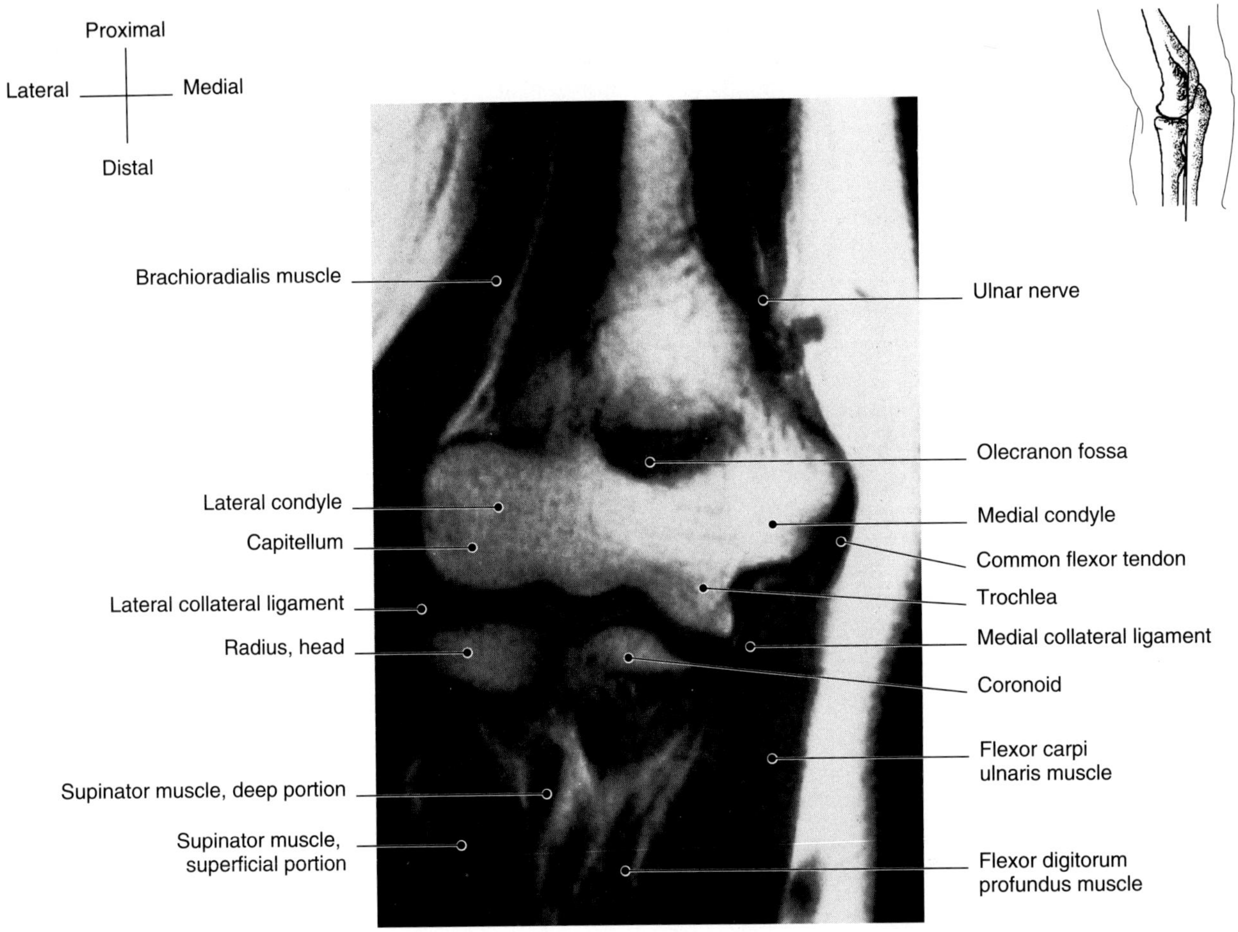

Figure 6–3
Posterior coronal magnetic-resonance image (TR, 600 ms; TE, 20 ms) of the elbow. (From Chan WP, Rauschning W, Wu CY, et al. Magnetic resonance imaging anatomy and cryomicrotome atlas. In *Chan WP, Lang P, Genant HK, eds. MRI of the Musculoskeletal System. Philadelphia: WB Saunders, 1994.)*

and attaches to the olecranon and coronoid process of the ulna. It is the major support of the elbow against valgus stress. It has three components: the anterior oblique ligament, which is the strongest and most important, the posterior oblique ligament, and the transverse ligament. The lateral (radial) collateral ligament is relatively weaker, originating from the lateral epicondyle and attaching predominantly to another ligament, the annular ligament. The annular ligament stabilizes the proximal radioulnar joint by surrounding the radial head and neck, attaching to the superior and inferior aspects of the radial notch of the proximal ulna. The ligaments are of low signal intensity on all pulse sequences. The medial and lateral collateral ligaments are best seen on the coronal and sagittal images. The annular ligament is visualized on the axial and coronal images. The gradient-recalled echo sequence is good at distinguishing ligament from adjacent bone because of the bright signal from cartilage. The olecranon bursa is situated over the dorsal aspect of the olecranon and develops at approximately 8 year of age.[3, 13, 19]

There are four muscle groups in the elbow constituting the medial, lateral, anterior, and posterior compartments. The pronator teres, flexor carpi radialis, palmaris longus, flexor digitorum superficialis, flexor carpi ulnaris, and flexor digitorum profundus constitute the medial compartment. The flexor muscles have a common tendon that originates from the medial humeral epicondyle. The brachioradialis, extensor carpi radialis longus, extensor carpi radialis brevis, extensor digitorum longus, extensor carpi ulnaris, and extensor digiti minimi constitute the lateral compartment and, except for the extensor carpi radialis longus, originate from the lateral humeral epicondyle along a common extensor tendon. The brachialis and biceps constitute the anterior compartment and provide elbow flexion. The brachialis inserts on the ulnar tuberosity, and the biceps inserts on the radial tuberosity. The triceps and anconeus constitute the posterior compartment. The triceps tendon appears heterogeneous as it inserts onto the olecranon because of fat between its fascicles. This normal heterogeneity should not be misinterpreted as a tear.[3, 13, 19]

The major vascular structures include the brachial artery, which travels medially to the biceps along the anterior superficial surface of the brachialis and divides into radial and ulnar arteries distal to the joint. The cephalic vein laterally and the basilic vein medially both reside anterior and superficial to the muscles. Three major nerves traverse the elbow joint: the ulnar, median, and radial nerves. The ulnar nerve passes superficially through the cubital tunnel behind the medial epicondyle. The arcuate ligament, posterior to the nerve, bridges the tunnel. The nerve can usually be seen in all three imaging planes. The median nerve is located anterior to the brachialis and parallels medially the brachial artery. The nerve is best seen on axial images. The radial nerve courses laterally between the brachialis and brachioradialis muscles. The nerve is best delineated on axial images. The radial nerve has superficial and deep divisions at the level of the radiocapitellar joint.[3, 13, 19]

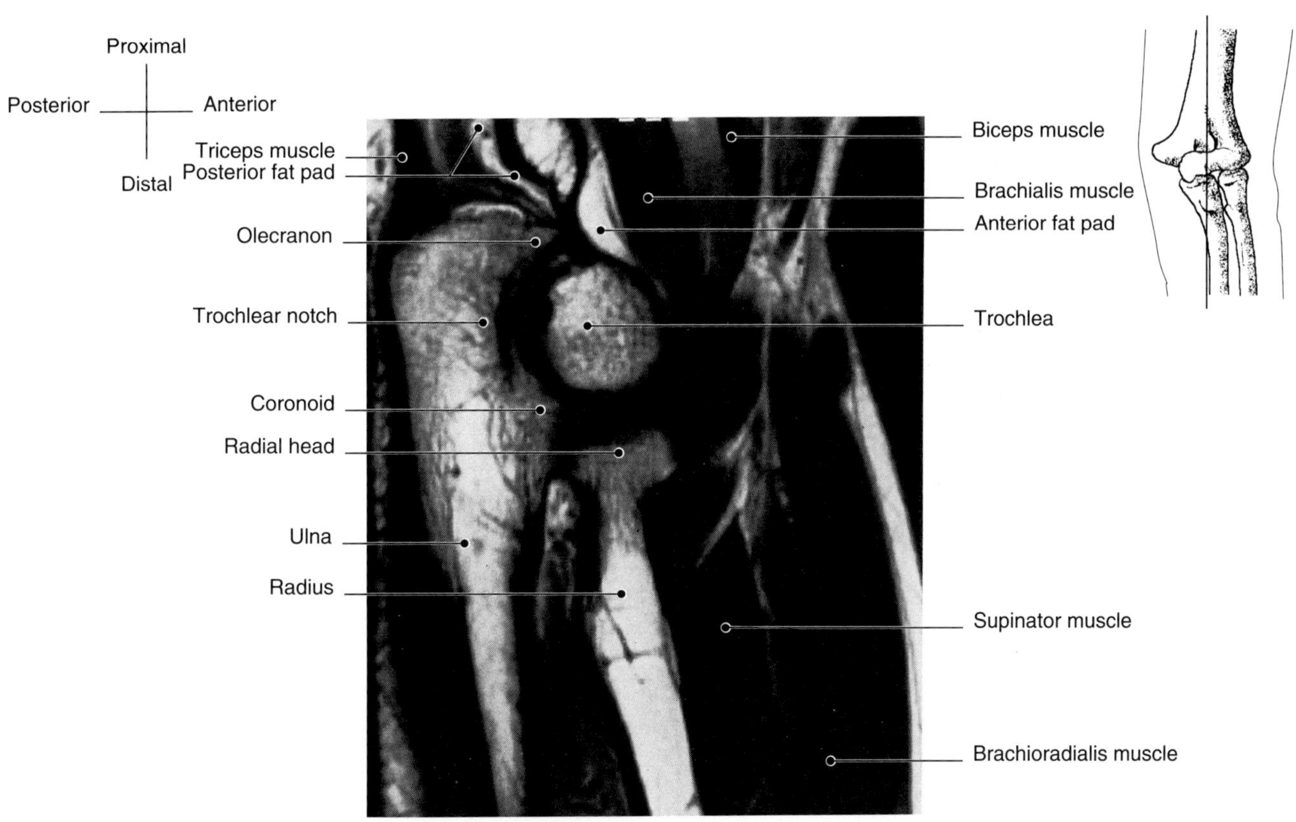

Figure 6–4
Paramedian sagittal magnetic-resonance image (TR, 600 ms; TE, 20 ms) of the elbow. (From Chan WP, Rauschning W, Wu CY, et al. Magnetic resonance imaging anatomy and cryomicrotome atlas. In *Chan WP, Lang P, Genant HK, eds. MRI of the Musculoskeletal System. Philadelphia: WB Saunders, 1994.)*

NORMAL VARIANTS AND INTERPRETATION PITFALLS

Numerous variants and interpretation pitfalls have been described, including the pseudodefect of the capitellum, transverse trochlear ridge, trochlear groove pseudodefect, and ulnar nerve dislocation.[17] The pseudodefect of the capitellum is a small notch at the junction of the capitellum with the lateral epicondyle that can be seen on sagittal and coronal images. This normal notch may simulate an osteochondral defect. The pseudodefect manifests as an apparently abrupt disruption of the posterolateral capitellar cortical surfaces. A true osteochondral impaction fracture or osteochondritis dissecans produces flattening and deformity of the capitellar curved articular surface. Bone-marrow abnormalities also are present.[17] A transverse trochlear ridge commonly traverses the trochlear groove in the proximal ulna that articulates with the trochlea of the humerus. This cartilage-free ridge is commonly seen on sagittal images as a central elevation of the articular surface of the trochlear groove[15] (Fig. 6–5). The trochlear groove pseudodefect is seen on the surface of the trochlear groove and is due to small medial and lateral indentations along the superior edges of the waist of the groove. They manifest themselves as normal cortical notches not to be mistaken for traumatic ulnar defects.[15] Finally, the ulnar nerve has been dislocated out of its groove in asymptomatic persons. The dislocated nerve is found immediately posterior or anteromedial to the tip of the medial epicondyle.[16]

PATHOLOGY

Biceps and Triceps Tendons

MRI is useful in the evaluation of these injuries because tendinosis, partial tears, and complete tears may be distinguished.[6, 7, 11, 12] The T2 sequence in the axial plane is best for determining the degree of biceps tendon tearing and must extend from the musculotendinous junction to the tendon's insertion on the radial tuberosity. MRI elucidates superficial and deep divisions, the degree of tearing, the size of the gap, and the location of the tear for preoperative planning (Fig. 6–6). The tendon typically tears from its attachment on the radial tuberosity as a result of resisted flexion of the elbow.

Injury to the triceps tendon is less common. The tendon typically avulses from its attachment on the olecranon (Fig. 6–7) secondary to a direct blow, a fall on an outstretched

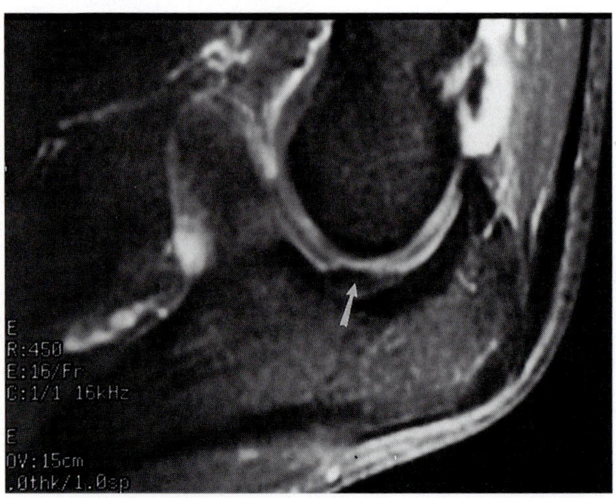

Figure 6–5
Sagittal T1 image. *Note cartilage-free central elevation of the articular surface of the trochlear groove* (arrow).

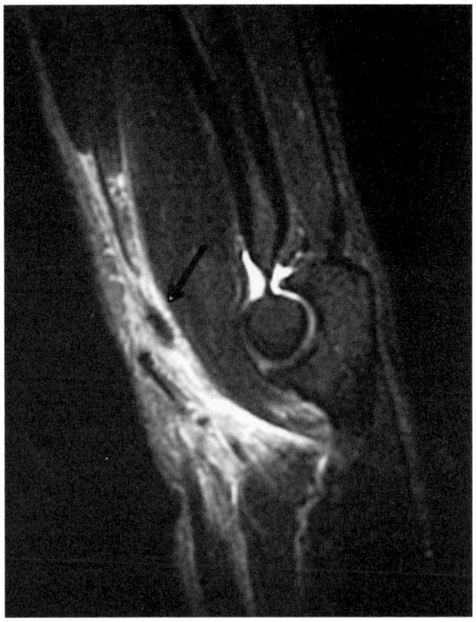

Figure 6–6
Sagittal fast spin-echo T2 image. *The biceps tendon is disrupted* (arrow) *with adjacent bright signal fluid.*

arm, or a decelerating counterforce during active extension.[11] Nevertheless, the injuries are well seen on MRI in the sagittal plane, but there are at least two potential pitfalls that should not be mistaken for pathology. The tendon may appear lax when imaged in full extension, but this resolves in mild flexion. Foci of increased signal intensity in the normal triceps tendon on the T1 sequence decrease in signal intensity on the T2 sequence.

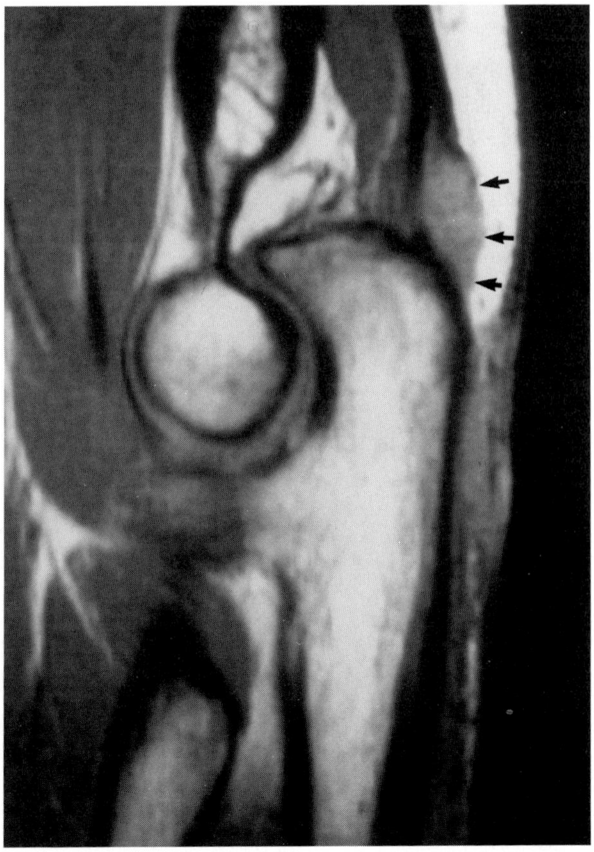

Figure 6–7
Sagittal T1 image. *Partial tear of the superficial fibers* (arrows) *of the triceps tendon at its olecranon insertion. (From Fritz RC, Steinbach LS. The elbow.* In *Chan WP, Lang P, Genant HK, eds. MRI of the Musculoskeletal System. Philadelphia: WB Saunders, 1994.)*

Lateral Epicondylitis

Lateral epicondylitis (tennis elbow) results from degeneration and tearing of the common extensor tendon. Tendinosis and tearing typically involve the extensor carpi radialis brevis portion of the common extensor tendon anteriorly (Fig. 6–8). MRI helps in assessing the degree of tendon damage. Tendinosis reveals tendon thickening and increased signal intensity on both T1 and T2 sequences without a progressive increase in signal intensity on the latter sequence. A partial tear reveals thinning of the tendon, which is outlined by fluid on the T2 sequence. A complete tear reveals a fluid-filled gap separating the tendon from its adjacent bony attachment site. Identification of tears helps management because significant partial tears and complete tears are unlikely to improve with rest and steroid injections. Unsuspected and associated ruptures of the lateral collateral ligament can also be detected on MRI. Lack of a significant abnormality may also prompt consideration of an alternative diagnosis such as radial nerve entrapment, which can mimic or accompany lateral epicondylitis.[9]

Valgus Stress Injury

Valgus stress injury is a result of acute trauma or chronic repetitive microtrauma. Flexor and pronator muscular strain, UCL strain, ulnar traction spurring, and ulnar neuropathy are typically the result of medial tension overload.[12] These are extra-articular injuries. Intra-articular injuries are typically the result of lateral compression overload, which include osteochondritis dissecans of the capitellum or radial head, loose bodies, and degenerative arthritis.[9]

Medial epicondylitis is a result of degeneration of the common flexor tendon. Overload of the flexor and pronator muscle groups arising from the medial epicondyle is the main etiology. MRI can assess tendinosis, a partial tear, or a complete tear.[8] The STIR sequence is particularly useful for the associated muscle and bone-marrow signal alteration. A therapeutic intramuscular injection in the past month for relief of medial epicondylitis can mimic this same signal alteration, which is seen in muscle strain.[14]

UCL injury secondary to degeneration or tearing can occur with or without concomitant injury of the common flexor tendon. An assessment of the anterior bundle of the UCL

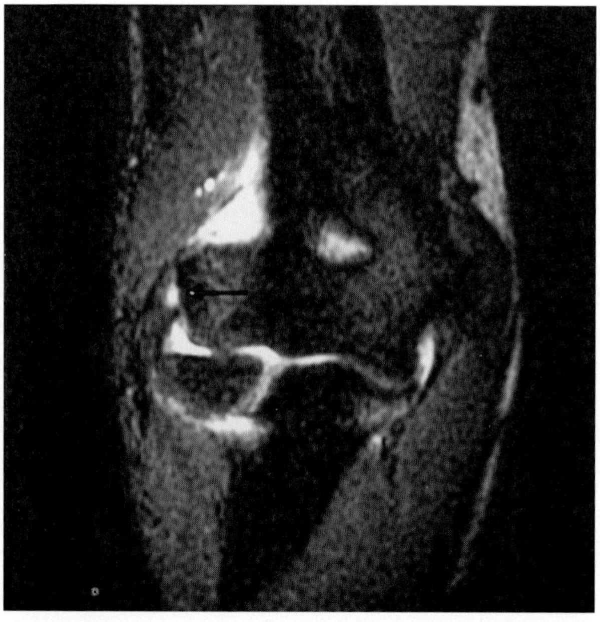

Figure 6–8
Coronal T2 image. *Partial disruption of the common extensor tendon is manifested by a focus of bright signal adjacent to the condyle* (arrow).

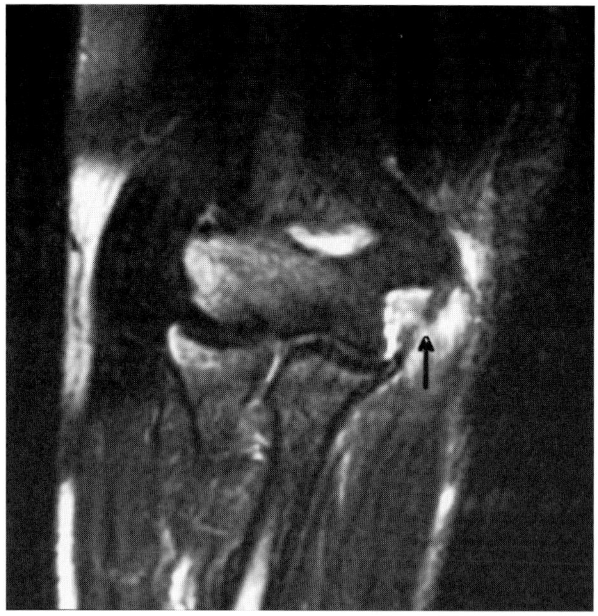

Figure 6–9
Coronal T2 image.
Midsubstance tear of the ulnar collateral ligament (arrow).

on the coronal and axial images can reveal partial tears of this ligament that spare the superficial fibers and that are, therefore, not visible to an open surgical approach.[9] Partial tears are better detected when intra-articular contrast is administered, which shows distal extension of contrast along the medial margin of the coronoid where the capsular fibers of the anterior bundle normally insert on the medial margin of the coronoid process.[18] Complete UCL tears are more commonly midsubstance in location (Fig. 6–9). Associated findings include strain of the flexor digitorum superficialis, which blends with the anterior bundle, and bone-marrow contusions. These findings manifest as bright signal on STIR images. Chronic degeneration of the UCL is characterized by ligamentous thickening.[4] Ulnar traction spurs occur at the UCL insertion on the coronoid process.

Ulnar nerve entrapment is easily identified on axial images as the nerve passes through the cubital tunnel. Thickening of the UCL, bone spurs, anatomic variations, and thickening of the cubital tunnel retinaculum can all contribute to ulnar neuropathy. The absence of this retinaculum can result in dislocation of the nerve.[9]

Osteochondritis dissecans is the result of chronic lateral impaction of the capitellum or radial head.[12] MRI can reliably detect and stage these lesions. Unstable lesions are characterized by bright fluid signal on the T2 sequence encircling the fragment (Fig. 6–10). Loose-body formation or residual deformity are concerns in this entity, which is most common in the teenage years. On the other hand, Panner's disease (Fig. 6–11), or osteochondrosis of the capitellum, typically occurs in childhood and does not usually result in these same complications.[9]

Loose bodies from unstable osteochondral lesions or incongruity between the medial olecranon and the medial olecranon fossa can grow in the joint and result in mechanical symptoms of locking and motion limitation, as well as result in premature degenerative arthritis. Effusion enhances their detection (Fig. 6–12).[9]

Bone Injury

T1, fat-suppressed T1 or proton-density, and STIR sequences are most sensitive to occult fractures, contusions, and other bone injuries. MRI can be used to detect subtle fractures of the anterior coronoid process and stress fractures of the olecranon, as well as to exclude radial head fractures in adults, supracondylar and lateral condylar fractures in children, and injury to a physis.[10]

Figure 6–10
Sagittal T2 image. *A fluid-filled cystic area in the anterior aspect of the capitellum* (arrow) *suggests instability of the overlying osteochondral fragment.*

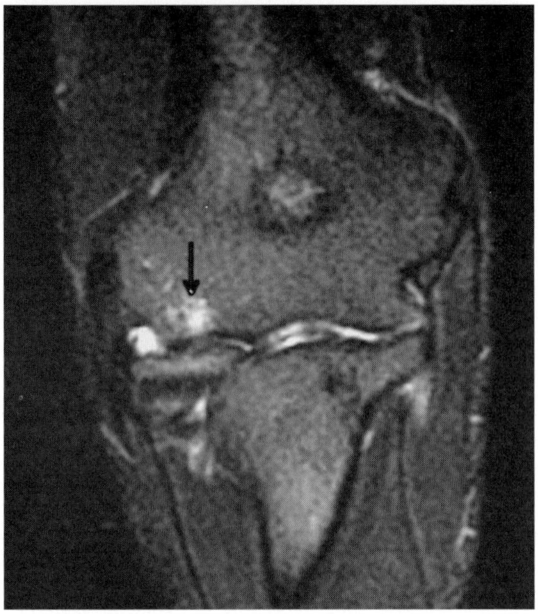

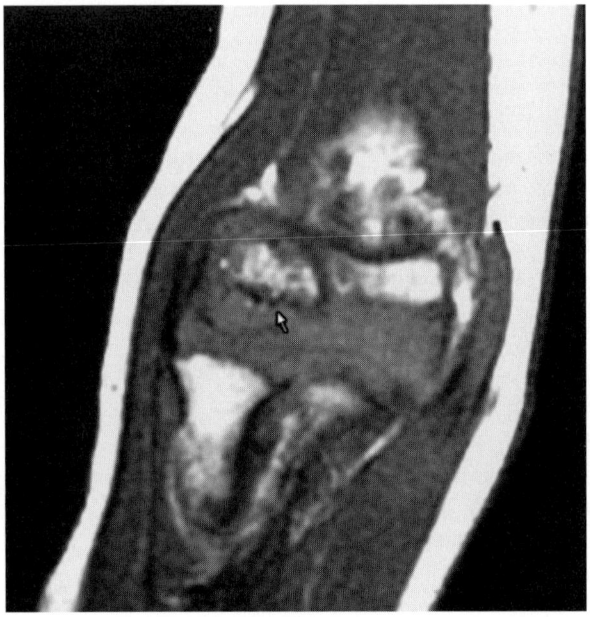

Figure 6–11
Coronal T1 image. *Note the characteristic low-signal region central to the capitellum* (arrow) *in this example of Panner's disease (i.e., osteochondrosis of the capitellum).*

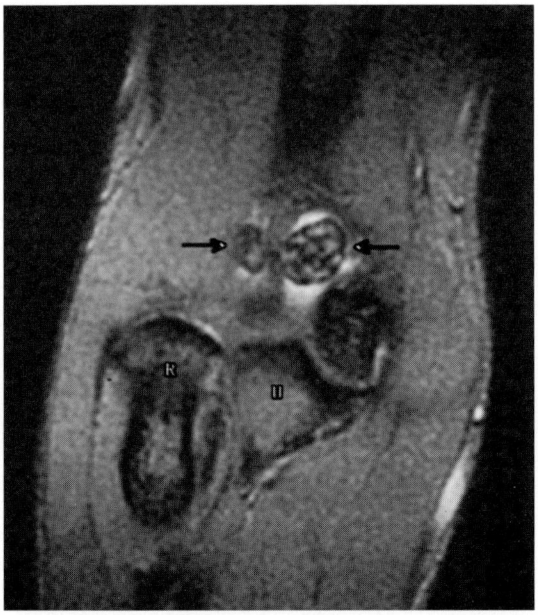

Figure 6–12
Coronal GRE image. *Two intra-articular loose bodies reside in the posterior recess* (arrows). *Joint fluid aids their visualization.*

References

1. Beltran J, Chandnani V, McGhee RA. Gadopentetate dimeglumine–enhanced MR imaging of the musculoskeletal system. AJR 1991; 156:457-466.
2. Berquist TH. The elbow and wrist. Top Magn Reson Imag 1989; 1(3):15-27.
3. Bunnell DH, Fisher DA, Bassett LW, et al. Elbow joint: Normal anatomy on MR images. Radiology 1987; 165:527-531.
4. Conway JE, Jobe FW, Glousman RE, et al. Medial instability of the elbow in throwing athletes. Treatment by repair or reconstruction of the ulnar collateral ligament. J Bone Joint Surg [Am] 1992; 74:67-83.
5. Ehman RL. MR imaging with surface coils. Radiology 1985; 157:549-550.
6. Falchook FS, Zlatkin MB, Erbacher GE, et al. Rupture of the distal biceps tendon: Evaluation with MR imaging. Radiology 1994; 190:659-663.
7. Fitzgerald SW, Curry DR, Erickson SJ, et al. Distal biceps tendon injury: MR imaging diagnosis. Radiology 1994; 191:203-206.
8. Fleckenstein JL, Shellock FG. Exertional muscle injuries: Magnetic resonance evaluation. Top Magn Reson Imaging 1991; 3:50-70.
9. Fritz CF, Steinbach LS. The elbow. *In* Chan WP, Lang P, Genant HK, eds. MRI of the Musculoskeletal System. Philadelphia: WB Saunders, 1994.
10. Jaramillo D, Hoffer FA. Cartilaginous epiphysis and growth plate: Normal and abnormal MR imaging findings. AJR 1992; 158:1105-1110.
11. Morrey BF. Tendon injuries about the elbow. *In* Morrey BF, ed. The Elbow and Its Disorders, 2nd ed. Philadelphia: WB Saunders, 1993.
12. Murphy BJ. MRI imaging of the elbow. Radiology 1992; 184:525-529.
13. Pitt MJ, Speer DP. Imaging of the elbow with an emphasis on trauma. Radiol Clin North Am 1990; 28(2):293-305.
14. Resendes M, Helms CA, Fritz RC, et al. MR appearance of intramuscular injections. AJR 1992; 158:1293-1294.
15. Rosenberg ZS. MRI of the elbow: Normal anatomy, variants and interpretation pitfalls. Postgrad Radiol 1994; 15:17-28.
16. Rosenberg ZS, Beltran J, Cheung Y, et al. The elbow: MR features of nerve disorders. Radiology 1993; 188:235-240.
17. Rosenberg ZS, Beltran J, Cheung Y. The pseudodefect of the capitellum: Potential MR imaging pitfall. Radiology 1994; 191:821-823.
18. Timmerman LA, Schwarz ML, Andrews JR. Preoperative evaluation of the ulnar collateral ligament by magnetic resonance imaging, computed tomography and arthrography: Evaluation in 25 baseball players with surgical confirmation. Am J Sports Med 1994; 22:26-32.
19. Weissman BNW, Sledge CB. Orthopedic Radiology. Philadelphia: WB Saunders, 1986.

Elbow Arthroscopy

Elbow arthroscopy, originally believed to be too dangerous to be of clinical use,[3] is now a well-accepted technique. Because of the shape of this joint and the proximity of important neurovascular structures, elbow arthroscopy can be a technically demanding procedure. Nevertheless, with an adequate appreciation of the anatomy of the region and arthroscopic skill, elbow arthroscopy can allow diagnostic and therapeutic intervention with minimal morbidity.[9]

INDICATIONS

Although the indications for elbow arthroscopy are still evolving, it is a well-accepted technique for removal of loose bodies, irrigation of an infected joint, synovectomy, osteophyte excision, and other uses. Loose or foreign bodies can be easily removed from the joint using the contralateral portal.[4, 7, 8] A septic joint can be irrigated with only two portals (proximal-medial and posterolateral).[9] Osteophytes can be removed using arthroscopic burrs and generous irrigation.[13] Synovectomy can be accomplished via both anterior and posterior portals and can provide considerable pain relief in patients with chronic synovitis.[2] Other proposed procedures include arthroscopic capsular release[6] and radial head excision.[9]

POSITIONING AND PORTAL PLACEMENT

Elbow arthroscopy can be done with the patient supine[1] or prone.[10] The prone position, which is more popular, allows improved arthroscopic manipulation and better visualization without the use of an overhead suspension device.[9]

The "soft spot," or anconeus triangle (Fig. 6–13), should be palpated, and 30 to 50 ml of fluid should be injected to distend the capsule prior to establishing arthroscopic portals. Three portals are commonly used for elbow arthroscopy: the proximal-medial, posterolateral, and anterolateral portals. A fourth portal, the direct posterior portal, can be established when posterior instrumentation is necessary. A final portal, the proximal lateral

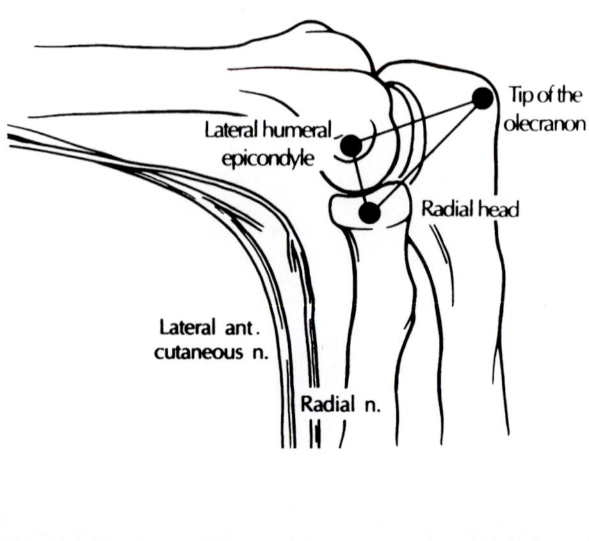

Figure 6–13
Anconeus triangle on the lateral aspect of the elbow (patient prone). (From Poehling GG, Ekman EF. Arthroscopy of the elbow. Instr Course Lect 1995; 44:217-223.)

portal, has recently been advocated for improved safety (Fig. 6–14).[5, 11, 12] The "nick and spread" method should be used when establishing all arthroscopic portals about the elbow because of the attendant neurovascular risk.

The proximal-medial portal is the primary diagnostic arthroscopic portal with the patient in the prone position.[9] It is located 2 cm proximal to the medial epicondyle, just anterior to the intermuscular septum. The arthroscopic sheath should contact the anterior surface of the humerus and is directed toward the radial head. The posterolateral portal is made in the anconeus triangle and can be used for inflow and outflow. The arthroscope can be introduced into this portal to allow visualization of the posterior joint. Some authors favor establishing this portal proximal and posterior to this location, 2 cm proximal to the tip of the olecranon and adjacent to the lateral edge of the triceps tendon.

The anterolateral portal is established 3 cm distal and 2 cm anterior to the lateral epicondyle with the elbow flexed 90 degrees. The portal can be established with an inside-out technique using a blunt rod. The radial nerve is at risk with this portal and is immediately adjacent to the portal in 50% of cases.[12]

The direct posterior portal is made 2 cm proximal to the tip of the olecranon, through the triceps tendon, and is used primarily for instrumentation in the posterior joint.

The proximal-lateral portal was developed to reduce the risk associated with other portals.[11] It is located 1 to 2 cm proximal to the lateral epicondyle, directly on the anterior surface of the humerus. As with the proximal-medial portal, the trocar is kept in direct contact with the anterior humerus during insertion. The proximal-lateral portal has been advocated in lieu of the more hazardous anterolateral portal.[12] The radial head and capitellum can be well visualized through this portal. The anteromedial portal, located 2 cm distal and

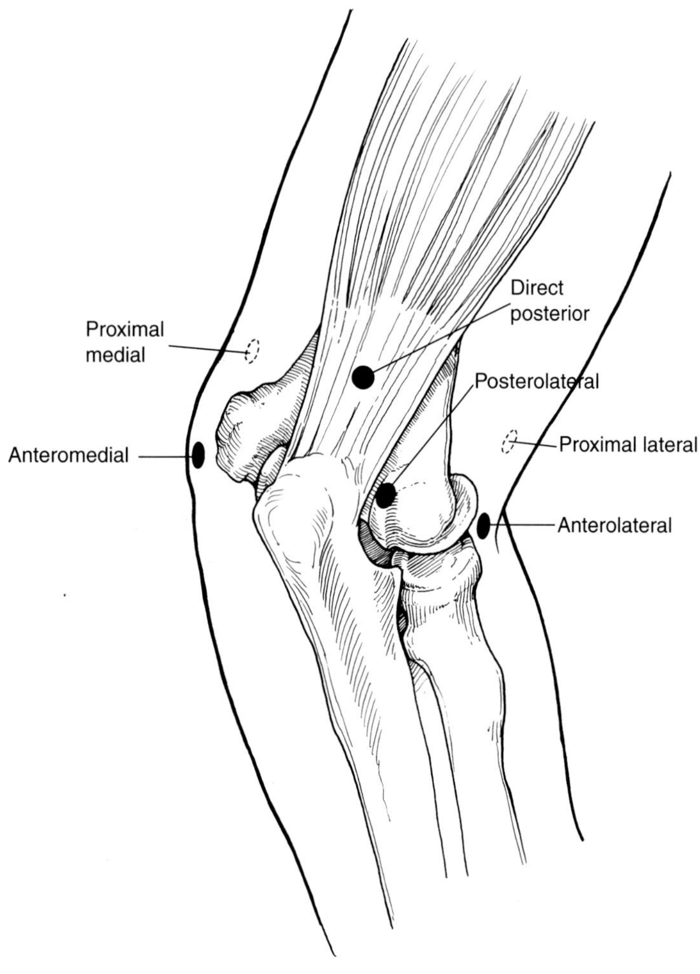

Figure 6–14
Arthroscopic portals.

2 cm anterior to the medial epicondyle, can jeopardize the anterior branch of the medial antebrachial cutaneous nerve and the median nerve and is not usually recommended. Therefore, the standard anterior portals used in elbow arthroscopy should be the proximal-medial and proximal-lateral portals. The anteromedial and anterolateral portals, if necessary, should be established using an inside-out technique, and the anterolateral portal should be established proximal to the radial head.

ARTHROSCOPIC ANATOMY

With the arthroscope placed in the proximal medial portal, the humeroulnar and radiocapitellar joints, the coronoid fossa, and the medial and lateral gutters can be well visualized (Fig. 6–15). The posterior joint (olecranon and olecranon fossa) can be well visualized through the posterolateral portal (Fig. 6–16).

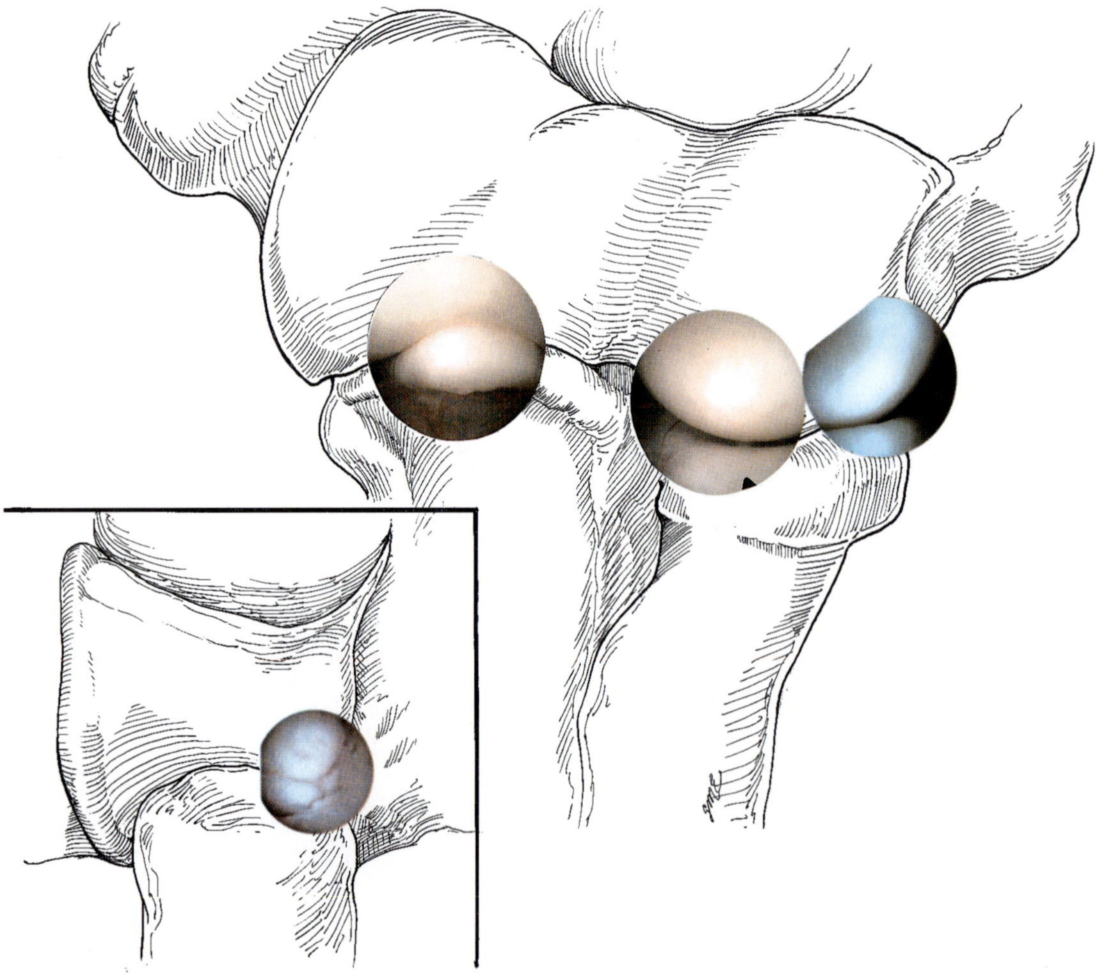

Figure 6–15
Arthroscopic anatomy of the elbow. Inset of posterior view.

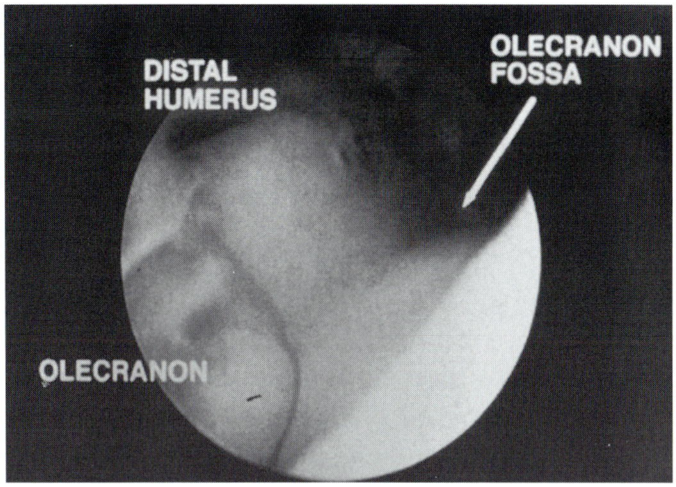

Figure 6–16
Arthroscopic view from the posterolateral portal demonstrates the olecranon, olecranon fossa, and distal humerus. (From Poehling GG, Ekman EF. Arthroscopy of the elbow. Inst Course Lect 1995; 44:217-223.)

COMPLICATIONS

The most distressing complication with elbow arthroscopy is neurovascular damage. Use of the proximal portals instead of anterior portals may reduce such risk. Other complications include infection, synovial fistula formation (anterolateral portal), and instrument breakage.

References

1. Andrews JR, Carson WG. Arthroscopy of the elbow. Arthroscopy 1985; 1:97-107.
2. Angelo RL. Advances in elbow arthroscopy. Orthopedics 1993; 16:1037-1046.
3. Burman MS. Arthroscopy or the direct visualization of joints. An experimental cadaver study. J Bone Joint Surg 1931; 669-695.
4. Cameron SE, Travis MT, Kruse RW. Foreign body arthroscopically retrieved from the elbow. Arthroscopy 1993; 9:220-221.
5. Field LD, Altchek DW, Warren RF, et al. Arthroscopic anatomy of the lateral elbow. A comparison of three portals. Arthroscopy 1994; 10:602-607.
6. Jones GS, Savoie FH III. Arthroscopic capsular release of flexion contractures (arthrofibrosis) of the elbow. Arthroscopy 1993; 9:277-283.
7. O'Driscoll SW. Elbow arthroscopy for loose bodies. Orthopedics 1992; 15:855-859.
8. Ogilvie-Harris DJ, Schemitwch E. Arthroscopy of the elbow for removal of loose bodies. Arthroscopy 1993; 9:5-8.
9. Poehling GG, Ekman EF. Arthroscopy of the elbow. Instr Course Lect 1995; 44:217-223.
10. Poehling GG, Whipple TL, Sisco I, et al. Elbow arthroscopy: A new technique. Arthroscopy 1989; 5:222-224.
11. Stothers K, Day B, Regan W. Arthroscopic anatomy of the elbow: An anatomical study and description of a new portal. Arthroscopy 1993; 9:362-363.
12. Stothers K, Day B, Regan WR. Arthroscopy of the elbow: Anatomy, portal sites, and a description of the proximal lateral portal. Arthroscopy 1995; 11:449-457.
13. Ward WG, Anderson TE. Elbow arthroscopy in a mostly athletic population. J Hand Surg [Am] 1993; 18:220-224.

Illustrative Cases—Elbow

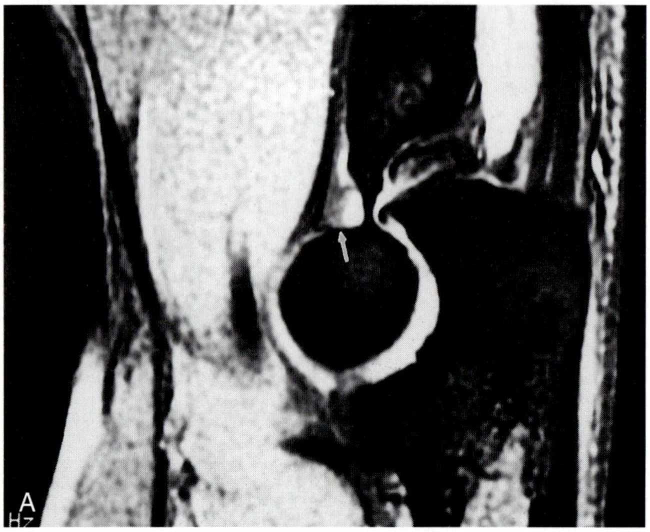

Figure 6–17. **Synovitis, Left Elbow**
A, *Sagittal fat-suppressed gradient recalled-echo image shows synovial nodular thickening* (arrow) *highlighted by adjacent joint fluid.*
B, *Arthroscopic view of hypertrophic synovium.*
Case courtesy of Ronald Jones, M.D.

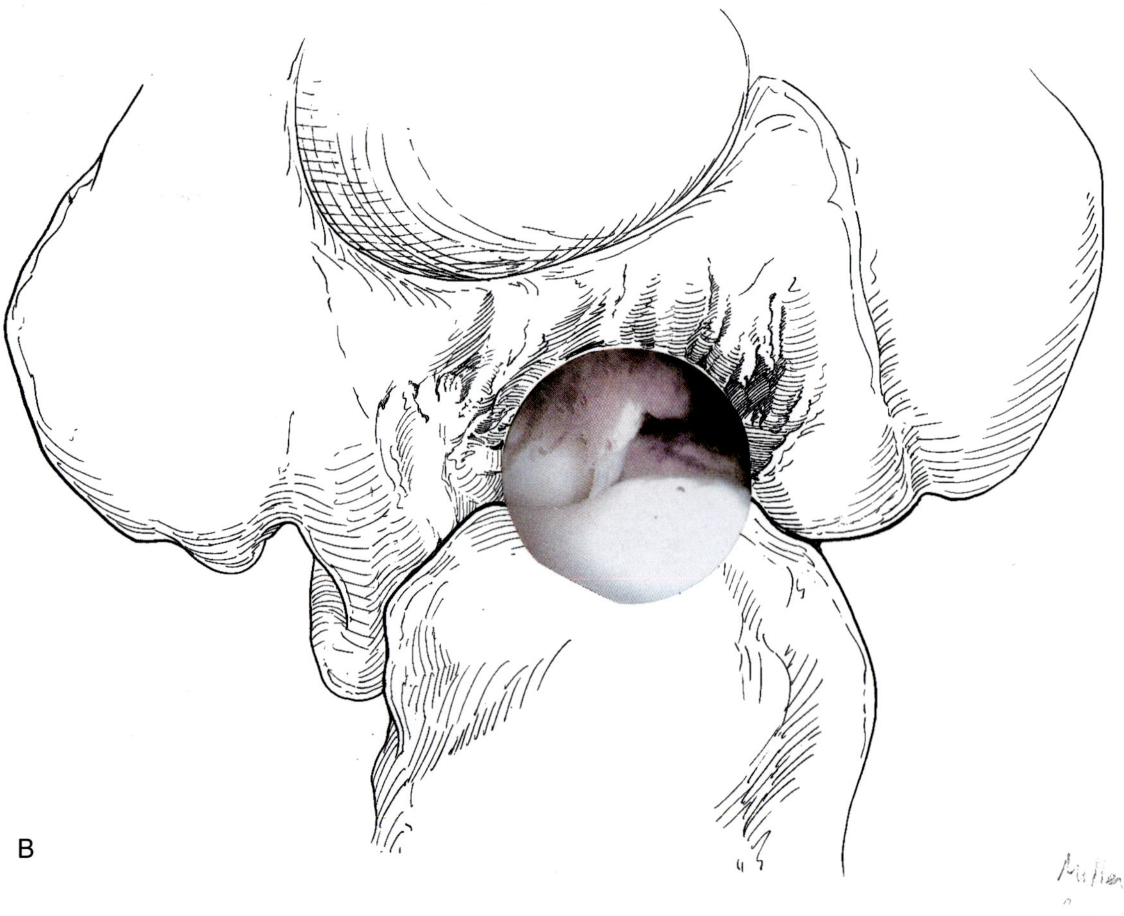

B

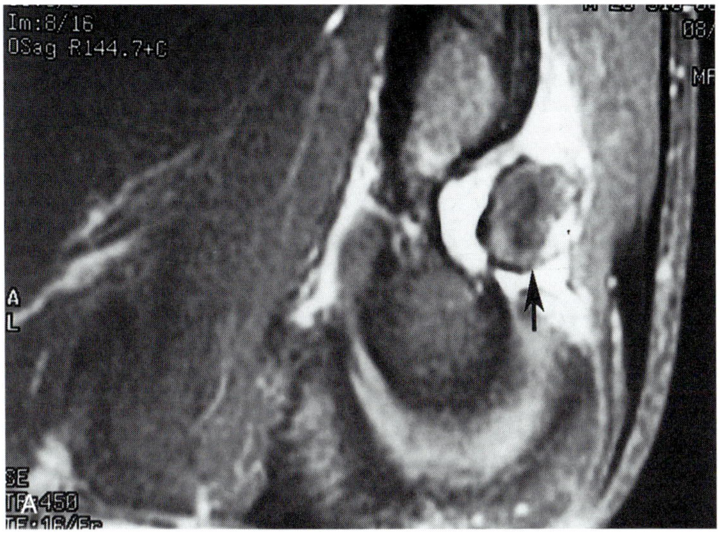

Figure 6–18. **Posterior Loose Body, Right Elbow**
A, *Sagittal SE T1-weighted fat-saturated image shows a 1-cm loose body* (arrow) *in the posterior recess.* B, *Arthroscopic view of loose body prior to removal.*

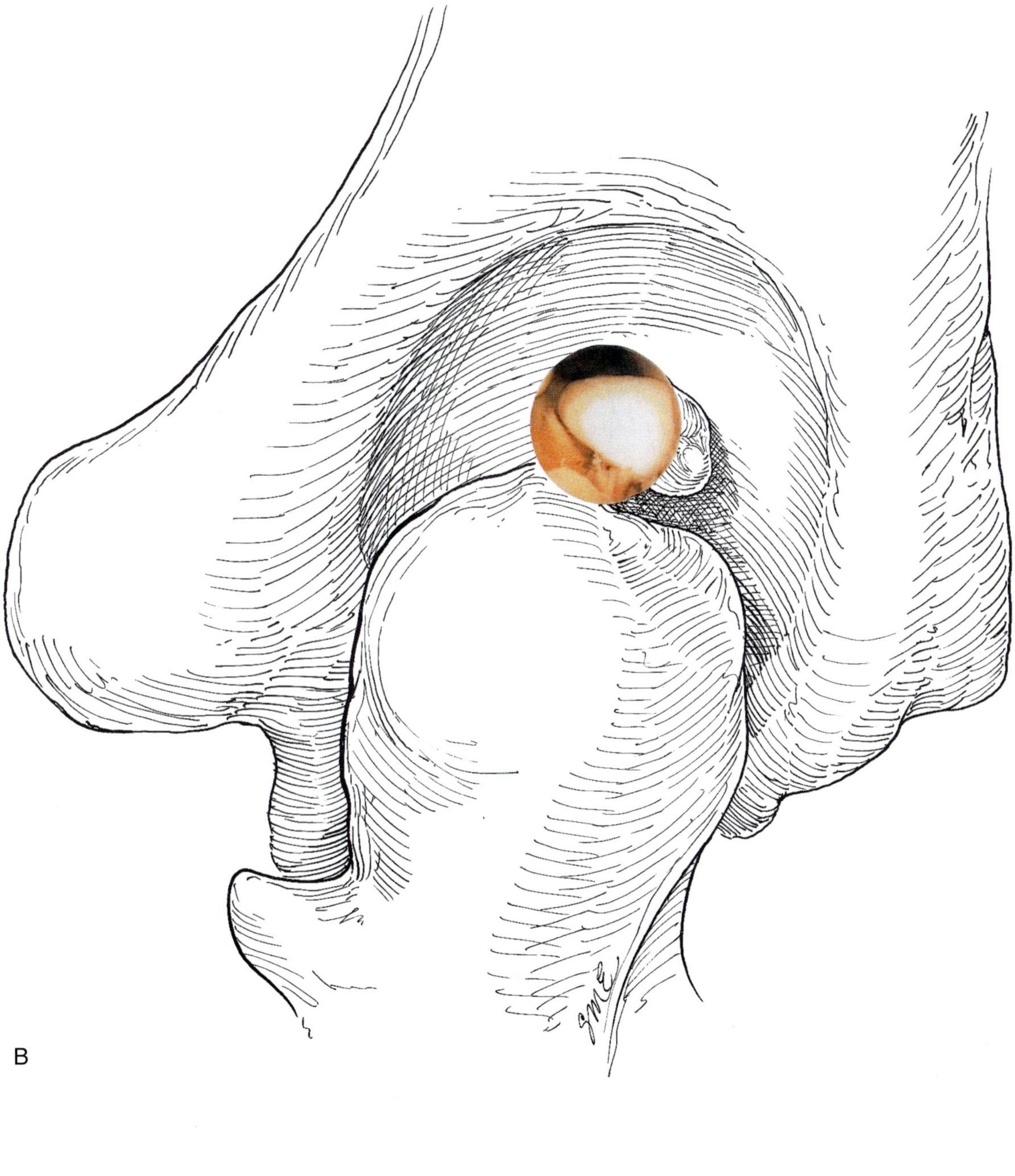

B

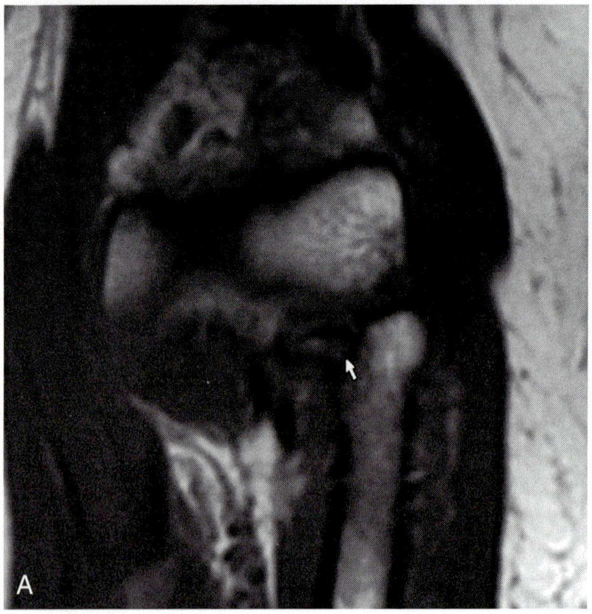

Figure 6–19. **Subacute Displaced Radial Head Fracture, Left Elbow**
A, *Coronal T1-weighted image demonstrates a displaced split compression fracture of the radial head* (arrow). B, *Arthroscopic view from the proximal medial portal demonstrates fracture through the head and neck of the radius. Note the displacement of the fracture and exposed subcortical bone* (inset).

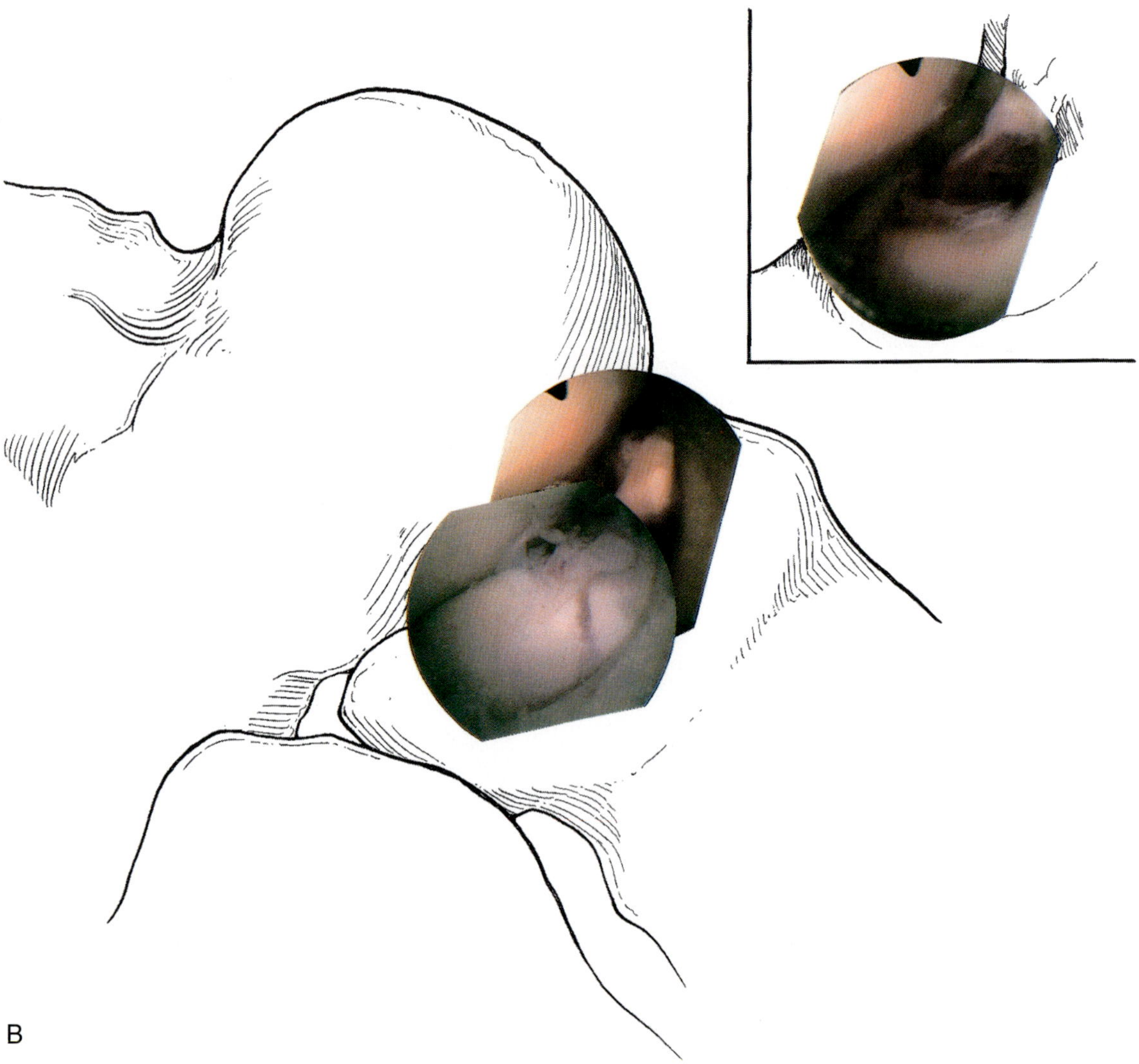

B

CHAPTER

7

Wrist

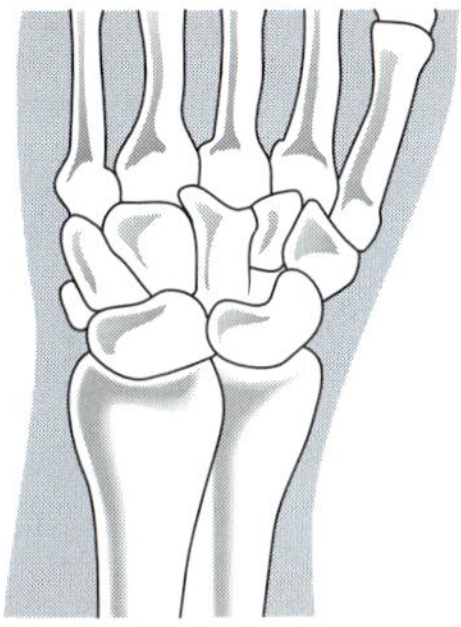

MRI of the Wrist

MRI has evolved as a versatile tool for imaging the wrist. As a single test, MRI provides diagnostic information that often exceeds that yielded by all pre-existing tests, such as standard radiography, bone scintigraphy, arthrography, and computed tomography. Applications include atypical carpal tunnel syndrome (CTS), carpal instability, triangular fibrocartilage complex (TFCC) tears and other intrinsic and extrinsic ligamentous injuries, tumors, synovial processes, tendon rupture, osteonecrosis, and fractures of the wrist.

TECHNIQUE

The wrist is ideally imaged on a high-field-strength magnet (1.5 Tesla). The wrist is scanned with a dedicated surface wrist coil (Figs. 7–1 and 7–2). Fingers should be kept straight so that the lumbrical muscles, which are attached to the flexor tendons, are not pulled into the carpal tunnel, which can mimic pathology. A small field of view is necessary, typically 8 to 10 cm. Slice thickness must also be small, 3 to 4 mm. One can interleave slices or use small gaps as well as multiple excitations. Three-dimensional volume acquisitions are possible with the gradient recalled-echo (GRE) sequence with a slice thickness of 1 mm or less. The imaging planes and sequences can be tailored to the patient's particular problem. For example, if the integrity of the scapholunate interosseous ligament is in question, coronal images would suffice. Examination is often more complex, however, to detect associated or unsuspected abnormalities. In general, a T1 sagittal sequence is obtained primarily to evaluate carpal alignment, extrinsic ligaments of the wrist, and bone-marrow signal of the carpal bones. A T2 coronal sequence best evaluates the TFCC and the intrinsic ligaments of the wrist. A GRE sequence provides a supplemental evaluation of these critical structures. T2-weighted axial images best evaluate the carpal tunnel and the extensor tendon compartments. They are particularly useful in the detection of ganglion cysts.[2]

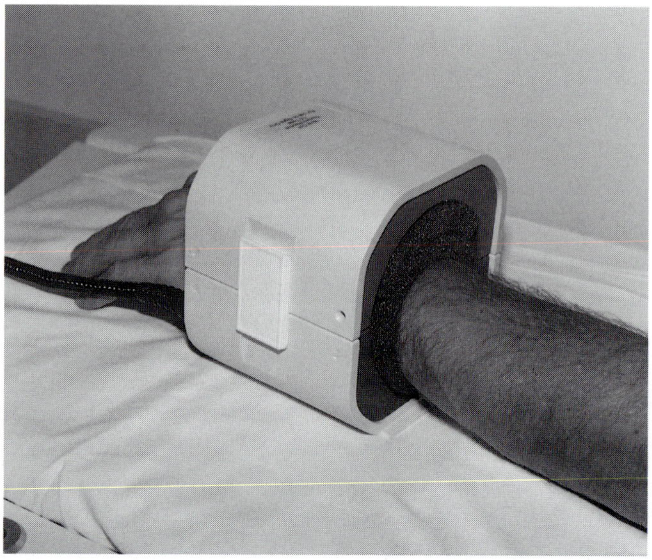

Figure 7–1
Dedicated transmit/receive wrist coil.

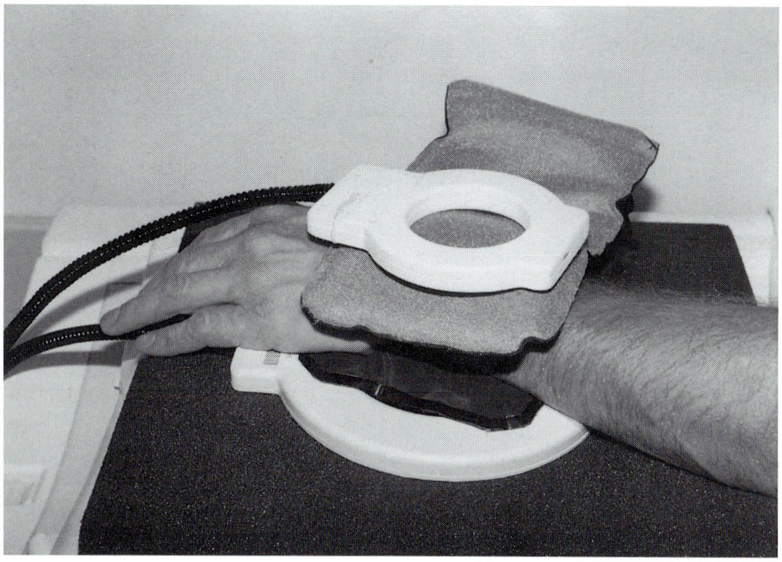

Figure 7–2
Three-inch and 5-in. circular coils coupled together for wrist imaging.

MRI ANATOMY

MRI anatomy of the wrist is well displayed in the axial, coronal, and sagittal planes (Figs. 7–3, 7–4, and 7–5).

The coronal sequence of the wrist best evaluates the TFCC. The triangular fibrocartilage (TFC), ulnocarpal ligament, and extensor carpi ulnaris tendon sheath make up the TFCC and provide stability to the ulnar side of the wrist. The TFC, a biconcave disk, is located in the ulnocarpal space attached to the base of the ulnar styloid and the ulnar side of the distal radius. It cushions the ulnar head and lunate during axial loading. Centrally, the TFC is low in signal intensity. It arises from the relatively high-signal hyaline cartilage at the ulnar aspect of the distal radius and inserts on the vascular ulnar fovea. Vascular connective tissue at this latter site may appear as interdigitated foci of increased signal. Both of these areas can display bright signal and should not be mistaken for a tear or perforation. The dorsal and volar radioulnar ligaments are thick fibrous structures that abut the dorsal and volar margins of the TFC and secure it at its attachments. Like the TFC, they are low in signal intensity. Their radial attachments, however, are to cortex, not hyaline cartilage. This is an important point because it helps identify these ligaments as separate structures, because they are often intact when the TFC is torn. The meniscus homologue is a bandlike structure of intermediate signal that is seen along the ulnar aspect of the TFC. It borders the openings of two extensions of the radiocarpal joint, namely the prestyloid recess and the pisiform recess. The meniscus homologue should not be mistaken for the TFC. The radial collateral ligament attaches the radial styloid process to the scaphoid. The ulnar collateral ligament extends from the ulnar styloid process to the triquetrum.[1, 2]

The position of the distal articular surface of the ulna relative to that of the radius is easily evaluated and is called "ulnar variance." This variance is positive if the ulna extends distally to the radius, negative if the radius extends more distally. Ulnar variance is neutral if the two articular surfaces are co-linear. The distribution of axially loading forces is altered when ulnar variance is not co-linear. Normally, the radius and ulnar bear 80% and 20% of axial loading, respectively. Kienböck's disease can be the result of an increase in forces borne by the radius and radial carpus when variance is negative.[3] Positive variance, on the other hand, is associated with TFC tears and chondromalacia of the ulnar head and lunate, a condition known as ulnolunate impingement syndrome.[4]

Text continues on page 208

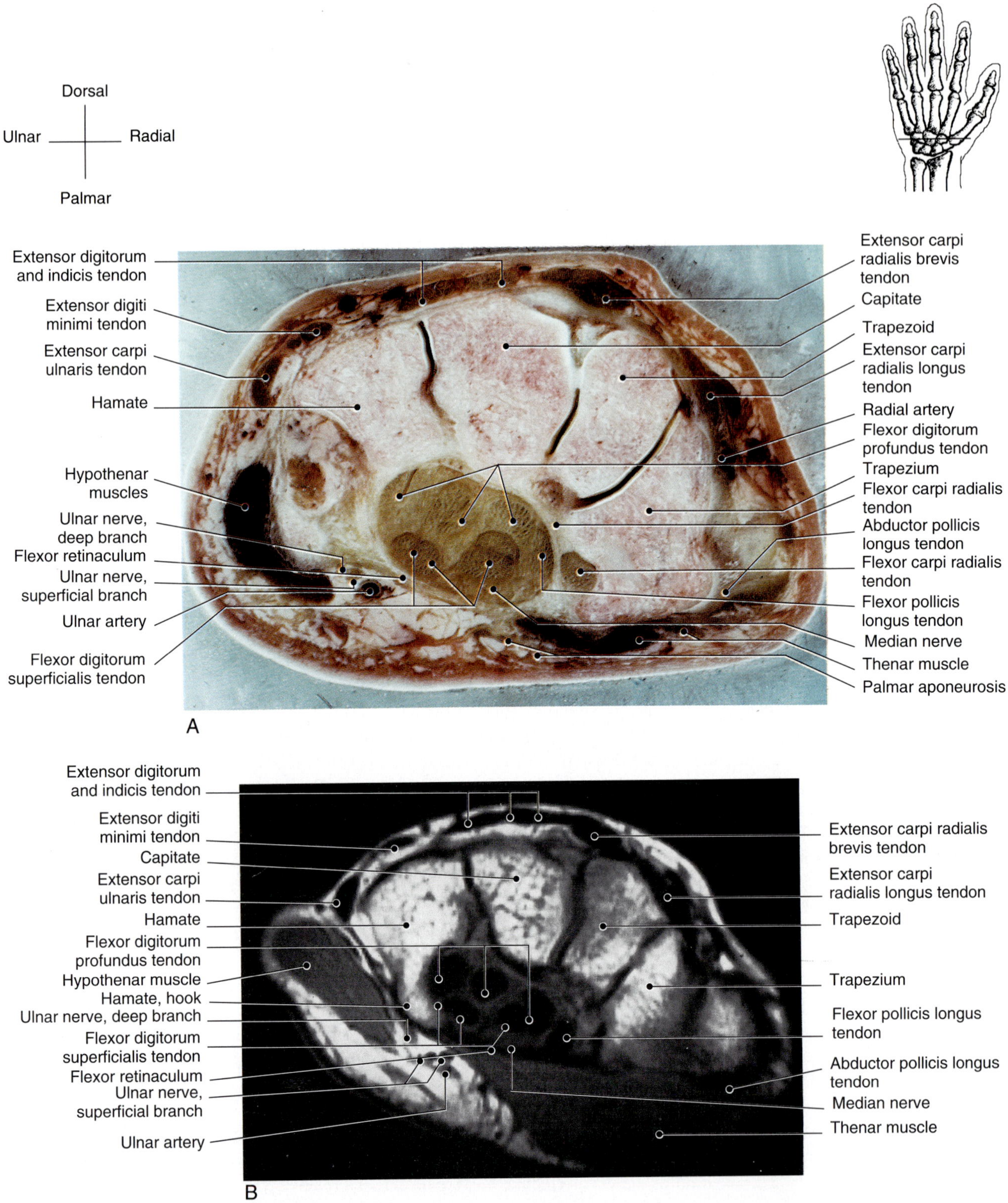

Figure 7–3

Axial cryoplaned section (A) *and magnetic-resonance image (TR, 700 ms; TE, 20 ms)* (B) *of the wrist at the level of the hamate and trapezium. (From Chan WP, Raushning W, Wu CY, et al. Magnetic resonance imaging anatomy and cryomicrotome atlas.* In *Chan WP, Lang P, Genant HK, eds. MRI of the Musculoskeletal System. Philadelphia: WB Saunders, 1994.)*

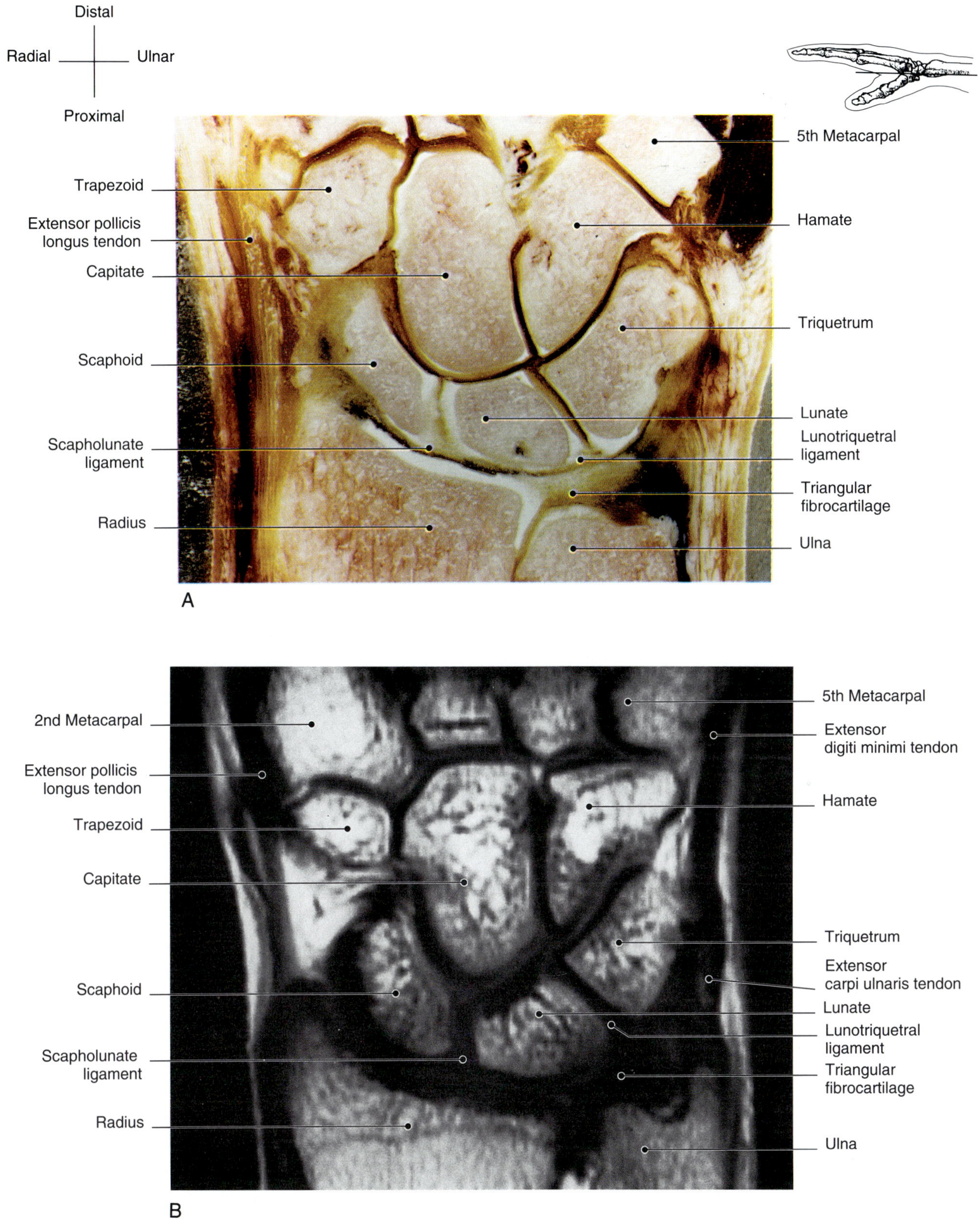

Figure 7–4

Midcoronal cryoplaned section (A) *and magnetic-resonance image (TR, 700 ms; TE, 20 ms)* (B) *of the wrist. (From Chan WP, Raushning W, Wu CY, et al. Magnetic resonance imaging anatomy and cryomicrotome atlas.* In *Chan WP, Lang P, Genant HK, eds. MRI of the Musculoskeletal System. Philadelphia: WB Saunders, 1994.)*

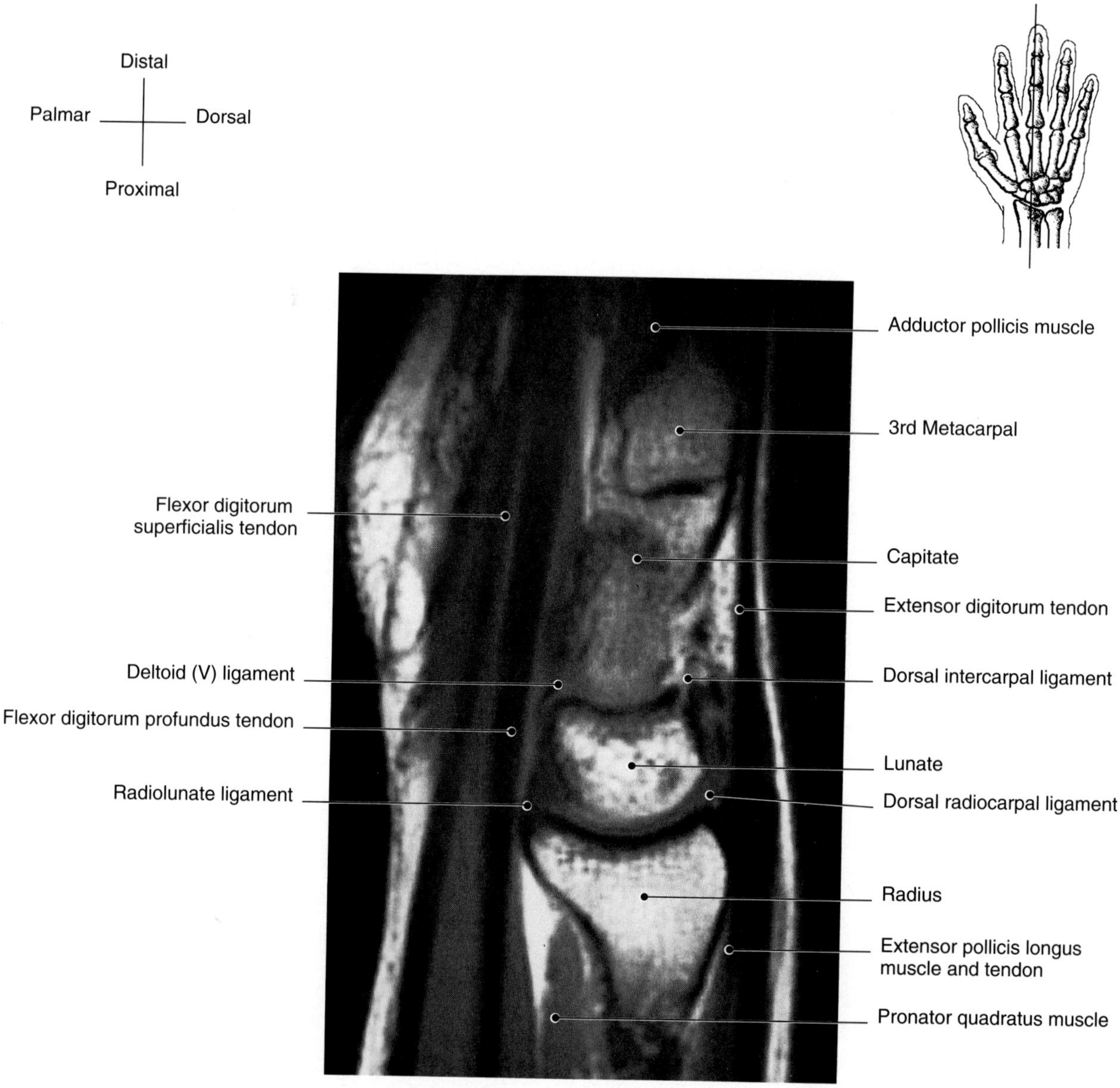

Figure 7–5
Sagittal magnetic-resonance image of the wrist (TR, 600 ms; TE, 20 ms) through the lunate. (From Chan WP, Raushning W, Wu CY, et al. Magnetic resonance imaging anatomy and cryomicrotome atlas. In *Chan WP, Lang P, Genant HK, eds. MRI of the Musculoskeletal System. Philadelphia: WB Saunders, 1994.)*

The ligaments of the wrist may be considered extrinsic or intrinsic. Extrinsic ligaments interconnect the radius and carpus (Fig. 7–6). Intrinsic ligaments interconnect carpal bones. The scapholunate ligament is the only intrinsic intercarpal ligament of the wrist that can be reliably seen on MRI. The lunatotriquetral ligament is seen only occasionally because of its small size. Disruption of one or both of these intrinsic ligaments has been associated with wrist pain and carpal instability. The scapholunate ligament is a low-signal, triangle-shaped structure. The lunatotriquetral ligament is a low-signal, more curved structure.[5, 7]

The sagittal sequence evaluates the dorsal and volar extrinsic radiocarpal ligaments, which maintain alignment of the carpal bones. A sagittal sequence through the scaphoid demonstrates two low-intensity, rounded structures along the volar aspect. These are the

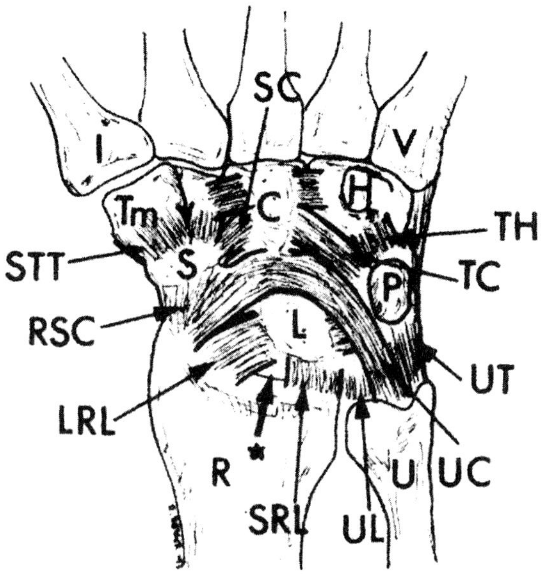

Figure 7–6
Palmar capsular ligaments. R = radius; U = ulna; S = scaphoid; L = lunate; P = pisiform; Tm = trapezium; C = capitate; H = hamate; I = first metacarpal; V = fifth metacarpal. The ligaments include RSC = radioscaphocapitate; LRL = long radiolunate; SRL = short radiolunate; UL = ulnolunate; UC = ulnocapitate; UT = ulnotriquetral; TH = triquetrohamate; TC = triquetrocapitate; SC = scaphocapitate; STT = scaphotrapeziotrapezoid. The asterisk marks the penetration of the neurovascular source of the radioscapholunate ligament. (From Berger RA. Anatomy and basic biomechanics of the wrist. In Hand Surgery Update. *Englewood, CO: American Society for Surgery of the Hand, 1994; 1:6–6.)*

radioscaphocapitate ligament, which resides more distally, and the long radiolunate ligament, which resides more proximally. The radioscaphocapitate ligament is more radial and originates from the radial styloid process. The long radiolunate ligament shares a similar origin and courses just ulnar to the radioscaphocapitate ligament. The short radiolunate can be seen on its long axis extending from the volar aspect of the radius to the volar surface of the lunate. The ulnolunate and ulnotriquetral ligaments secure the TFC to the lunate, lunotriquetral ligament, and triquetrum.[1]

Carpal instability is best evaluated in the sagittal plane (Fig. 7–7). The longitudinal axis through the radius, the lunate, the capitate, and the third metacarpal are normally within 10 degrees of each other. The scaphoid normally is tilted to the volar aspect between 30 and 60 degrees relative to the long axis of the radius.[6, 8]

The axial plane reveals the carpal tunnel. The volar border of the carpal tunnel is formed by the flexor retinaculum, also called the transverse carpal ligament. The retinaculum attaches to the hook of the hamate and pisiform on the ulnar side of the wrist and to

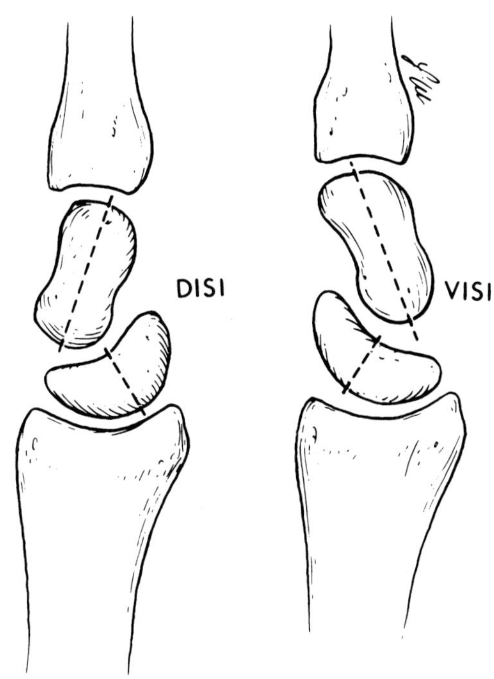

Figure 7–7
Diagram of dorsal intercalated segmental instability versus volar intercalated segmental instability (dorsal is on the reader's left). (From Kellerhouse LE, Reicher MA, Kursunoglu-Brahme S, et al. MR imaging of the wrist. In Edelman RR, Hesselink JR, eds. Clinical Magnetic Resonance Imaging. Philadelphia: WB Saunders, 1990.)

the tubercle of the trapezium and scaphoid on the radial aspect. The retinaculum may be flat or slightly bowed. This feature is best appreciated at the level of the hook of the hamate, where it is thickest. The contents of the carpal tunnel are the median nerve and nine flexor tendons, which are the flexor pollicis longus, the four superficial flexor digitorum tendons, and the four deep flexor digitorum tendons. These are surrounded by synovial sheaths, which are not readily appreciated unless distended with fluid. Fat is sparse, but when present it is located dorsal to the deep flexor tendons. The volar arch of the distal row of carpal bones has a more rounded contour than that of the proximal row, which provides more room distally. This has implications in disorders that cause wrist shortening, such as rheumatoid arthritis with carpal involvement, which may lead to CTS.[9]

The median nerve is normally an ovoid structure of intermediate signal on both T1 and T2 images. Its position and configuration vary somewhat. Usually the median nerve is interposed between the flexor retinaculum and the superficial flexor digitorum tendon of the index finger and the pollicis longus. Guyon's canal, which contains the ulnar nerve and artery, is a potential site for entrapment. It is bounded by the flexor retinaculum, the pisiform medially, and a fascial layer superficially.[9]

The extensor tendons are seen in cross-section on the dorsum of the wrist (Fig. 7–8). The tendons, from the medial to lateral aspects, are the extensor carpi ulnaris on the dorsum of the ulna, extensor digiti minimi (small finger), digitorum communis and extensor indicis proprius tendons (ring, middle, and index fingers), extensor pollicis longus adjacent to the radial, or Lister's, tubercle (a bony prominence on the posterior aspect of the radius), extensor carpi radialis longus and brevis on the other side of Lister's tubercle, and extensor pollicis brevis and abductor pollicis longus adjacent to the radial styloid.[9]

In summary, normal anatomy best displayed in the coronal plane includes the carpal bones, TFCC, radial collateral and ulnar collateral ligaments, and interosseous ligaments. Consequently, TFCC perforations, scapholunate ligament tears, and osseous abnormalities of the carpus are delineated in this plane. Normal anatomy best displayed in the sagittal plane includes alignment of the carpal bones and extrinsic ligaments. Consequently, carpal instability and extrinsic ligament ruptures are delineated in this plane. Finally, normal anatomy best displayed in the axial plane includes the flexor and extensor tendons, median nerve, ulnar nerve and artery in Guyon's canal, flexor retinaculum, and distal radioulnar joint. Consequently, soft tissue masses, tendon abnormalities, CTS, and distal radioulnar joint disruption are delineated in this plane.

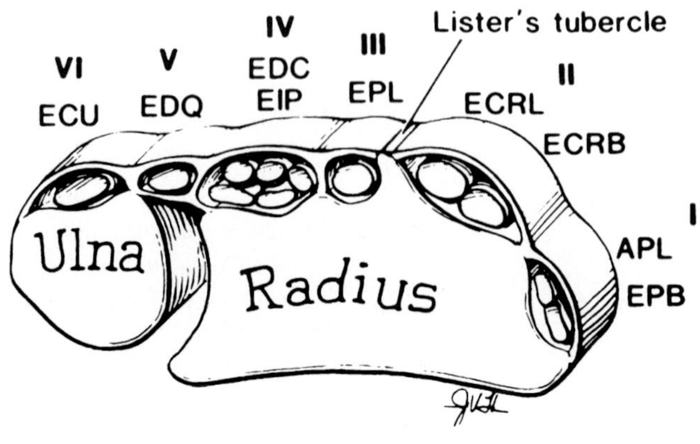

Figure 7–8
Diagram of the six extensor tendon compartments. *ECU, extensor carpi ulnaris; EDQ, extensor digiti quinti; EDC, extensor digitorum communis; EIP, extensor indicis proprius; EPL, extensor pollicis longus; ECRL, extensor carpi radialis longus; ECRB, extensor carpi radialis brevis; APL, abductor pollicis longus; EPB, extensor pollicis brevis. (From Kellerhouse LE, Reicher MA, Kursunoglu-Brahme S, et al. MR imaging of the wrist.* In *Edelman RR, Hesselink JR, eds. Clinical Magnetic Resonance Imaging. Philadelphia: WB Saunders, 1990.)*

PATHOLOGY

Carpal Tunnel Syndrome

CTS is a compressive neuropathy of the median nerve as it passes through the carpal tunnel. There are a variety of underlying causes, including a volumetric increase or decrease of the tunnel or a space-occupying lesion. The most common cause of CTS is tenosynovitis of the flexor tendons from overuse of the hands as commonly seen in typists and cashiers. Additional causes include narrowing of the tunnel from osseous deformity (callous, displaced fracture fragments, malalignment of carpal bones) or increased volume of the contents (which has multiple causes, including fat from obesity, muscular hypertrophy, anomalous lumbrical muscle origins, persistent median artery, synovitis, ganglions, neuromas (Fig. 7–9), hematoma, and tumor). Signs of CTS reported by MRI include (1) focal or segmental swelling of the median nerve, which is subjectively determined by comparing its size at the distal radius and at the pisiform, (2) flattening or angulation of the median nerve, which is best seen at the distal tunnel at the hook of the hamate (Fig. 7–10), (3) bowing of the flexor retinaculum because of increased volume of the tunnel contents, which is also best seen at the level of the hook of the hamate, and (4) increased signal intensity of the median nerve on T2 images. MRI often shows both the cause of CTS and occasional failure of a carpal tunnel release. The latter can include fibrotic scarring, neuroma development, and incomplete excision of the flexor retinaculum.[10]

Ligamentous Injury

Tears of the TFC are either degenerative or traumatic (Fig. 7–11). Degenerative tears are common after the age of 50 and rare below the age of 30. Traumatic tears occur at any age. The distinction of these tears is important because they are treated differently and the associated injuries may be different. Degenerative tears result from the "wear and tear" of repetitive axial loading. This is especially true in association with positive ulnar variance. An early sign of TFC degeneration is thinning of the horizontal midportion of the disk, which eventually progresses to a large, central tear. Without proper functioning of the TFC, chondromalacia of the ulnar head and ulnar aspect of the lunate develops, resulting in the ulnolunate impingement syndrome. Treatment of degenerative tears is conservative or, in some cases, corrected with ulnar shortening. Traumatic tears of the TFC are slitlike and usually occur about 2 mm ulnar to the TFC radial attachment. The radial or ulnar attachment rarely avulses. These tears do not tend to respond to conservative therapy and may undergo debridement or reattachment. The TFC is best evaluated on the proton-density spin-echo or the GRE coronal sequences. Focal bright signal within the disk tends to correlate with perforation. Bright fluid signal traversing the disk correlates with a complete tear.[1, 11]

The diagnosis of scapholunate interosseous ligament disruptions is highly reliable (Fig. 7–12). Abnormalities that indicate such an injury include discontinuity, distorted morphology, complete absence, elongation with an increased intercarpal space (Fig. 7–13), and the inability to identify the ligament on at least two contiguous images. Accuracy is good. Visualization of lunotriquetral interosseous ligamentous tears and injury to the extrinsic ligaments is less reliable.[7, 11]

Avascular Necrosis

MRI is an exquisitely sensitive indicator of marrow ischemia (Fig. 7–14) and necrosis and has been useful in the study of suspected cases of avascular necrosis (AVN) of the carpal bones. Foci of AVN are seen as regions of decreased signal on the T1 sequence and of

Text continues on page 214

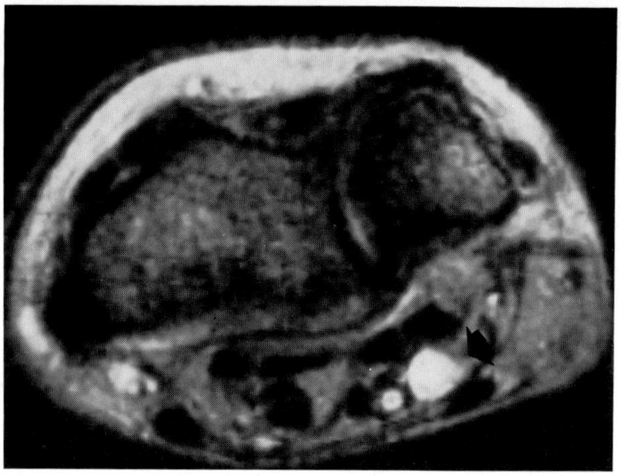

Figure 7–9
Axial GRE image. *A high-signal neuroma involves the ulnar nerve* (arrow). *(From Steinbach LS, Fritz RC. The wrist and hand.* In *Chan WP, Lang P, Genant HK, eds. MRI of the Musculoskeletal System. Philadelphia: WB Saunders, 1994.)*

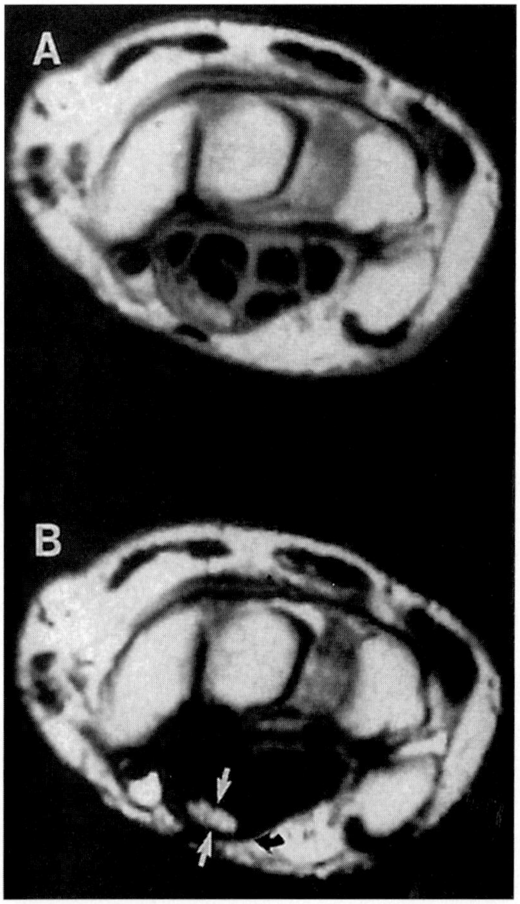

Figure 7–10
A, *Axial proton density–weighted spin-echo image of the carpal tunnel.* B, *Axial T2-weighted spin-echo image reveals bowing of the flexor retinaculum* (curved black arrow) *and bright signal intensity of the median nerve* (straight white arrows). *(From Stoller DW. The wrist. Semin Roentgenol 1995; 30:265-276.)*

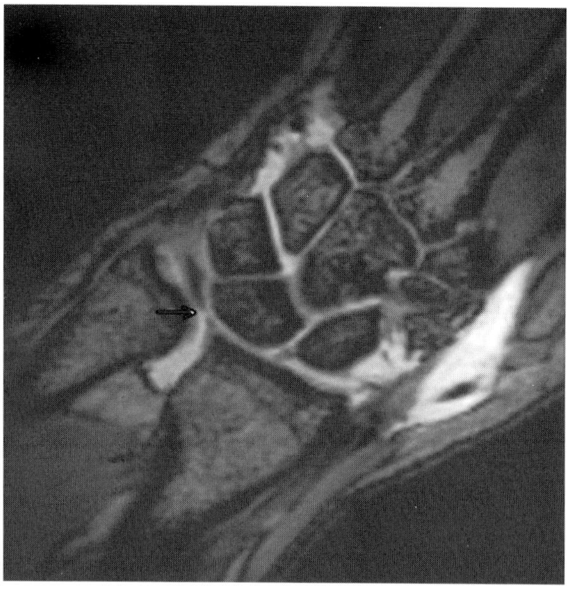

Figure 7–11
Coronal GRE image after intra-articular contrast injection. *Note the complete tear of the triangular fibrocartilage filled with fluid* (arrow).

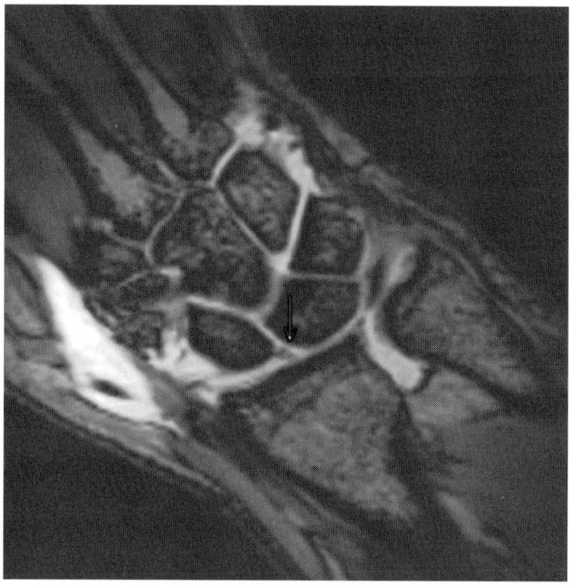

Figure 7–12
Coronal GRE image after intra-articular contrast injection. *Note the complete disruption of the scapholunate ligament* (arrow) *at the lunate attachment.*

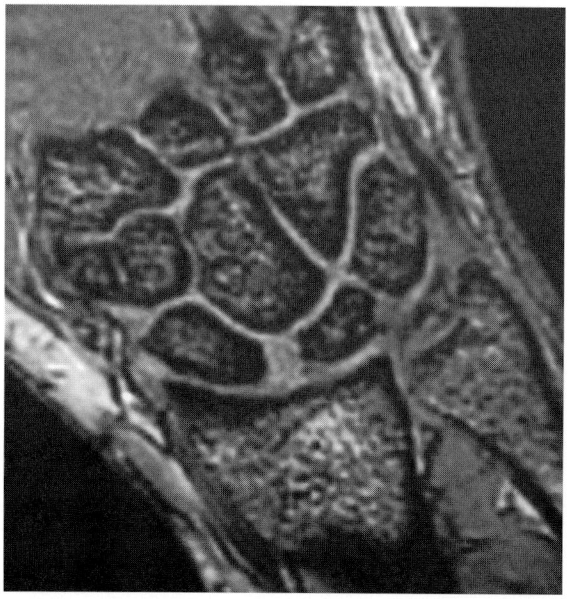

Figure 7–13
Coronal GRE image. *The scapholunate interval is widened secondary to disruption of the interosseous ligament.*

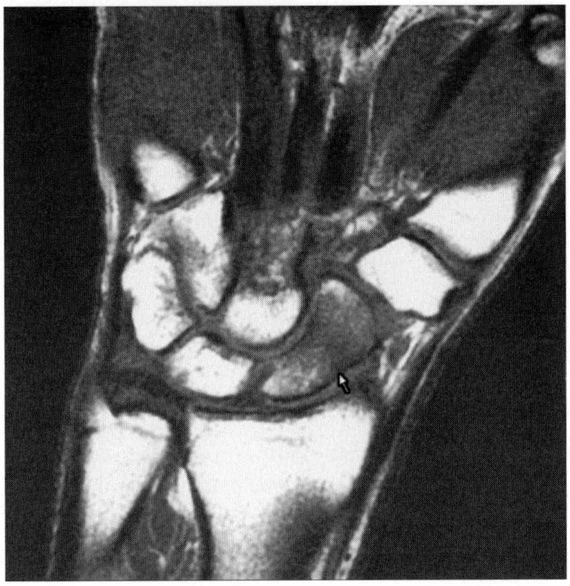

Figure 7–14
Coronal T1 spin-echo image. *Signal is diminished within the bone marrow of the scaphoid* (arrow) *because of marrow ischemia.*

varying signal on the T2 sequence. Degenerative changes may be confusing, and correlation with plain films is recommended. The scaphoid has the second highest incidence of AVN in the body; approximately 30% of the middle third scaphoid fractures and nearly all of the proximal scaphoid fractures are associated with AVN of the proximal pole.

AVN of the lunate, or Kienböck's disease, is a post-traumatic condition and commonly associated with negative ulnar variance. The disease often occurs in young adult males, and it is usually unilateral and involves the dominant hand.[3] MRI findings include focal thinning of the articular cartilage on the proximal, radial aspect of the lunate early; diminished signal on the T1 sequence; and eventual shortening, scaphoid rotary subluxation, and capitate migration. Both osteochondral defects and fractures can mimic these earlier alterations. Also, these defects and fractures are often associated with lunate AVN, which further complicates the diagnosis.[12]

Carpal Instability

Carpal alignment is maintained by the intrinsic and extrinsic ligaments of the wrist. Furthermore, the radius, lunate, and capitate form the central column of alignment for wrist flexion and extension. The scaphoid and its associated ligaments help link this relationship. Disruption of normal alignment between the carpal bones is called carpal instability. It is generally due to post-traumatic or inflammatory injury to the ligaments. Two common types of carpal instability are scapholunate dissociation and dorsal intercalated segmental instability.

Scapholunate dissociation results from scapholunate and radioscaphocapitate ligamentous injury. The scaphoid loses its function as a carpal row stabilizer, which often leads to coexistent dorsal intercalated segmental instability. The scapholunate interval is wide, and the ligament is not visualized, abnormal in configuration, or marked by increased signal on the coronal T2 sequence. The distal scaphoid tilts volarly, and configuration is abnormal, usually thickening or increased signal, within the radioscaphocapitate ligament on the sagittal T2 sequence.

Dorsal intercalated segmental instability is defined as a dorsal rotation of the lunate with loss of the familiar radius, lunate, and capitate alignment (Fig. 7–15). This results from disruption of the long radiolunate ligament. The T2 sagittal sequence shows the dorsal tilting of the lunate and abnormal configuration or signal to the ligament.

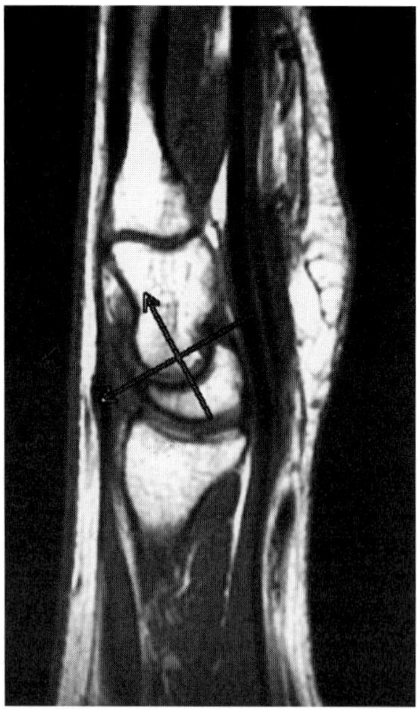

Figure 7–15
Sagittal T1 spin-echo image. *Note the dorsal rotation of the lunate with loss of the familiar radius, lunate, and capitate alignment, characteristic of dorsal intercalated segmental instability.*

References

1. Gilula LA. Carpal injuries: Analytic approach and case exercises. AJR 1979; 133:503-517.
2. Gilula LA, Weeks PM. Post-traumatic ligamentous instabilities of the wrist. Radiology 1978; 129:641-651.
3. Golimbu CN, Firooznia H, Melone CP, et al. Tears of the triangular fibrocartilage of the wrist: MR imaging. Radiology 1989; 171:749-754.
4. Mesgarzadeh M, Schneck CD, Bonakdarpour A. Carpal tunnel: MR imaging. Part II: Carpal tunnel syndrome. Radiology 1989; 171:749-754.
5. Palmer AK, Werner FW. The triangular fibrocartilage complex of the wrist: Anatomy and function. J Hand Surg 1981; 6:153-161.
6. Reicher MA, Kellerhouse LE. Carpal tunnel disease, flexor and extensor tendon disorders. In Reicher MA, Kellerhouse LE, eds. MRI of the Wrist and Hand. New York: Raven Press, 1990, pp 49-57.
7. Reicher MA, Kellerhouse LE. Normal wrist anatomy, biomechanics, basic imaging protocol, and normal multiplanar MRI of the wrist. In Reicher MA, Kellerhouse LE, eds. MRI of the Wrist and Hand. New York: Raven Press, 1990, pp 17-48.
8. Reinus WR, Conway WF, Totty WG, et al. Carpal avascular necrosis: MR anatomy. Radiology 1986; 160:689-693.
9. Schweitzer ME, Brahme SK, Hodler J, et al. Chronic wrist pain: Spin-echo and short tau inversion recovery MR imaging and conventional and MR arthrography. Radiology 1992; 182:205-211.
10. Taleisnik J. Kienböck's disease. In Taleisnik J, ed. The Wrist. New York: Churchill Livingstone, 1985, pp 169-194.
11. Totterman SM, Miller RJ. MRI of the wrist and hand. In Gilula LA, Yin Y, eds. Imaging of the Wrist and Hand. Philadelphia: WB Saunders, 1995, pp 441-478.
12. Zlatkin MB, Chao PC, Osterman AL, et al. Chronic wrist pain: Evaluation with high-resolution MR imaging. Radiology 1987; 173:723-729.

Wrist Arthroscopy*

The advent of enhanced optics and smaller arthroscopes in the 1980s made small joint arthroscopy feasible. Since that time, wrist arthroscopy has emerged as the diagnostic method of choice and is the standard against which other methods are compared.[1,2] As with arthroscopy of larger joints, the principal advantages lie in minimizing capsular injury and obtaining a clear magnified view of joint pathology. Arthroscopy also allows a dynamic evaluation of complex, three-dimensional anatomic structures.[3] Further advances in small joint instrumentation have made operative wrist arthroscopy more productive, and new indications continue to emerge.[4,5]

INDICATIONS

Arthroscopy of the wrist is more accurate than arthrography and at least as sensitive and specific as arthrotomy in establishing the etiology of chronic and acute wrist pain.[1] Data that compare the merits of MRI with those of arthroscopy are not available. MRI has become a very useful tool for the diagnoses of disorders of the wrist, particularly when the pathology involves diseased bone. Experienced surgeons and radiologists are becoming quite adept at interpreting MR images of ligament injuries and TFCC pathology. MRI presents data in a two-dimensional static format. Arthroscopy, in contrast, has the advantage of providing a three-dimensional dynamic evaluation.

The dynamic evaluation afforded by arthroscopy allows for correlation with the preoperative evaluation and for identification of biomechanically significant ligament or TFCC perforations or tears. The principal disadvantage of arthroscopy compared with MRI is the obvious risk surrounding an invasive procedure.

In addition to confirming a diagnosis, wrist arthroscopy is very useful in preoperative planning. It allows a careful evaluation of the joint prior to selection of appropriate open intervention. A good example is determining the character of the articular cartilage on the proximal pole of the capitate when deciding on proximal row carpectomy or scaphoid excision and four-corner fusion for scapholunate advanced collapse (SLAC). Another example is during the decision to base treatment for instability on the degree of intercarpal ligament injury. Geissler and colleagues[6] have classified these ligamentous injuries based on the degree of instability as defined by arthroscopic dynamic evaluation (Table 7–1).

*Steven M. Topper, M.D., co-author.

Table 7–1 • Ligament Instability by Arthroscopic Dynamic Evaluation

Grade	Description
I	Attenuation or hemorrhage of interosseous ligament as seen from radiocarpal space. No incongruity of carpal alignment in midcarpal space.
II	Attenuation or hemorrhage of interosseous ligament as seen from radiocarpal space. Incongruity or step-off of carpal space. There may be a slight gap (less than the width of a probe) between the carpal bones.
III	Incongruity or step-off of carpal alignment as seen from both radiocarpal and midcarpal space. Probe may be passed through the gap between carpal bones.
IV	Incongruity or step-off of carpal alignment as seen from both radiocarpal and midcarpal space. There is gross instability with manipulation. A 2.7-mm arthroscope may be passed through the gap between the carpal bones.

From Geissler WB, Freeland AE, Savoie FH, et al. Intracarpal soft tissue lesions associated with an intraarticular fracture of the distal end of the radius. J Bone Joint Surg 1996; 78A:357-365.

Different grades of ligament instability can be managed successfully with different techniques. Grade I lesions generally respond to debridement of frayed inflamed edges.[7] Grade II and III lesions have been managed successfully with the multiple pinning technique advocated by Whipple.[3,8] This method theoretically creates a fibrous synostosis that stabilizes the interval. Grade IV lesions require open repair, reconstruction, or stabilization based on the surgeon's preference.

The primary employment of operative wrist arthroscopy to date has been in managing TFCC lesions. The classification of these injuries has been described by Palmer (Fig. 7–16).[9] Type 1A lesions are generally managed by debridement of the unstable flap back to a stable rim.[10] Repairs in this region of the TFCC are not likely to be successful because it is avascular. The peripheral rim of the TFCC is well vascularized and amenable to repair. Type 1B lesions can be repaired arthroscopically with either an inside-out technique, using a Tuohy needle, or an outside-in technique, using commercially available TFCC repair instrumentation (Linvatec Inc., Largo, FL). Success has been reported utilizing these techniques.[11]

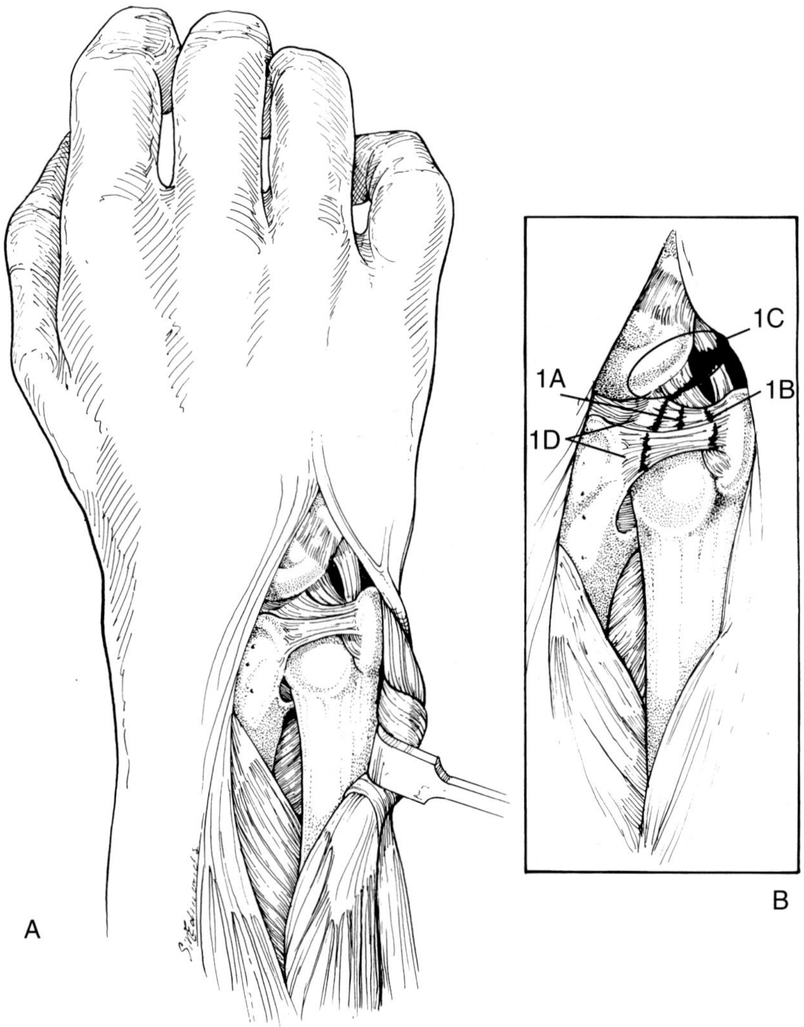

Figure 7–16
A, *Triangular fibrocartilage complex (TFCC) anatomy.* B, *TFCC injuries include radial side horizontal tears (1A), avulsion from the ulna (1B), avulsion from the carpus with ulnolunate and ulnotriquetral ligament injury (1C), and avulsion from the radius (1D), as well as a variety of degenerative (Type-2) tears with or without chondromalacia* (not shown). *(Adapted from Palmer AK. Triangular fibrocartilage disorders: Injury patterns and treatment. Arthroscopy 1990; 6:125-132.)*

Type 1C volar rim tears of the TFCC that involve the origins of the ulnotriquetral (UT) and ulnolunate (UL) ligaments are managed with an open procedure after arthroscopic identification. The treatment of these injuries is controversial, but two good choices currently exist. Osterman and colleagues[11] have advocated direct repair augmented with a strip of the flexor carpi ulnaris tendon. The other option is to advance the origin of the UT and UL ligaments into the triquetrum with a bone anchor (author's preferred technique).

Type 1D tears of the radial attachment of the TFCC by definition involve either the dorsal radioulnar ligament (DRUL) or the volar radioulnar ligament (VRUL) or both. Tears close to the radial attachment of the TFCC, which spare the DRUL and VRUL, are best considered Type 1A tears and are treated with debridement.

Tears that are true Type 1D lesions can be associated with instability of the distal radioulnar joint (DRUJ) based on concomitant injury of other stabilizing elements.[12] Good results have been reported with open repairs of these lesions.[13] Jantea and colleagues[14] have reported on the early results of an arthroscopic technique that involves the drilling of suture tracks from the radial aspect of the radius to the radial attachment site of the TFCC. Spinal needles are then used as suture passers to accomplish repair of a Type 1D tear. Although the early experience is positive, this procedure appears technically demanding. The added benefit of doing this procedure arthroscopically remains speculative.

Degenerative perforations of the TFCC have also been classified (Table 7–2) by Palmer.[9] In the early stages, the changes can result from normal age-related wear of the TFCC.[15] When associated with symptoms and positive ulnar variation, the sequence of pathologic changes in the TFCC is secondary to ulnocarpal impaction syndrome. Degenerative tears of the TFCC respond well to arthroscopic debridement. In order to prevent recurrence or progression of chondromalacia, it is important to decompress the ulnocarpal articulation. Osterman[10] has reported success with arthroscopic ulnar shortening, done with a burr through the hole in the TFCC. The other options include open wafer resection of the ulnar head, as described by Feldon and colleagues,[16] and standard diaphyseal ulnar shortening.

The arthroscope has also been utilized effectively for "ectomy" procedures in the wrist joint. These include synovectomy, synovial biopsy, removal of loose bodies, and proximal row carpectomy.[17]

Chondral defects are a common cause of occult wrist pain and are easily identified with the arthroscope. Whipple[8] has had success in relieving symptoms with abrasion chondroplasty for defects less than 5 mm in diameter. Savoie[18] has also reported on the benefit of abrasion chondroplasty in selected cases.

Arthroscopic reduction and fixation of intra-articular distal radius fracture is becoming more frequently employed. In the search for the most appropriate and beneficial treatment for this difficult injury, the arthroscope has some important potential advantages.[19, 20]

Table 7–2 • Degenerative TFCC Tear Classification

Type	Description
2A	Thinning of the articular disc
2B	2A + chondromalacia of the ulnar head and proximal ulnar pole of the lunate
2C	Perforation of the articular disc and chondromalacia of the lunate and ulnar head
2D	2C + disruption of the lunatotriquetral interosseous ligament
2E	2D + arthritis of the DRUJ and ulnar carpus

From Palmer AK. Triangular fibrocartilage disorders: Injury patterns and treatment. Arthroscopy 1990; 6: 125-132.

Reduced scarring in the skin and tendon compartments may lead to improved postoperative motion. By avoiding open exposure, fewer comminuted fragments should be devitalized. The magnified view of the joint allows for a highly accurate reduction. Concomitant intercarpal ligament injuries and fractures can also be readily identified, which allows for treatment of the total injury. Optimizing recovery and rehabilitation should provide for better functional outcome and earlier return to work.

After the radius, the scaphoid is the next most frequently seen intra-articular fracture in the wrist. Whipple[21] has devised an instrument for arthroscopically assisted reduction and internal fixation of scaphoid fractures. In 20 fractures treated with this technique, he reported union in 19 and an average of only 3 to 4 weeks of cast immobilization. This technique may diminish the wrist stiffness and atrophy seen after open reduction and fixation with its prolonged postoperative immobilization.

Dorsal carpal ganglia is a common cause of wrist pain and patient concern. Operative treatment of these lesions, however, can be associated with stiffness and recurrence. Patients often seek treatment for cosmetic reasons and are presented with the less than satisfactory choice of trading a bump for a scar. The key to preventing recurrence of dorsal carpal ganglia is obliterating the stalk that usually emanates from the scapholunate interval. An arthroscopic approach to this problem has the potential advantages of a magnified accurate identification and an obliteration of the stalk through two very small incisions—with less capsular damage than an open procedure. Osterman and Raphael[22] have reported preliminary success with this technique in an ongoing prospective trial.

POSITIONING AND PORTAL PLACEMENT

Wrist arthroscopy is performed with the patient supine. Wrist distraction (10 to 12 lb.) is usually accomplished with a commercially available traction device (Fig. 7–17). A small 1.9- to 2.7-mm arthroscope and small joint instruments with a maximum diameter of 3.0 mm are used.

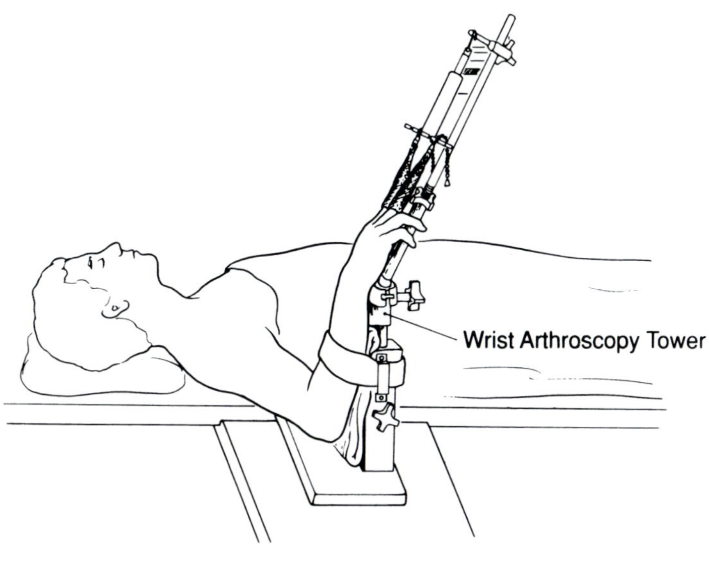

Figure 7–17
Commercially available traction tower allows distraction and wrist flexion. (From Whipple TL, Poehling GG, Roth JH. Surgical technique for wrist arthroscopy. In *McGinty JB, ed. Operative Arthroscopy. New York: Raven Press, 1991, p 626.)*

Arthroscopic portals about the wrist are designated based on their location in reference to the dorsal extensor compartments (Fig. 7–18). The standard portals for any diagnostic wrist arthroscopy are the 3-4, the 4-5, and the radial midcarpal portal. Accessory radiocarpal portals include the 1-2, 6R, and 6U. The 3-4 is the primary portal for arthroscopic visualization. Inflow is usually established through the scope. Outflow can be done with an 18-gauge catheter through either the 1-2 or 6U portal. Alternatively, a pressure sensitive inflow-outflow pump device can be utilized. The 4-5 and 6R portals are primarily for instrumentation. The optimum configuration for working on the TFCC is to place the arthroscope in the 4-5 portal and to introduce instruments through the 6R portal.

The midcarpal portals include the midcarpal radial (MR), midcarpal ulnar (MU), and scaphotrapezio-trapezoid (STT) portals. The MR portal is 1 cm distal to the 3-4 portal, and the MU portal is 1 cm distal to the 4-5 portal. Generally, visualization is accomplished through the MR portal. Instruments are then introduced through the MU portal, although the steps can certainly be reversed. The STT portal is located just ulnar to the extensor pollicus longus tendon over the STT joint. When debriding the STT joint, visualization is accomplished through the MR portal. Instruments are introduced through the STT portal.

Abrams and colleagues[23] have studied the anatomy of wrist arthroscopy portals to assess the risk of injuring adjacent soft tissue. This is obviously a densely packed area of anatomy. Careless technique can lead to vascular, nerve, or tendon damage. They found that the portals that presented the greatest risk were the 1-2, 6R, and 6U because of the proximity of the radial artery and dorsal sensory branches of the radial and ulnar nerves. The technique of establishing portals is particularly important in protecting the anatomy and avoiding injury to the underlying structures. The recommended technique is to sharply incise the skin only. Then, using a hemostat clamp, bluntly dissect down to the capsule ("nick-and-spread" method). At this point, a blunt trocar is used to puncture through the capsule into the joint that should have been previously distended with fluid.

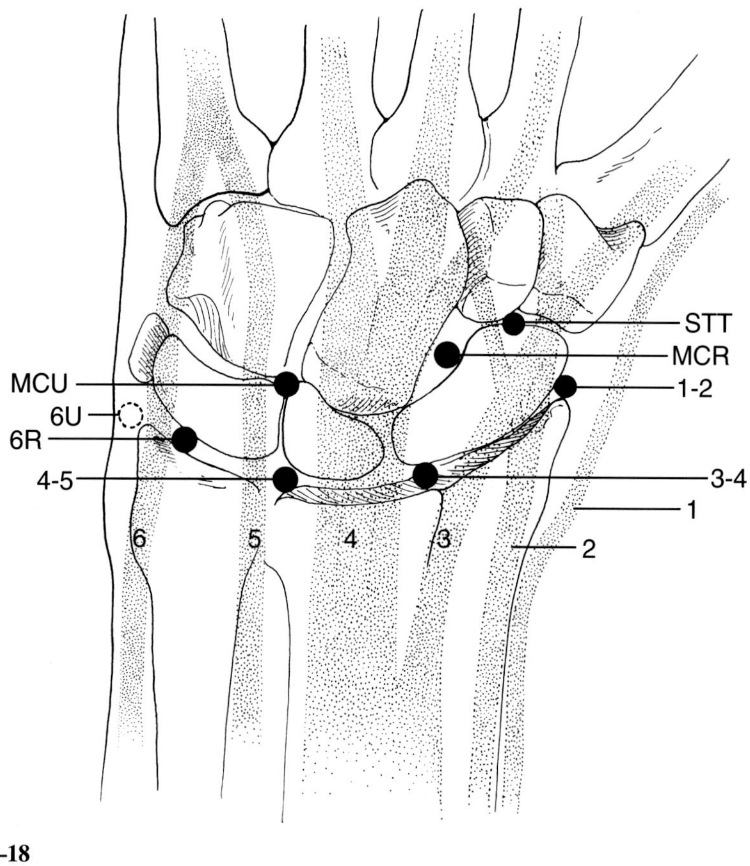

Figure 7–18
Arthroscopic wrist portals. Numbers indicate wrist extensor compartments and associated portals. R = radial; U = ulnar; MCU = midcarpal ulnar; MCR = midcarpal radial; STT = scaphotrapezio-trapezoid.

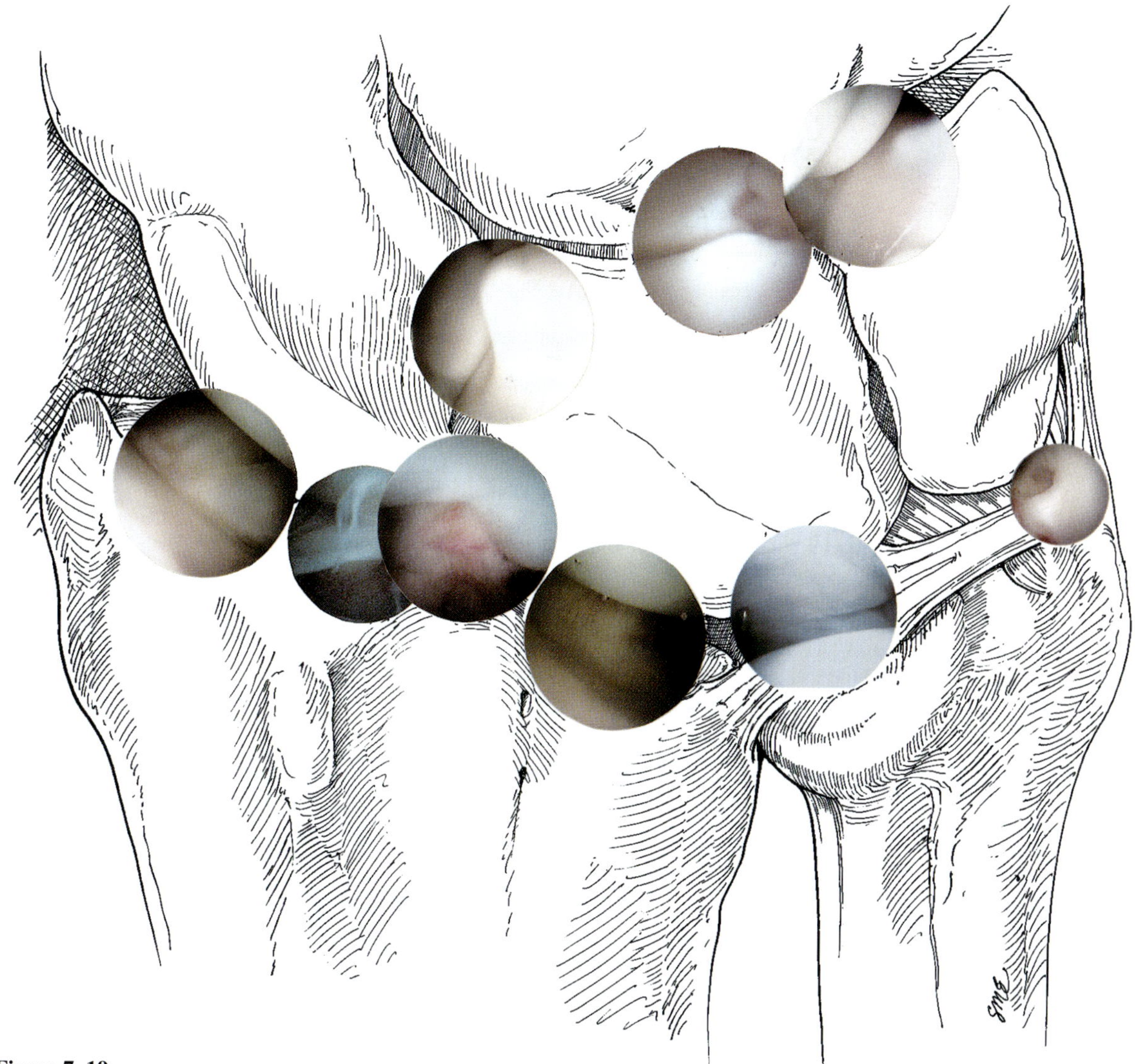

Figure 7–19
Arthroscopic wrist anatomy.

ARTHROSCOPIC ANATOMY

A thorough and complete wrist arthroscopy details the anatomy of the articular surfaces, intrinsic carpal ligaments, extrinsic carpal ligaments, and TFCC (Fig. 7–19). Proceeding from radial to ulnar in the radiocarpal joint the following structures are observed: radial styloid, radioscaphocapitate ligament, long radiolunate ligament, scaphoid proximal pole, radius scaphoid facet, scapholunate interosseous ligament, radioscapholunate ligament (ligament of Testut), lunate proximal pole, radius lunate facet, short radiolunate ligament, TFCC (including the dorsal and volar radioulnar ligaments), ulnolunate ligament, ulnotriquetral ligament, lunatotriquetral interosseous ligament, and triquetrum proximal pole.

Proceeding from radial to ulnar in the midcarpal joint, examination of the following structures is accomplished: STT, capitate proximal pole, scaphoid distal pole, scapholunate interval stability, lunate distal pole, lunatotriquetral interval stability, triquetrum distal pole, capitohamate interval, hamate proximal pole.

The ligaments that cross the midcarpal joint are often difficult to visualize because of overlying synovium. If a midcarpal instability is suspected, visualization can be accomplished by debriding the synovium carefully. The ligaments in question include the radioscaphocapitate, ulnocapitate, triquetrocapitate, and triquetrohamate.

COMPLICATIONS

Perhaps the most common complication with wrist arthroscopy is articular cartilage damage as a result of traumatic arthroscopy. Injury to tendons, nerves, and vascular structures is also possible with inexact or careless portal placement. Infection, however, is infrequent.

References

1. Cooney WP. Evaluation of chronic wrist by arthrography, arthroscopy, and arthrotomy. Hand Surg 1993; 18:815-822.
2. Koman LA, Poehling GG, Toby EB, et al. Chronic wrist pain: Indications for wrist arthroscopy. Arthroscopy 1990; 6:116-119.
3. Whipple TL. The role of arthroscopy in the treatment of wrist injuries in the athlete. Clin Sports Med 1992; 11:227-238.
4. De Smet L, Dauwe D, Fortems Y, et al. The value of wrist arthroscopy: an evaluation of 129 cases. J Hand Surg 1996; 21B:210-212.
5. Rettig ME, Amadio PC. Wrist arthroscopy: Indications and clinical applications. J Hand Surg 1994; 19B:774-777.
6. Geissler WB, Freeland AE, Savoie FH, et al. Intracarpal soft tissue lesions associated with an intra-articular fracture of the distal end of the radius. J Bone Joint Surg 1996; 78A:357-365.
7. Ruch DS, Poehling GG. Arthroscopic management of partial scapholunate and lunotriquetral injuries of the wrist. J Hand Surg 1996: 21A:412-417.
8. Whipple TL. Arthroscopic Surgery: The Wrist. Philadelphia: JB Lippincott, 1992; pp 125-128.
9. Palmer AK. Triangular fibrocartilage disorders: Injury patterns and treatment. Arthroscopy 1990; 6:125-132.
10. Osterman AL. Arthroscopic debridement of triangular fibrocartilage complex tears. Arthroscopy 1990; 6:120-124.
11. Bednar JM, Osterman AL. The role of arthroscopy in the treatment of traumatic triangular fibrocartilage injuries. Hand Clin 1994; 10:605-614.
12. Kihura H, Palmer AK, Werner FW, et al. The effect of dorsally angulated distal radius fractures on distal radioulnar joint congruency and forearm rotation. J Hand Surg 1996; 21A:40-47.
13. Cooney WP, Linschied RL, Dobyns JH. Triangular fibrocartilage tears. J Hand Surg 1994; 19A:143-154.
14. Jantea CL, Baltzer A, Ruther W. Arthroscopic repair of radial-sided lesions of the fibrocartilage complex. Hand Clin 1995; 11:31-36.
15. Mikic ZD. Age changes in the triangular fibrocartilage of the wrist joint. J Anat 1978; 126:367-384.
16. Feldon P, Terrano AL, Belsky MR. Wafer distal ulna resection for triangular fibrocartilage tears and/or ulna impaction syndrome. J Hand Surg 1992; 17A:731-737.
17. Roth JH, Poehling GG. Arthroscopic "ectomy" surgery of the wrist. Arthroscopy 1990; 6:141-147.
18. Savoie FH. The role of arthroscopy in the diagnosis and management of cartilaginous lesions of the wrist. Hand Clin 1995; 11:1-5.
19. Cooney WP, Berger RA. Treatment of complex fractures of the distal radius. Combined use of internal and external fixation and arthroscopic reduction. Hand Clin 1993; 9:603-612.
20. Geissler WE. Arthroscopically assisted reduction of intra-articular fractures of the distal radius. Hand Clin 1995; 11:19-29.
21. Whipple TL. The role of arthrotomy in the treatment of intra-articular wrist fractures. Hand Clin 1995; 11:13-18.
22. Osterman AL, Raphael J. Arthroscopic resection of dorsal ganglion of the wrist. Hand Clin 1995; 11:7-12.
23. Abrams RA, Petersen M, Botte MJ. Arthroscopic portals of the wrist: An anatomic study. J Hand Surg 1994; 19A:940-944.

Illustrative Cases—Wrist

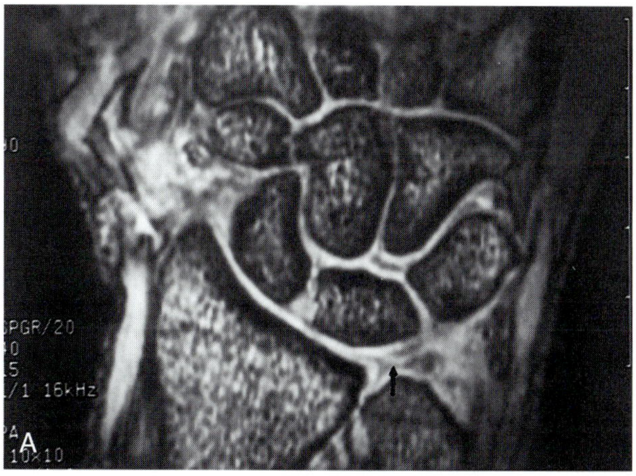

Figure 7–20. **Type-IA TFCC Tear, Right Wrist**
A, *Coronal three-dimensional GRE image shows linear bright signal* (arrow) *near the radial attachment of the TFCC.* B, *Arthroscopic view of a radial TFCC tear.*
Case courtesy of Steven M. Topper, M.D.

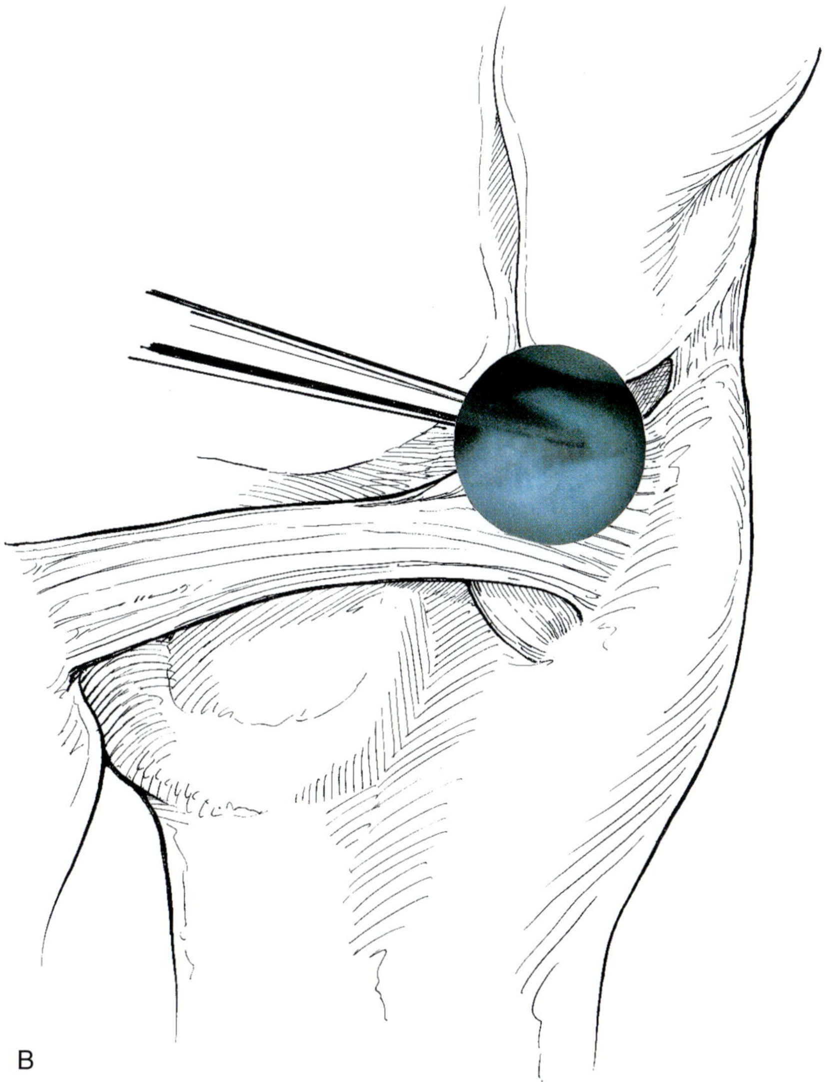

B

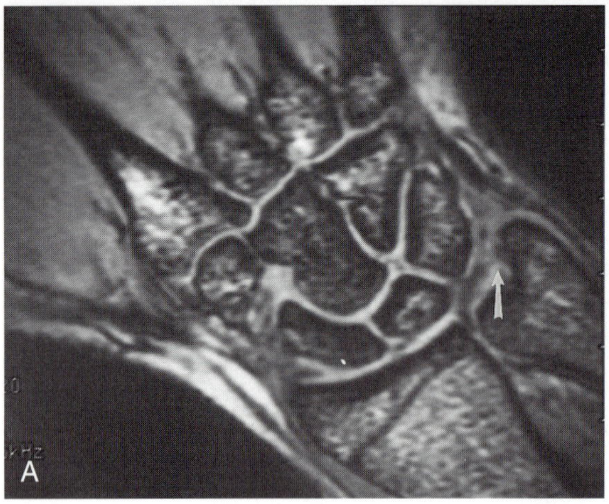

Figure 7–21. **Type-IB TFCC Tear, Right Wrist**
A, *Coronal three-dimensional GRE image shows linear bright signal* (arrow) *indicative of TFCC disruption at its ulnar attachment.* B, *Arthroscopic view of ulnar TFCC detachment.*
Case courtesy of Steven M. Topper, M.D.

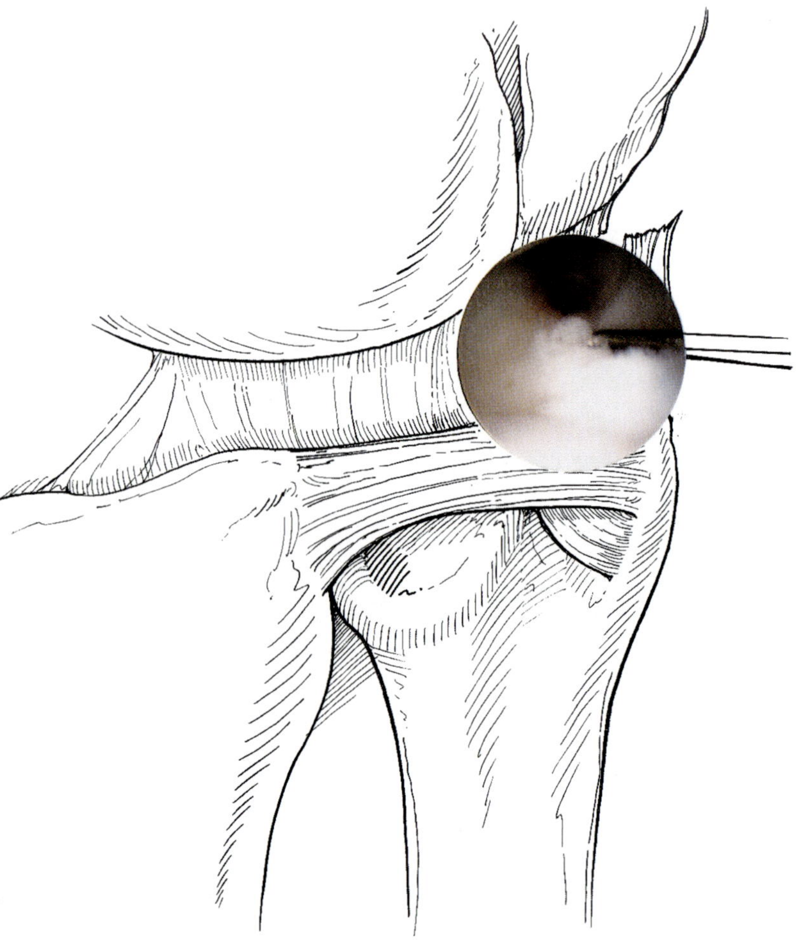

B

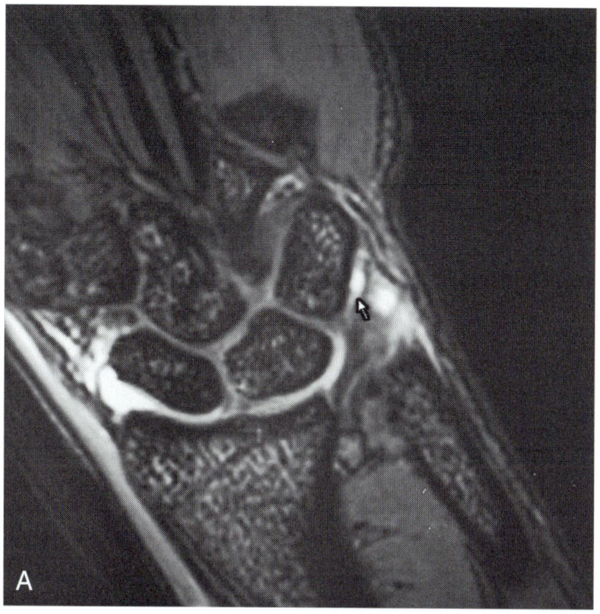

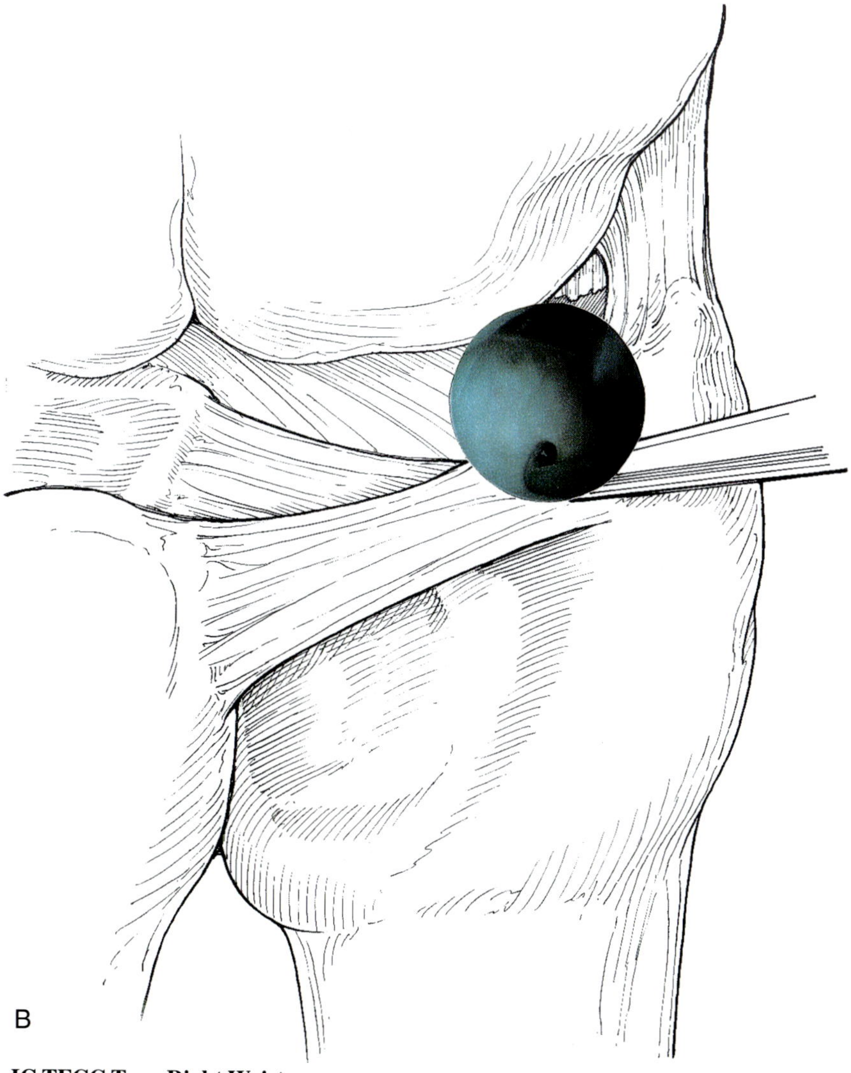

Figure 7–22. **Type-IC TFCC Tear, Right Wrist**
A, *Coronal three-dimensional GRE image following intra-articular administration of gadolinium shows discontinuity of the ulnotriquetral ligament* (arrow). B, *Arthroscopic view demonstrates disruption of the ulnotriquetral ligament.*
Case courtesy of Steven M. Topper, M.D.

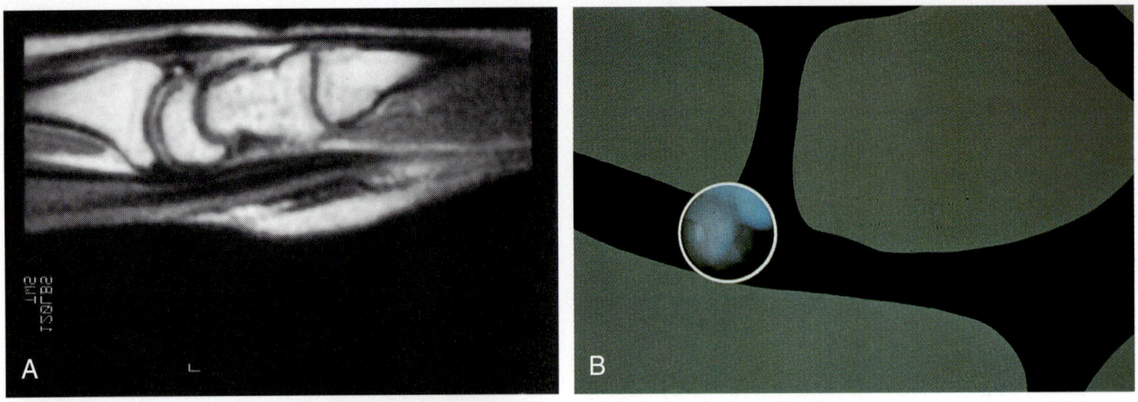

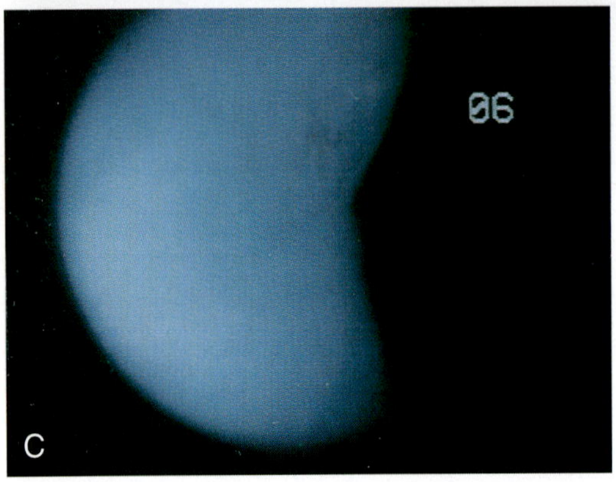

Figure 7–23. **Occult Dorsal Carpal Ganglion, Right Wrist**
A, *Sagittal spin-echo proton density–weighted image demonstrates a small round focus of bright signal at the dorsal aspect of the lunate.* B, *Arthroscopic view of dorsal carpal ganglion arising from the scapholunate interval.* C, *Oblique view across the dorsal aspect of the scaphoid and lunate shows the intra-articular occult ganglion at the upper portion of the figure next to the "06" label.*
Case courtesy of Steven F. Viegas, M.D.

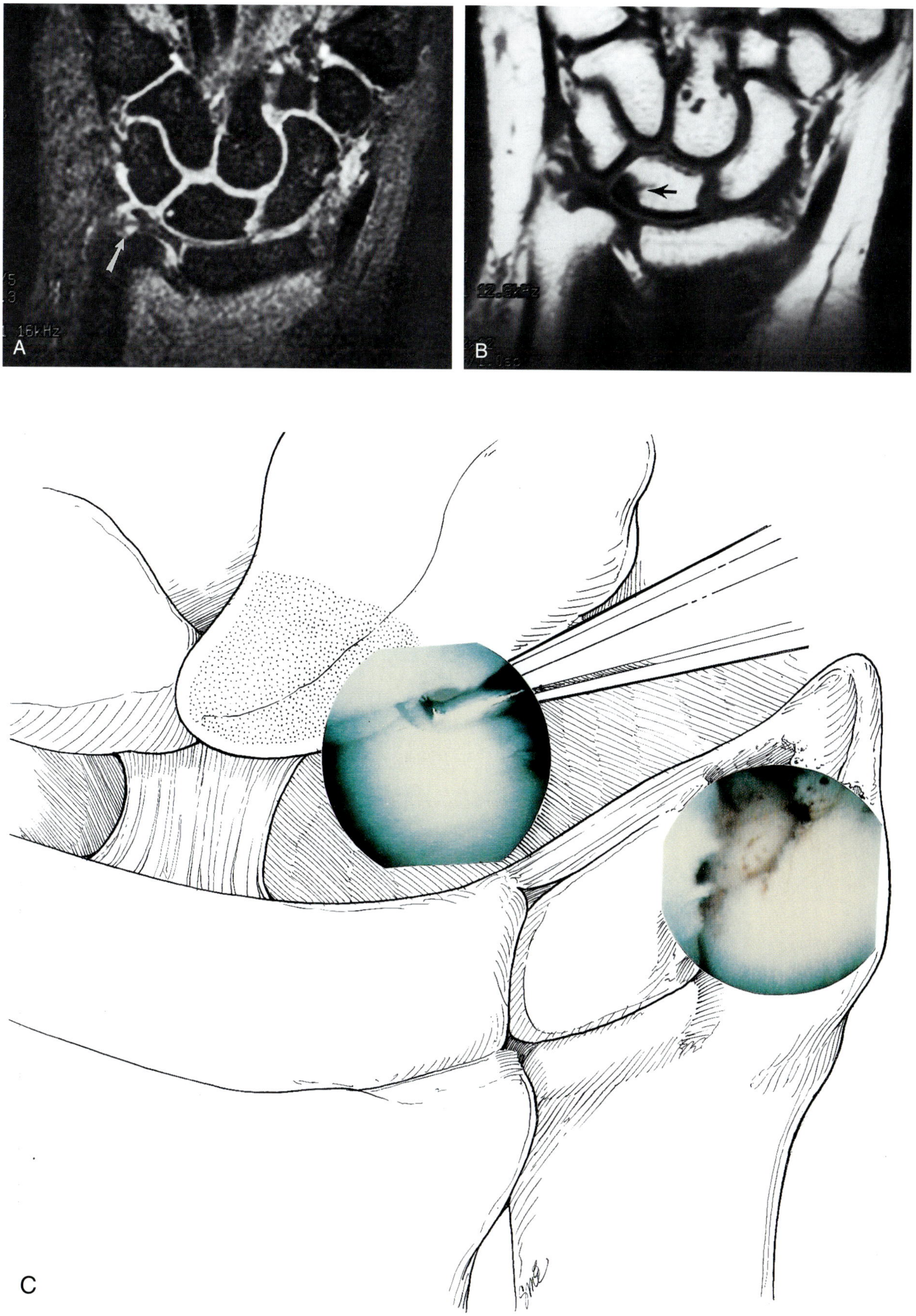

Figure 7–24. **Ulnar Impaction Syndrome with Lunate Chondromalacia and TFCC Tear**
A, *Coronal GRE three-dimensional acquisition image shows a region of bright signal* (arrow) *indicative of disruption of the TFCC near its ulnar attachment.* B, *Coronal spin-echo T1-weighted image shows a geographic region of low signal intensity within the ulnar side of the lunate* (arrow), *consistent with subchondral injury.* C, *Arthroscopic view demonstrates softening of the lunate and an associated TFCC tear.*
Case courtesy of William B. Geissler, M.D.

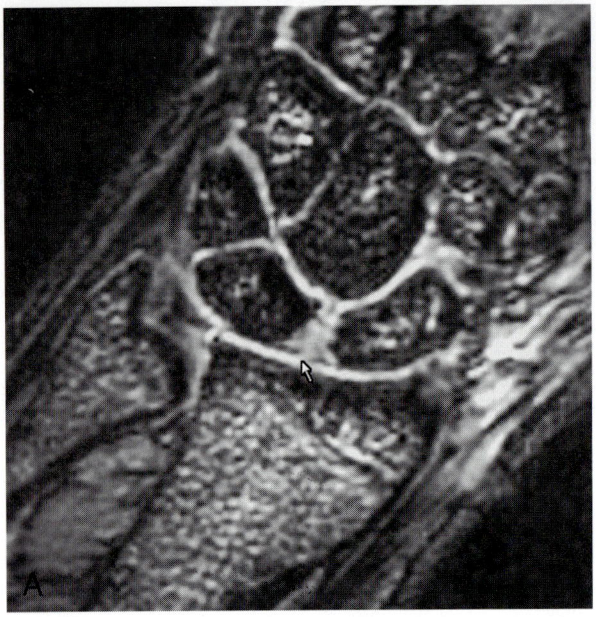

Figure 7–25. **Scapholunate Injury, Right Wrist**
A, *Coronal three-dimensional GRE image reveals increased space between the scaphoid and lunate carpal bones and complete disruption of the scapholunate ligament* (arrow). B, *Arthroscopic view from radiocarpal and midcarpal portals demonstrates complete disruption of the scapholunate ligaments. Note that midcarpal visualization is necessary to confirm this diagnosis.*
Case courtesy of Steven M. Topper, M.D.

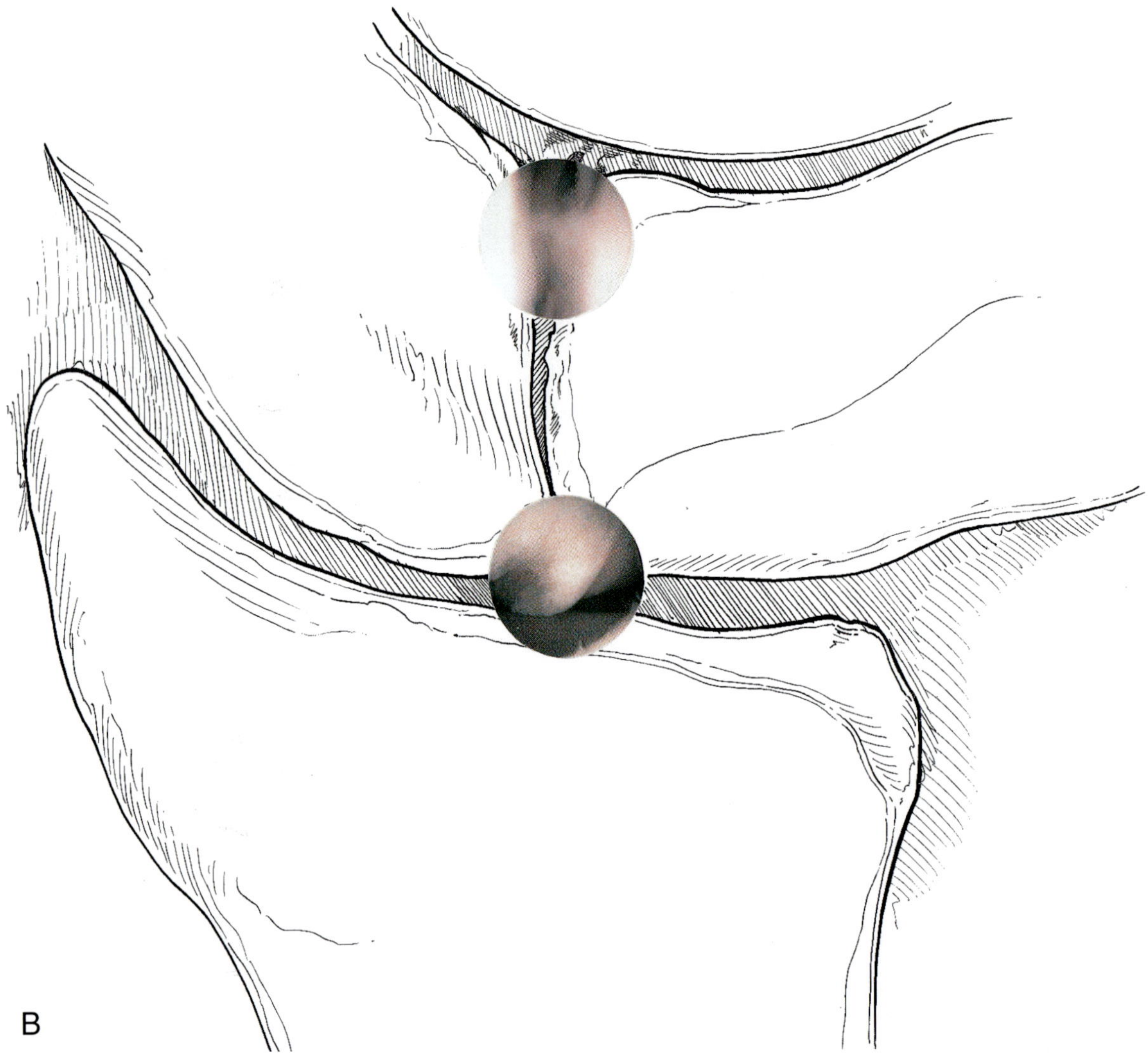

B

Index

Note: Page numbers in *italics* refer to illustrations; page numbers followed by t refer to tables.